Fracture Reduction and Fixation Techniques

Peter V. Giannoudis
Editor

Fracture Reduction and Fixation Techniques

Upper Extremities

Springer

Editor
Peter V. Giannoudis
School of Medicine
University of Leeds
Leeds
Yorkshire
United Kingdom

ISBN 978-3-030-09843-8 ISBN 978-3-319-68628-8 (eBook)
https://doi.org/10.1007/978-3-319-68628-8

Softcover re-print of the Hardcover 1st edition 2018

Printed on acid-free paper

This Springer imprint is published by Springer Nature
The registered company is Springer International Publishing AG
The registered company address is: Gewerbestrasse 11, 6330 Cham, Switzerland

Preface

Fracture fixation techniques have continued to evolve since their introduction in the 1950s by the AO Group in Switzerland. Advances made in metallurgy, implant design, targeting devices, surgical instruments, radiology and functional anatomy and the better understanding of fracture healing led to the modern practising techniques. Preoperative planning became a routine step of every fixation case. Moreover, it was recognised that optimal fracture reduction prior to fixation is a key element facilitating bone repair and a satisfactory anatomical and functional outcome. There is plenty of scientific evidence available that suboptimal fracture reduction is often associated with complications such as implant failure, impaired healing, malunion and early onset of osteoarthritis, amongst others.

This highly illustrated textbook is written by a panel of experts in the upper limb, who share tips and tricks that will aid in achieving an optimal reduction and fixation of different fracture types whilst avoiding common pitfalls.

Each technique is clearly demonstrated using a stepwise approach with real-time intraoperative photographs, improving the understanding and ensuring the production of an easy-to-read, memorable textbook.

Each chapter in this book includes an outline of useful techniques for fracture reduction. Its objective is to provide orthopaedic surgeons and especially those still in training with a quick reference to common reduction techniques becoming an essential guide to their practice. The ultimate goal is to improve the standards of care of our patients.

Leeds, UK Peter Giannoudis

Contents

Part I

General Considerations

1 Fracture Healing: Back to Basics and Latest Advances

Ippokratis Pountos and Peter V. Giannoudis

The research on bone biology and healing over the last decades has been intense. The reason for this high research output can be attributed to two elements: firstly, the discovery of mesenchymal stem cells (MSCs), a population of multipotent stem cells found to reside in bone marrow (and in many other tissues within the body), which opened new avenues in tissue engineering approaches for bone regeneration, and secondly, the discovery and commercialization of molecules that can upregulate bone repair mechanisms. The aim of this chapter is to present the key aspects of bone healing biology, factors that can influence it adversely, and key strategies found to enhance the healing of fractures.

Types of Bone Healing

Bone healing is a well-orchestrated complex process that results in the reconstitution of bone continuity without the formation of scar tissue. It prerequisites the coordinated interplay of multiple cell types with local and systemic cytokines, chemokines, and growth factors. This local milieu is influenced and often regulated by the mechanical forces exerted locally. Bone healing can be divided into primary and secondary types of healing.

Primary

Primary bone healing occurs when there is a small fracture gap and absolutely no movement at the fracture site. The discovery of this type of healing occurred over a century ago with the introduction of stable internal fixation [1]. It was initially called "healing by primary intention" and subsequently "soudure autogène," but following histopathologic studies, the terms "direct" and "primary" bone healing were established [2]. Primary bone healing is the same process as the normal bone remodeling. Bone production and apposition to fill the fracture gap occur by the osteoblasts, in the same way that the Howship lacunae are filled after the action of "cutting cones." It occurs in cases where anatomic reduction and rigid internal fixation are achieved or in incomplete stable cracks of the bone. Fragment end resorption does not occur and no callus is formed. This form of bone healing is less frequent. The majority of fractures heal through secondary bone healing.

I. Pountos, M.B., M.D., E.E.C.
Academic Department of Trauma and Orthopaedics, School of Medicine, University of Leeds, Leeds, UK

P.V. Giannoudis, M.D., F.R.C.S. (✉)
Academic Department of Trauma and Orthopaedics, School of Medicine, University of Leeds, Leeds, UK

NIHR, Leeds, UK

Musculoskeletal Biomedical Research Center, Chapel Allerton Hospital, Leeds, UK
e-mail: pgiannoudi@aol.com

P.V. Giannoudis (ed.), *Fracture Reduction and Fixation Techniques*,
https://doi.org/10.1007/978-3-319-68628-8_1

Secondary Bone Healing

Secondary bone healing is the type of healing that occurs in the absence of rigid fixation. It represents an organized pattern of interlinked events that aim to activate a number of different cell types to prepare the fracture site for its consolidation, to restore the vascularity, to produce a stable mechanical environment, and once successful to conclude with the ossification of the area. It has been previously proposed that this type of healing occurs in three phases: the inflammatory, reparative, and remodeling phases. These generalized phases include a number of events, which are often overlapping. A more comprehensive description is that of the six stages of bone healing. Based on this descriptive system, healing starts at the time of the injury with the formation of fracture hematoma, followed by the inflammatory stage, which concludes with the formation of granulation tissue. Then, the formation of the soft callus occurs that eventually calcifies and remodels (Figs. 1.1 and 1.2).

Fracture Hematoma

The formation of fracture hematoma represents a distinct stage of the bone healing process. It is the first and possibly the most important determinant of the healing outcome. Several animal studies have shown that removing the fracture hematoma leads to an arrest of the healing process. Equally, when fracture hematoma is injected in ectopic sites, osteogenesis follows.

During fracture hematoma formation, a number of changes of the local microenvironment occur. The disruption of blood supply leads to a significant drop of the oxygen availability. The low local oxygen saturation changes the genetic expression of osteoprogenitor cells, promoting their proliferation, formation of extracellular matrix, and differentiation toward chondrocytes [3, 4]. This environment also induces the release of several inflammatory molecules, collagen, as well as angiogenic and osteogenic growth factors. In addition to the hypoxia, the CO_2 exudation from the dead and dying cells, the production of lactic acid, and the conversion of blood sugars make the local microenvironment acidic. This acidic environment favors osteoclast resorptive activity, and the levels of calcium increase by tenfold compared to peripheral circulating levels. Phosphorous, alkaline phosphatase, lactic acid, and beta and gamma globulins are also elevated in fracture hematoma [5].

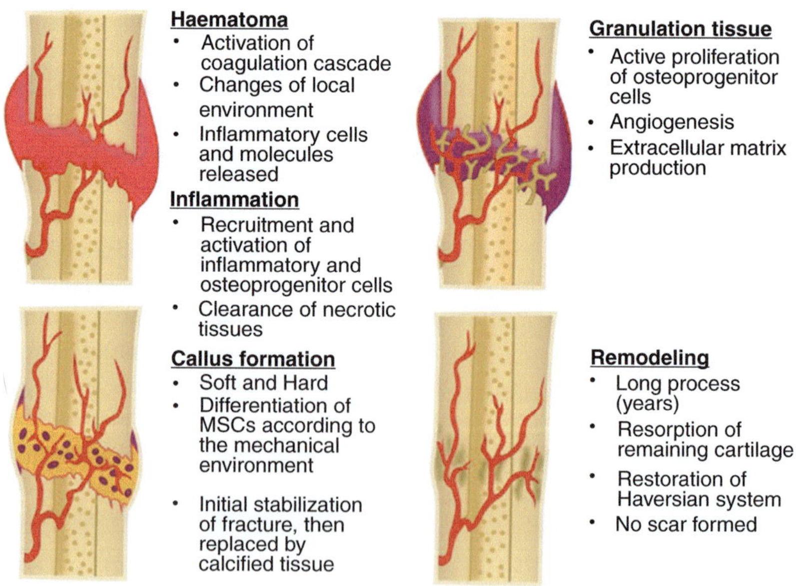

Fig. 1.1 The stages of secondary bone healing

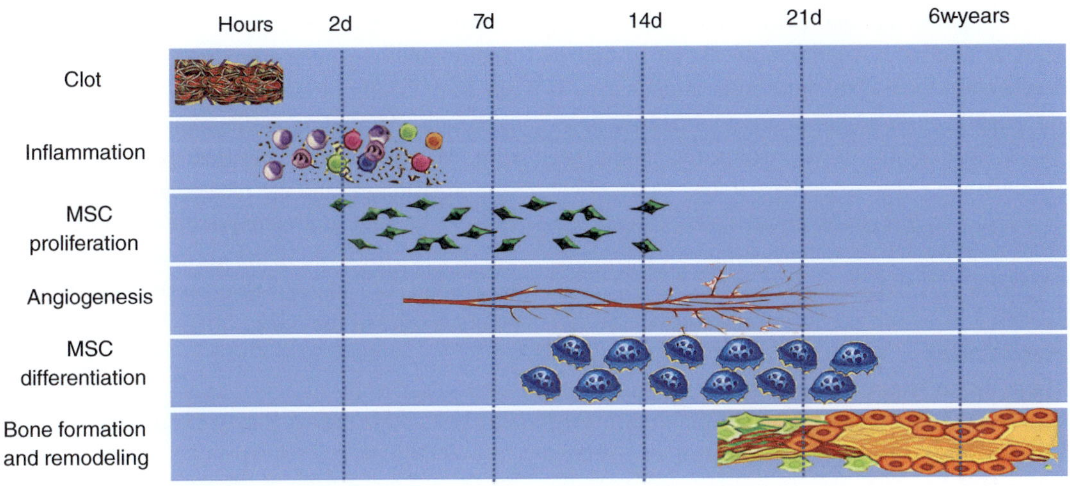

Fig. 1.2 Evolution of fracture healing over time

Inflammatory Stage

An adequate inflammatory phase is a prerequisite for successful bone healing [6, 7]. The inflammatory stage is activated after the hematoma formation and serves mainly two purposes. Firstly, it prepares the site for the upcoming healing process and secondly elicits pain that forces the individual to immobilize the affected limb. A large number of cells invade the fracture site attracted by the numerous inflammatory molecules. Polymorphonuclear leukocytes, lymphocytes, blood monocytes, and macrophages are present and release cytokines. They exert chemotactic effect, recruiting further inflammatory and mesenchymal cells, and stimulate angiogenesis, enhancing extracellular matrix synthesis. RUNX1 (runt-related transcription factor 1) expression predominates which is important for the proliferation of the hematopoietic stem cells and osteoprogenitor cells [8]. TNF-α plays an important role in the inflammatory stage, as it is significantly upregulated. Absence of TNF-α delays fracture healing, while excessive amounts destroy the bone [9, 10]. A number of cytokines are present, but their exact role is still largely obscure. Interleukin-17 (IL-17) has a dual effect enhancing osteogenic output but also bone resorption by the osteoclasts [11]. The levels of many inflammatory (IL-6, IL-8, IL-12) and anti-inflammatory (IL-10) molecules are significantly increased. Within the first week after the fracture, the fracture site develops an osteogenic identity.

Granulation Tissue

Once the inflammatory stage expires, the area of the fracture site is organized forming the granulation tissue. The granulation tissue is a loose aggregate of cells (mainly mesenchymal, endothelial, and immune cells) scattered inside an extracellular matrix. Mesenchymal stem cells from the periosteum and adjacent tissues are seen in the granulation tissue [12]. The fibrin deposits are removed by macrophages and through the actions of fibrinolytic enzymes. There is a significant mitogenic activity at the area, which is supported by the formation of new small blood vessels.

Soft Callus

Soft callus is closely related to the formation of cartilage through endochondral ossification. Endochondral ossification can be seen as an attempt of the body to improve the stability at the fracture site, allowing the ossification process to commence. The soft callus extends throughout the fracture gap connecting the ends of the bone. This process is similar to the bone growth observed in the growth plate. Chondrocytes start preparing cartilage and extracellular matrix. The cellular density is significantly higher to that of healthy articular cartilage but its organization is different [13]. In addition to chondrocytes, fibroblasts start laying down stroma that helps and supports vascular ingrowth. It has been previously shown that smoking adversely affects this particular aspect of bone healing, i.e., vascular ingrowth [14, 15].

Hard Callus

Hard callus is synonymous to the formation of woven bone. Depending on the stability of the fracture site, woven bone can be formed immediately after the formation of granulation tissue through intramembranous ossification (stable fracture), or it can follow the endochondral ossification. During the intramembranous ossification, osteoprogenitor cells differentiate directly to osteoblasts, without the formation of cartilage as an intermediate step. In less stable fractures, the cartilage previously formed by chondrocytes is replaced by the bone. Irrespectively of the route followed, osteoblasts release vesicles that contain calcium phosphate complexes into the matrix [16]. They also release enzymes that degrade the proteoglycan-rich matrix and hydrolyze phosphate esters to provide phosphate ions for precipitation with calcium [17]. The transition from cartilage formation to bone formation is not yet fully elucidated. The simplest theory is based on the property of cells of mesenchymal origin to swap fates and become a different cell types. It was previously shown that fully differentiated osteoblasts with detectable alkaline phosphatase activity and elaboration of calcified extracellular matrix can redifferentiate to other cell types like adipocytes and vice versa. This phenomenon is termed genetic reprogramming or transdifferentiation. Another hypothesis suggests that chondrocytes became engulfed in the newly formed matrix, stop producing cartilage, and eventually die [18]. Chondrocyte cell death seems to occur at the border of the soft callus, just within the newly produced matrix [18].

Remodeling

The remodeling stage is the final stage of secondary bone healing that can last for many years. It represents a gradual modification of the architecture that ultimately reestablishes the typical osteon structure and the haversian system of the bone [19]. This is done under the same mechanical stresses involved in the normal remodeling of the bone [20]. The end result resembles the prefracture state of the bone.

Factors Affecting Bone Healing

The last century was characterized by a revolution in our understanding of bone biology and fracture management. Among the pioneers are the members of the Arbeitsgemeinschaft für Osteosynthesefragen (AO) group who identified some of the key principles governing fracture management, such as (1) accurate anatomical reduction, (2) rigid internal fixation, (3) sound atraumatic surgical technique, and (4) respect for the soft tissue envelope. A number of factors have been found to interrupt the normal flow of the bone healing process. These factors can be broadly divided in fracture or injury dependent and patient dependent (Table 1.1).

Table 1.1 Factors affecting bone healing

Local factors	Systemic factors
• Location • Type of the fracture • Fracture gap • Bone loss—comminution • Degree of local trauma (injury and iatrogenic) • Blood supply • Method of fixation • Level of fracture stability • Presence of infection, foreign material, debris, dead tissue	• Age • Metabolic state and nutrition • Vitamins and mineral deficiencies • Smoking, alcohol • Systemic diseases – Diabetes – Vascular disease – Cancer—radiotherapy • Drug • Corticosteroids • NSAIDs • Antibiotics • Anticoagulants • Antineoplastic

Patient Dependent

Age and Gender

Patient's gender does not increase the risk of delayed healing or non-union. Males, however, have an increased risk of complications with healing due to the higher incidence of high-energy fractures.

Children heal faster than adults and a non-union is a rare occurrence [21, 22]. Children have a higher regeneration potential and thick periosteum and form large subperiosteal hematoma [21]. These factors contribute to the rapid formation of callus (seen in children) [21, 22]. In adults, animal and experimental models have shown that bone healing potential declines with age [23]. Some clinical studies have shown that age is a negative predictor for healing in specific fracture types like fractures of the clavicle and hip [24, 25]. However, whether this increased risk is related to the age per se or is related to the increased number of comorbidities seen in elderly is yet to be further elucidated [26].

Comorbidities

Malnutrition and metabolic deficiencies represent major risk factors for unsuccessful bone healing. In addition to the general health state, the patient's body should be able to cope with the increased metabolic requirements [27]. Deficiencies in calcium, phosphorus, vitamins C and D, albumin, and proteins were all shown to affect bone healing and functional recovery following a fracture [28, 29]. These parameters should be checked and corrected in all high-risk patients.

Following a fracture, the local trauma and swelling impair the blood supply to the fracture site. In patients with peripheral vascular disease, blood supply is already compromised resulting in a critical supply to the bone and soft tissue envelope. The oxygen transport can be reduced as well as the cellular flow to the fracture site. Nutrient and systemically released molecule availability can be compromised. Literature has shown that in such situations, i.e., compromised peripheral blood supply, inhibition of the bone healing process can occur [30]. A circulatory assessment should always be performed in patients that have sustained a fracture especially those with vascular disease.

Increased healing times and higher risk of non-union have been demonstrated in patients with diabetes. Growth factors like the VEGF and TGF-β were found to be reduced in diabetes, and insulin availability seems to be an important factor during bone healing [31]. The effective management of diabetes in these patients is critical to minimize the potential complications [32].

Hypothyroidism has been found to inhibit endochondral ossification and delay bone healing [33]. As undiagnosed hypothyroidism is quite prevalent in the general population (approximately 5%), screening in high-risk patients should be performed [34].

Anemia is associated with significant deficiencies in bone healing. This has been evident in both clinical and animal studies [35]. These findings have been attributed to the availability of oxygen at the fracture site and the impairment of cellular functions like the production of collagen [36].

Other comorbidities that have been associated with an impairment of bone healing include renal disease, rheumatoid arthritis (possibly related to the use of steroids), and obesity [37].

Drug Administration

The antineoplastic drugs have strong antiproliferative and cytotoxic properties. They inhibit angiogenesis and callus formation and result in higher non-union rates [38]. Similarly, antiangiogenesis agents have a detrimental effect on fracture healing, and the final outcome resembles atrophic non-union [39].

Corticosteroid administration leads to osteoblast apoptosis, osteocyte apoptosis, and inhibition of osteoblastogenesis. Patients on long-term steroids are likely to suffer of low bone mass and have a higher incidence of fractures [40]. During bone healing the length of corticosteroid administration and dose are two critical parameters. Prolonged administration and high doses seem to be detrimental for bone healing. Smaller doses can downregulate fracture healing as well; hence, the clinicians should decide on risks versus the benefits basis [41]. In addition to corticosteroids, disease-modifying drugs like methotrexate are widely used for the treatment of chronic diseases. The available evidence is limited and mainly related to methotrexate. Methotrexate seems to have a dose-dependant effect on experimental studies with low doses being relatively safe [42]. The clinical case series presenting bone healing complications are related to higher doses similar to the ones used in cancer treatment [43]. There is limited evidence in regard to the remaining disease-modifying drugs [42].

Nonsteroidal anti-inflammatory drugs (NSAIDs) are effective medications for the management of acute musculoskeletal pain. They block the cyclooxygenase activity and inhibit the synthesis of prostaglandins, which are potent mediators of pain and inflammation [20]. Their analgesic effect in patients with fractures has been graded equal to that of stronger opiates [20]. The numerous experimental studies available are inconclusive and present diverse and contradicting results [20]. With regard to the clinical studies, there is sufficient evidence to suggest that NSAIDs can inhibit bone healing and the formation of heterotopic bone [44, 45]. Non-union risk was shown to double or even triple among various studies [46]. In balance of evidence, it seems judicious to avoid exposure to NSAIDs in patients with fractures.

Antibiotics play an important role in trauma care and fracture management. They are most frequently administered systemically but also applied locally, usually loaded onto the bone cement. Current literature is rather insufficient to allow a clear statement on whether they inhibit bone healing. Fluoroquinolones at therapeutic doses were found to interfere with the early stages of bone healing in small animal models [47]. Other drugs like tobramycin, rifampicin, and gentamicin were also found to downregulate the functions of osteoblasts [48]. Combinations of antibiotics could be detrimental in osteoprogenitor proliferation and differentiation, although the same antibiotics in isolation do not exhibit significant effects. Often underestimated are the kinetics of antibiotics loaded on cement which can reach concentrations 1000-fold higher that the systemically applied ones. Such high doses were shown to have detrimental effects on bone cells biology.

Anticoagulants are prescribed in the majority of hospitalized and non-weight-bearing patients to prevent deep venous thrombosis. Studies that evaluate their direct effect on human osteoprogenitor cells, quite uniformly, suggest that they reduce the proliferation and differentiation potential of osteoprogenitor cells and several osteogenic markers like BMP-2 and IGFs [49]. With regard to the in vivo experimental studies, contradictory results exist; some studies suggest that anticoagulants can impair bone healing, while others contradict these results [50]. At present there are no clinical studies to address this in humans [53].

Smoking and Alcohol

Smoking has several adverse effects on the human skeleton. It decreases the proliferative capacity of osteoblasts, reduces the overall bone mineral density, increases the rate of hip fractures, and decreases its healing capacity [51]. Currently several hypotheses exist for the mode of action of tobacco smoking on the skeleton; reduced blood supply, increase of oxygen intermediates, interference with arteriole receptors, and inhibition of vitamins are all potential pathways [52]. The vast majority of orthopedic literature highlights the importance of ceasing smoking with clinical studies uniformly showing that smoking delays bone healing, significantly increases the risk of non-union and, and at least doubles the risk of infection in patients undergoing surgery [53].

Chronic alcohol consumption induces osteopenia and increases the risk of falls. Alcohol is found to downregulate bone formation through a dose-dependant adverse effect on the functions of osteoblasts. It is of great interest that Saville have shown that the bone density measured in the left iliac crest of alcoholics below 45 years of age was similar to that of nonalcoholic men and women older than 70 years [54]. In addition, alcohol inhibits the proliferation and differentiation of MSCs as well as the production of ossified bone matrix [55]. Clinical studies have shown that alcoholism is associated with osteomalacia, impaired fracture healing, and aseptic necrosis (primarily necrosis of the femoral head) [55].

In addition to smoking and alcohol consumption, the use of recreational drugs also impairs bone mineral density and bone healing capacity. The available literature is limited, but the available studies clearly highlight an adverse effect [56].

Genetic Predisposition

A significant number of patients with an atrophic non-union do not have any of the aforementioned risk factors. These patients are most often young, active, fit and well, and without any conditions that are known to interfere with bone healing. The theory of "genetic predisposition" to equation of fracture non union has been supported by a number of authors. Animal studies have shown that a downregulated expression of various bone morphogenetic proteins, bone morphogenetic protein inhibitors, fibroblast growth factor signaling pathway, and insulin-derived growth factor can result in non-union [57]. In humans, an association between the CCG haplotype of PDGF-A, specific variants of the TLR4 (mutated 1/W) and TGF-β (mutated homozygote T and heterozygote C/T), and the occurrence of non-unions has been shown [58]. In addition Dimitriou et al. showed that two specific polymorphisms of two inhibitors of the BMP pathway, the noggin (the G/G genotype of the rs1372857 SNP) and Smad6 (the T/T genotype of the rs2053423 SNP), were associated with a greater risk of fracture non-union [59].

Fracture Dependent

In addition to the patient-dependent factors, local factors related to the injury are important. Among them, the fracture personality, location, extent of soft tissue damage, and fixation method are critical elements for the bone healing process.

Fracture Personality and Location

The orientation of the fracture line and the underlying bone are two factors that can influence the bone healing process. The orientation of the fracture line influences the surface areas of bony contact and can influence the healing. The differences in the repair process between undisplaced and displaced fractures are well documented. They involve retardation of the rate as well as an increase in the amount of cartilage formed and a decrease in the amount of primary bone formation between the fracture ends [60]. The location of the fracture can be also an important factor. Different healing rates are reported between different bones. For instance, reported non-union rates ranged from up to 18% in tibial diaphysis but 1.7% in the femoral shaft after reamed nailing [61].

The fracture gap can directly influence the healing process. A gap of 2 mm or higher can adversely affect the bone healing process [62]. Claes et al. compared three different gap sizes: small, medium, and large [62]. Comparing the small to the medium fracture gaps, a large callus was noted with lower fracture stiffness in the group with medium fracture gap. The group with the large gap produced little callus and had low stiffness. In addition to the amount of callus formation, the fracture gap influences the revascularization of the fracture site [63]. Other factors that can influence the fracture healing process include the amount of bone loss, the fracture comminution, and the presence of debris or necrotic tissue or other foreign materials [64]. Finally, the presence of infection has devastating outcomes on the overall healing process.

Soft Tissue Envelope

The degree of local trauma is crucial for fracture healing. An intact soft tissue envelope will prevent the escape of fracture hematoma, provide osteoprogenitor cells, and contribute to the angiogenesis of the fracture site. It will also act as a barrier against pathogen invasion. The amount of trauma and the condition of the soft tissue envelope are related to the amount of callus that is formed. Moderate soft tissue trauma delays new bone formation but only in the early phase of fracture healing [65]. The latter occurs because the surrounding soft tissues are the primary sites to support the bone healing by acting as an important vascular source to deliver oxygen, nutrients, and osteoprogenitor cells to the fracture area. Vascular damage accompanying skeletal injury increases the rate of non-union by fourfold [66]. It requires muscle flap coverage that increases the local bone blood flow and the rate of osteotomy union compared to skin repair, thus supporting the vascular role of muscle in bone regeneration [67]. In addition to the blood flow, the surrounding soft tissue contributes in terms of osteogenic growth factors, cytokines, and chemokines [67]. Reverte et al. demonstrated that tibial fractures with associated soft tissue injury significantly impaired fracture healing [68]. They showed that the rate of delayed union or non-union in tibial fractures with associated compartment syndrome was 55%, in comparison to 17.8% in patients with tibial fracture without associated compartment syndrome [68].

Iatrogenic damage to the bones' soft tissue envelope is a parameter often overlooked. The surgical approach used, the manipulation to reduce the fracture, and the preparation for the application of the implant are all factors that can lead to a vascular compromise of the fracture site. Another factor often underestimate is the excessive stripping of the periosteum during plating and the pressure of the plates on the on the periosteal surfaces. A sound surgical technique and the use of low contact implants help to reduce the area of contact. Today's LC-DCP plates use a trapezoidal cross section, which varies along the length of the plate, to reduce the impact on the periosteum.

Fixation Method and Mechanical Stability

The mechanical stability is closely related to the fracture itself and the method used for fixation. It has been previously shown that small interfragmentary movement is beneficial to fracture healing but small interfragmentary movement is critical. Claes et al. have shown that the fate and output of osteogenic cells are related to the mechanical environment [69]. In particular, intramembranous ossification found to occur with small strain and small hydrostatic pressures, while endochondral ossification occurred with higher hydrostatic pressures. Large strains were found to lead to connective tissue formation. The proliferation and transforming growth factor beta production of osteoblasts were increased for strains up to 5% but decreased for larger strains. In addition to the in vitro models, it has been shown that excessive macroscopic movement can arrest the fracture healing process or result in the refracture of the hard callus [70]. On the other hand, the absence of any strains can result in the remodeling mechanisms to prevail over the modeling drifts, and the net result would be removal of callus with delayed or failed bone healing [70].

The fracture fixation can significantly change the biology of bone healing. Fractures treated with the AO principles of absolute stability heal through primary bone healing without the formation of callus. On the other hand, if the same fracture is fixed through the relative stability principle, the fracture will heal with indirect bone healing with callus formation (Fig. 1.3). In addition to the mode of healing, the type of fracture fixation used can alter the outcome. It has been shown, for example, that humeral shaft fractures treated with an intramedullary device carry worse outcome in comparison to those treated with plating [71]. Another example is the different union rates between reamed and unreamed femoral nail with regard to the delayed union and non-union rate [72]. Even minor adaptations of the principles can alter the outcome. In a study by Krettek et al., for instance, 99 open tibial shaft fractures were treated with external fixation, which was complemented with a lag screw [73].

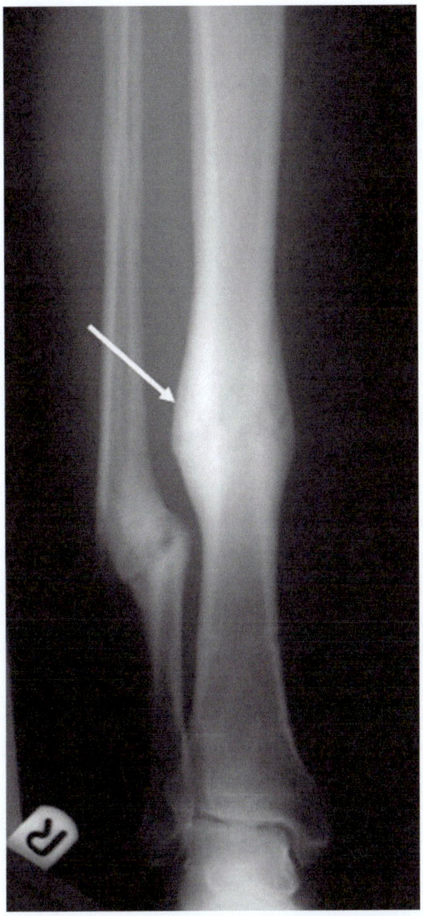

Fig. 1.3 Anteroposterior right tibia radiograph 14 months after originally the fracture was fixed with an intramedullary nail which was removed at 12 months following fracture union. The arrow demonstrates that union occurred with indirect/secondary bone healing (callus formation)

The result was a significant reduction in fracture consolidation. In a similar study, good union rates were documented with external fixation alone [74].

Approaches to Enhance Bone Healing

A number of different approaches have been described to enhance the bone repair response (Table 1.2). Moreover, the conceptual framework of the diamond concept has been described to assist the clinicians to appreciate the most important components of fracture healing that must be present for a successful outcome (Fig. 1.4) [75].

Bone Grafting

Autologous bone grafting from the iliac crest contains all the required elements for bone healing [76]. It has osteoinductive, osteoconductive, and osteogenic properties. It can be harvested with a simple technique; it has low cost and no risk of disease transmission or immunorejection. On the other hand, autologous bone grafting is associated with significant donor site morbidity, often with persistent pain at the harvest site. It can be of limited volume, and the isolated graft, unless tricortical, does not offer any structural support [77].

Table 1.2 Potential applications for the upregulation of bone healing

Application of osteogenic materials

- Autologous bone
- Autologous bone marrow
- Reamer-irrigation aspiration graft
- Combined grafts (Diamond concept)

Systemic enhancement

- Parathyroid hormone
- Biphosphonates
- Anti-sclerostin antibodies
- Anti-Dickkopf-related protein 1 antibodies

Local growth factor applications

- Bone morphogenetic proteins (BMPs)
- Fibroblast growth factors (FGF)
- Vascular Endothelial growth factor (VEGF)
- Platelet-derived growth factors (PDGF)
- Molecules involved in Wnt pathway

Biophysical Stimulation

- Electromagnetic field stimulation
- Low-intensity pulsed ultrasound stimulation
- Etracorporeal shock wave therapy

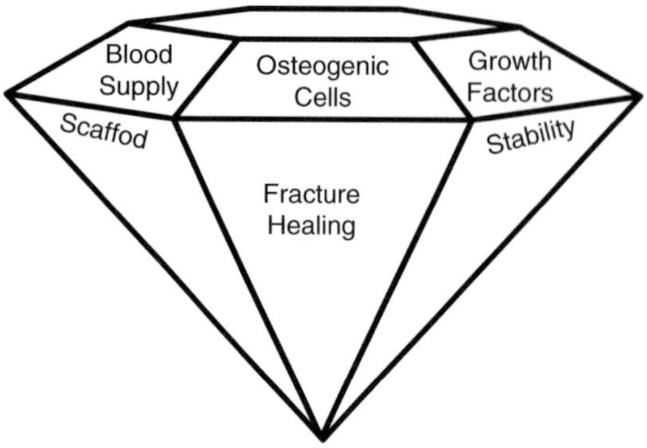

Fig. 1.4 Diamond concept of fracture healing demonstrating the key players that must be present for a successful bone repair response

In addition to the autologous grafting from the iliac crest, grafts obtained with the use of the reamer-irrigator-aspirator (RIA) system (Synthes®, Inc. West Chester, Philadelphia) have gained popularity over the years. A larger volume of graft material can be harvested, capable to fill large bone defects. Unfortunately, RIA grafts contain no or little osteoprogenitor cells (most contained in the waste water) [78] and are associated with a number of complications. Significant intraoperative blood loss with need for transfusion as well as thinning of the cortex and iatrogenic fractures can occur [74]. A large number of bone graft materials are currently commercially available; none, however, is found to outperform the autologous bone grafts.

Application of Cells

Bone marrow aspirates contain MSCs, which are renowned of their osteogenic and angiogenic properties. These cells have the capacity of self-regenerating and are able to produce some of the key molecules involved in bone healing (BMPs, VEGF, etc.). Several authors have shown that a simple bone marrow injection in the fracture or non-union site can result in healing in approximately 90% of cases [79]. Hernigou et al. found that there was a significant correlation between the numbers of MSCs with the clinical outcome. Techniques to concentrate the bone marrow aspirates exist; however, difficulties regarding the high volume of the injectable formulation and the technical issues resulting in inconsistencies in the number of MSCs and the volume of the bone marrow require further research.

Application of Growth Factors

Bone morphogenetic proteins (BMPs) are molecules involved in many functions of the body including development, repair, and regeneration. BMP-2 and BMP-7 have become commercially available for clinical applications including open tibial fractures and lumbar spine fusion or under a humanitarian device exception [80]. However, their off-label application has been diverse. BMP-2 and BMP-7 are potent osteoinductive molecules; both upregulate the osteogenic differentiation and osteogenic output. Clinical results of studies investigating the bone healing have been favorable [80, 81].

Platelet-rich plasma (PRP) is an increased concentration of autologous platelets suspended in a small amount of plasma after centrifugation. The activation of platelets results in the release of several molecules involved in the clotting cascade but also growth factors stored in the platelet α-granules. Such molecules include the platelet-derived growth factor (PDGF), insulin-like growth factor (IGF), vascular endothelial growth factor (VEGF), platelet-derived angiogenic factor (PDAF), and transforming growth factor beta (TGF-β) [82]. This technique is relatively safe and of low cost. The experimental studies have been favorable; however, in a recent meta-analysis including 23 RCTs and 10 prospective studies, the authors questioned its overall effectiveness in fracture healing [83].

Platelet-derived growth factor is a potent promoter of osteogenic cell proliferation, differentiation, and osteogenic output. It also regulates chemotaxis and angiogenesis at the fracture site [84]. A prospective RCT including 434 patients undergoing hindfoot or ankle arthrodesis has shown that PDGF with beta-tricalcium (Augment® Bone Graft, Wright Medical) results in comparable fusion rates as autologous grafting but with less side effects and less complaints of pain [85].

Systemic Biological Factors

Parathyroid hormone (PTH) is a naturally occurring hormone that is known to increase the bone density. Its effect seems to be directly related to the osteogenic cell lineages and through interaction with the Wnt pathway. Experimental and clinical results have been encouraging [86]. In elderly patients with pelvic fractures, PTH administration resulted in a faster time to union compared to controls [86, 87]. In a similar study, faster healing times were also noted in patients suffering of distal radial fractures [88].

Bisphosphonates are inhibitors of osteoclastic activity. Experimental studies have shown however that they could also enhance fracture healing [89]. Despite the fact that the clinical studies are very limited, some of the data presented seem promising [90].

Physical Stimulation

Several devices nowadays are marketed as bone stimulators. They are appealing as they are noninvasive and with minimal complications. These devices can be broadly divided into three categories: electrical stimulators, low-intensity pulsed ultrasonography, and extracorporeal shock wave therapy.

Electrical stimulators are devices capable of generating an electrical potential at the fracture site. It was previously found that during fracture compression an electronegative potential is created which can trigger bone formation [91]. On the contrary an electropositive potential leads to bone loss. Therefore, applying the appropriate electrical potential can result in bone formation at the fracture site. Experimental studies were in the majority in favor of this theory [91]. Clinical studies have been inconclusive. A recent meta-analysis has concluded that there was no significant impact of electromagnetic stimulation on delayed unions or ununited long bone fractures. However, some uncertainty exists due to the methodological limitations and the high between-study heterogeneity [91].

The low-intensity pulsed ultrasonography (LIPUS) principle is based on the production of its sound waves that generate micro-stresses at the fracture site. The cells present at the fracture site can be stimulated by these stresses and increase their osteogenic output. LIPUS was found to accelerate mineralization in vitro through the upregulation of the expression of osteocalcin, alkaline phosphatase, VEGF, and MMP-13 [92]. In vivo evidence also suggests that LIPUS can accelerate all stages of the fracture repair process (inflammation, soft callus formation, hard callus formation). However, in a recent meta-analysis of the available evidence, it was suggested that LIPUS does not improve outcomes and probably has no effect on radiographic bone healing [93].

Extracorporeal shock wave therapy produces a single high-amplitude sound wave that propagates through the fracture site. These shock waves stimulated cellular changes promoting the production of several osteogenic growth factors. Some evidence that extracorporeal shock wave therapy is effective for hypertrophic non-unions than atrophic non-unions exists, but most of the current knowledge is based on level 4 evidence, and further studies are needed to confirm whether any benefit exists [94, 95].

Conflict of Interest No benefits in any form have been received or will be received from a commercial party related directly or indirectly to the subject of this chapter.

References

1. Lane WAL. The operative treatment of fractures. 2nd ed. London: The Medical Publishing Co. Ltd; 1914.
2. Danis R. Théorie et pratique de l'ostéosynthèse. Paris: Masson; 1949.
3. Kolar P, Gaber T, Perka C, Duda GN, Buttgereit F. Human early fracture hematoma is characterized by inflammation and hypoxia. Clin Orthop Relat Res. 2011;469(11):3118–26.
4. Burke D, Dishowitz M, Sweetwyne M, Miedel E, Hankenson KD, Kelly DJ. The role of oxygen as a

regulator of stem cell fate during fracture repair in TSP2-null mice. J Orthop Res. 2013;31(10):1585–96.
5. Wray JB. The biochemical characteristics of the fracture hematoma in man. Surg Gynecol Obstet. 1970;130(5):847–52.
6. Mountziaris PM, Mikos AG. Modulation of the inflammatory response for enhanced bone tissue regeneration. Tissue Eng Part B Rev. 2008;14(2):179–86.
7. Xing Z, Lu C, Hu D, Miclau T 3rd, Marcucio RS. Rejuvenation of the inflammatory system stimulates fracture repair in aged mice. J Orthop Res. 2010;28(8):1000–6.
8. Friedman AD. Cell cycle and developmental control of hematopoiesis by Runx1. J Cell Physiol. 2009;219(3):520–4.
9. Karnes JM, Daffner SD, Watkins CM. Multiple roles of tumor necrosis factor-alpha in fracture healing. Bone. 2015;78:87–93.
10. Mountziaris PM, Spicer PP, Kasper FK, Mikos AG. Harnessing and modulating inflammation in strategies for bone regeneration. Tissue Eng Part B Rev. 2011;17(6):393–402.
11. Nam D, Mau E, Wang Y, Wright D, Silkstone D, Whetstone H, Whyne C, Alman B. T-lymphocytes enable osteoblast maturation via IL-17F during the early phase of fracture repair. PLoS One. 2012;7(6):e40044.
12. Einhorn TA. The cell and molecular biology of fracture healing. Clin Orthop Relat Res. 1998;(355 Suppl):S7–21.
13. Bianco P, Cancedda FD, Riminucci M, Cancedda R. Bone formation via cartilage models: the "borderline" chondrocyte. Matrix Biol. 1998;17(3):185–92.
14. Daftari TK, Whitesides TE Jr, Heller JG, Goodrich AC, McCarey BE, Hutton WC. Nicotine on the revascularization of bone graft. An experimental study in rabbits. Spine (Phila Pa 1976). 1994;19(8):904–11.
15. Rubenstein I, Yong T, Rennard SI, Mayhan WG. Cigarette smoke extract attenuates endothelium-dependent arteriolar dilatation in vivo. Am J Phys. 1991;261(6 Pt 2):H1913–8.
16. Brighton CT, Hunt RM. Histochemical localization of calcium in the fracture callus with potassium pyroantimonate. Possible role of chondrocyte mitochondrial calcium in callus calcification. J Bone Joint Surg Am. 1986;68(5):703–15.
17. Einhorn TA, Hirschman A, Kaplan C, Nashed R, Devlin VJ, Warman J. Neutral protein-degrading enzymes in experimental fracture callus: a preliminary report. J Orthop Res. 1989;7(6):792–805.
18. Ford JL, Robinson DE, Scammell BE. The fate of soft callus chondrocytes during long bone fracture repair. J Orthop Res. 2003;21(1):54–61.
19. Claes L, Recknagel S, Ignatius A. Fracture healing under healthy and inflammatory conditions. Nat Rev Rheumatol. 2012;8(3):133–43. https://doi.org/10.1038/nrrheum.2012.1.
20. Pountos I, Georgouli T, Calori GM, Giannoudis PV. Do nonsteroidal anti-inflammatory drugs affect bone healing? A critical analysis. Sci World J. 2012;2012:606404.
21. Lindaman LM. Bone healing in children. Clin Podiatr Med Surg. 2001;18:97–108.
22. Wilkins KE. Principles of fracture remodeling in children. Injury. 2005;36(Suppl 1):A3–11.
23. Aho AJ. Electron microscopic and histologic studies on fracture repair in old and young rats. Acta Chir Scand Suppl. 1966;357:162–5.
24. Parker MJ. Prediction of fracture union after internal fixation of intracapsular femoral neck fractures. Injury. 1994;25(Suppl 2):B3–6.
25. Robinson CM, Court-Brown CM, McQueen MM, Wakefield AE. Estimating the risk of nonunion following nonoperative treatment of a clavicular fracture. J Bone Joint Surg Am. 2004;86-A(7):1359–65.
26. Zura R, Braid-Forbes MJ, Jeray K, Mehta S, Einhorn TA, Watson JT, Della Rocca GJ, Forbes K, Steen RG. Bone fracture nonunion rate decreases with increasing age: A prospective inception cohort study. Bone. 2017;95:26–32.
27. Hayda RA, Brighton CT, Esterhai JL Jr. Pathophysiology of delayed healing. Clin Orthop Relat Res. 1998;(355 Suppl):S31–40.
28. Einhorn TA, Gerstenfeld LC. Fracture healing: mechanisms and interventions. Nat Rev Rheumatol. 2015;11(1):45–54.
29. Einhorn TA, Bonnarens F, Burstein AH. The contributions of dietary protein and mineral to the healing of experimental fractures. A biomechanical study. J Bone Joint Surg Am. 1986;68(9):1389–95.
30. Brinker MR, Bailey DE Jr. Fracture healing in tibia fractures with an associated vascular injury. J Trauma. 1997;42(1):11–9.
31. Bibbo C, Lin SS, Beam HA, Behrens FF. Complications of ankle fractures in diabetic patients. Orthop Clin North Am. 2001;32(1):113–33.
32. Gorter EA, Krijnen P, Schipper IB. Vitamin D status and adult fracture healing. J Clin Orthop Trauma. 2017;8(1):34–7.
33. Kowalewski K, Yong S. Bone and urinary hydroxyproline in normal and hypothyroid rat with a long bone fracture. Acta Endocrinol. 1967;56(3):547–53.
34. Bilous RW, Tunbridge WM. The epidemiology of hypothyroidism-an update. Bailliere Clin Endocrinol Metab. 1988;2(3):531–40.
35. Dix B, Grant-McDonald L, Catanzariti A, Saltrick K. Preoperative Anemia in Hindfoot and Ankle Arthrodesis. Foot Ankle Spec. 2017;10(2):109–15.
36. Gruson KI, Aharonoff GB, Egol KA, Zuckerman JD, Koval KJ. The relationship between admission hemoglobin level and outcome after hip fracture. J Orthop Trauma. 2002;16(1):39–44.
37. Chakkalakal DA, Novak JR, Fritz ED, Mollner TJ, McVicker DL, Lybarger DL, McGuire MH, Donohue TM Jr. Chronic ethanol consumption results in deficient bone repair in rats. Alcohol Alcohol. 2002;37(1):13–20.

38. Hazan EJ, Hornicek FJ, Tomford W, Gebhardt MC, Mankin HJ. The effect of adjuvant chemotherapy on osteoarticular allografts. Clin Orthop Relat Res. 2001;385:176–81.
39. Hausman MR, Schaffler MB, Majeska RJ. Prevention of fracture healing in rats by an inhibitor of angiogenesis. Bone. 2001;29(6):560–4.
40. Aaron JE, Francis RM, Peacock M, Makins NB. Contrasting microanatomy of idiopathic and corticosteroid-induced osteoporosis. Clin Orthop Relat Res. 1989;243:294–305.
41. Pountos I, Georgouli T, Blokhuis TJ, Pape HC, Giannoudis PV. Pharmacological agents and impairment of fracture healing: what is the evidence? Injury. 2008;39(4):384–94.
42. Pountos I, Giannoudis PV. Effect of methotrexate on bone and wound healing. Expert Opin Drug Saf. 2017;16(5):535–45.
43. Gerster JC, Bossy R, Dudler J. Bone non-union after osteotomy in patients treated with methotrexate. J Rheumatol. 1999;26:2695–7.
44. Neal BC, Rodgers A, Clark T, Gray H, Reid IR, Dunn L, MacMahon SW. A systematic survey of 13 randomized trials of non-steroidal anti-inflammatory drugs for the prevention of heterotopic bone formation after major hip surgery. Acta Orthop Scand. 2000;71(2):122–8.
45. Miller GK. Editorial Commentary: The Efficacy of Nonsteroidal Anti-inflammatory Drugs for Prophylaxis of Heterotopic Ossification in Hip Arthroscopy-Do We Treat Patients or X-rays? Arthroscopy. 2016;32(3):526–7.
46. Jeffcoach DR, Sams VG, Lawson CM, Enderson BL, Smith ST, Kline H, Barlow PB, Wylie DR, Krumenacker LA, McMillen JC, Pyda J, Daley BJ, University of Tennessee Medical Center, Department of Surgery. Nonsteroidal anti-inflammatory drugs' impact on nonunion and infection rates in long-bone fractures. J Trauma Acute Care Surg. 2014;76(3):779–83.
47. Perry AC, Prpa B, Rouse MS, Piper KE, Hanssen AD, Steckelberg JM, Patel R. Levofloxacin and trovafloxacin inhibition of experimental fracture-healing. Clin Orthop Relat Res. 2003;414:95–100.
48. Miclau T, Edin ML, Lester GE, Lindsey RW, Dahners LE. Bone toxicity of locally applied aminoglycosides. J Orthop Trauma. 1995;9(5):401–6.
49. Pilge H, Fröbel J, Prodinger PM, Mrotzek SJ, Fischer JC, Zilkens C, Bittersohl B, Krauspe R. Enoxaparin and rivaroxaban have different effects on human mesenchymal stromal cells in the early stages of bone healing. Bone Joint Res. 2016;5(3):95–100.
50. Street JT, McGrath M, O'Regan K, Wakai A, McGuinness A, Redmond HP. Thromboprophylaxis using a low molecular weight heparin delays fracture repair. Clin Orthop Relat Res. 2000;(381): 278–89.
51. Melhus H, Michaëlsson K, Holmberg L, Wolk A, Ljunghall S. Smoking, antioxidant vitamins, and the risk of hip fracture. J Bone Miner Res. 1999;14(1):129–35.
52. Porter SE, Hanley EN Jr. The musculoskeletal effects of smoking. J Am Acad Orthop Surg. 2001;9(1):9–17.
53. Castillo RC, Bosse MJ, MacKenzie EJ, Patterson BM, LEAP Study Group. Impact of smoking on fracture healing and risk of complications in limb-threatening open tibia fractures. J Orthop Trauma. 2005;19(3):151–7.
54. Saville PD. Changes in bone mass with age and alcoholism. J Bone Joint Surg Am. 1965;47:492–9.
55. Arlot ME, Bonjean M, Chavassieux PM, Meunier PJ. Bone histology in adults with aseptic necrosis. Histomorphometric evaluation of iliac biopsies in seventy-seven patients. J Bone Joint Surg Am. 1983;65:1319–27.
56. Nogueira-Filho Gda R, Cadide T, Rosa BT, Neiva TG, Tunes R, Peruzzo D, Nociti FH Jr, César-Neto JB. Cannabis sativa smoke inhalation decreases bone filling around titanium implants: a histomorphometric study in rats. Implant Dent. 2008;17(4):461–70.
57. Dimitriou R, Kanakaris N, Soucacos PN, Giannoudis PV. Genetic predisposition to non-union: evidence today. Injury. 2013;44(Suppl 1):S50–3.
58. Zeckey C, Hildebrand F, Glaubitz LM, Jürgens S, Ludwig T, Andruszkow H, Hüfner T, Krettek C, Stuhrmann M. Are polymorphisms of molecules involved in bone healing correlated to aseptic femoral and tibial shaft non-unions? J Orthop Res. 2011;29(11):1724–31. https://doi.org/10.1002/jor.21443.
59. Dimitriou R, Carr IM, West RM, Markham AF, Giannoudis PV. Genetic predisposition to fracture non-union: a case control study of a preliminary single nucleotide polymorphisms analysis of the BMP pathway. BMC Musculoskelet Disord. 2011;12:44.
60. Rhinelander FW, Baragry RA. Microangiography in bone healing: Undisplaced closed fractures. J Bone Joint Surg. 1962;44A:1273.
61. Fong K, Truong V, Foote CJ, Petrisor B, Williams D, Ristevski B, et al. Predictors of nonunion and reoperation in patients with fractures of the tibia: an observational study. BMC Musculoskelet Disord. 2013;14:103.
62. Claes L, Augat P, Suger G, Wilke HJ. Influence of size and stability of the osteotomy gap on the success of fracture healing. J Orthop Res. 1997 Jul;15(4):577–84.
63. Claes L, Eckert-Hübner K, Augat P. The fracture gap size influences the local vascularization and tissue differentiation in callus healing. Langenbeck's Arch Surg. 2003;388(5):316–22.
64. Riehl JT, Connolly K, Haidukewych G, Koval K. Fractures Due to Gunshot Wounds: Do Retained Bullet Fragments Affect Union? Iowa Orthop J. 2015;35:55–61.
65. Claes L, Maurer-Klein N, Henke T, Gerngross H, Melnyk M, Augat P. Moderate soft tissue trauma delays new bone formation only in the early phase of fracture healing. J Orthop Res. 2006;24(6):1178–85.

66. Lu C, Miclau T, Hu D, Marcucio RS. Ischemia leads to delayed union during fracture healing: a mouse model. J Orthop Res. 2007;25(1):51–61.
67. Reverte MM, Dimitriou R, Kanakaris NK, Giannoudis PV. What is the effect of compartment syndrome and fasciotomies on fracture healing in tibial fractures? Injury. 2011;42(12):1402–7.
68. Claes LE, Heigele CA, Neidlinger-Wilke C, Kaspar D, Seidl W, Margevicius KJ, Augat P. Effects of mechanical factors on the fracture healing process. Clin Orthop Relat Res. 1998;(355 Suppl):S132–47.
69. Mavčič B, Antolič V. Optimal mechanical environment of the healing bone fracture/osteotomy. Int Orthop. 2012;36(4):689–95.
70. Hu X, Xu S, Lu H, Chen B, Zhou X, He X, Dai J, Zhang Z, Gong S. Minimally invasive plate osteosynthesis vs conventional fixation techniques for surgically treated humeral shaft fractures: a meta-analysis. J Orthop Surg Res. 2016;11(1):59.
71. Duan X, Li T, Mohammed AQ, Xiang Z. Reamed intramedullary nailing versus unreamed intramedullary nailing for shaft fracture of femur: a systematic literature review. Arch Orthop Trauma Surg. 2011;131(10):1445–52.
72. Krettek C, Haas N, Tscherne H. The role of supplemental lag-screw fixation for open fractures of the tibial shaft treated with external fixation. J Bone Joint Surg Am. 1991;73(6):893–7.
73. Claes L, Grass R, Schmickal T, Kisse B, Eggers C, Gerngross H, Mutschler W, Arand M, Wintermeyer T, Wentzensen A. Monitoring and healing analysis of 100 tibial shaft fractures. Langenbeck's Arch Surg. 2002;387(3–4):146–52.
74. Pountos I, Panteli M, Georgouli T, Giannoudis PV. Neoplasia following use of BMPs: is there an increased risk? Expert Opin Drug Saf. 2014;13(11):1525–34.
75. Giannoudis PV, Einhorn TA, Marsh D. Fracture healing: the diamond concept. Injury. 2007;38(Suppl 4):S3–6.
76. Crist BD, Stoker AM, Stannard JP, Cook JL. Analysis of relevant proteins from bone graft harvested using the reamer irrigator and aspirator system (RIA) versus iliac crest (IC) bone graft and RIA waste water. Injury. 2016;47(8):1661–8.
77. Marchand LS, Rothberg DL, Kubiak EN, Higgins TF. Is This Autograft Worth It?: The Blood Loss and Transfusion Rates Associated With Reamer Irrigator Aspirator Bone Graft Harvest. J Orthop Trauma. 2017;31(4):205–9.
78. Pountos I, Georgouli T, Kontakis G, Giannoudis PV. Efficacy of minimally invasive techniques for enhancement of fracture healing: evidence today. Int Orthop. 2010;34(1):3–12.
79. Kanakaris NK, Calori GM, Verdonk R, Burssens P, De Biase P, Capanna R, Vangosa LB, Cherubino P, Baldo F, Ristiniemi J, Kontakis G, Giannoudis PV. Application of BMP-7 to tibial non-unions: a 3-year multicenter experience. Injury. 2008;39(Suppl 2):S83–90.
80. Anitua E, Andia I, Ardanza B, Nurden P, Nurden AT. Autologous platelets as a source of proteins for healing and tissue regeneration. Thromb Haemost. 2004;91(1):4–15.
81. Sheth U, Simunovic N, Klein G, Fu F, Einhorn TA, Schemitsch E, Ayeni OR, Bhandari M. Efficacy of autologous platelet-rich plasma use for orthopaedic indications: a meta-analysis. J Bone Joint Surg Am. 2012;94(4):298–307.
82. Pountos I, Georgouli T, Henshaw K, Bird H, Jones E, Giannoudis PV. The effect of bone morphogenetic protein-2, bone morphogenetic protein-7, parathyroid hormone, and platelet-derived growth factor on the proliferation and osteogenic differentiation of mesenchymal stem cells derived from osteoporotic bone. J Orthop Trauma. 2010;24(9):552–6.
83. DiGiovanni CW, Lin SS, Baumhauer JF, Daniels T, Younger A, Glazebrook M, Anderson J, Anderson R, Evangelista P, Lynch SE, North American Orthopedic Foot and Ankle Study Group. Recombinant human platelet-derived growth factor-BB and beta-tricalcium phosphate (rhPDGF-BB/β-TCP): an alternative to autogenous bone graft. J Bone Joint Surg Am. 2013;95(13):1184–92.
84. Tzioupis CC, Giannoudis PV. The Safety and Efficacy of Parathyroid Hormone (PTH) as a Biological Response Modifier for the Enhancement of Bone Regeneration. Curr Drug Saf. 2006;1(2):189–203.
85. Peichl P, Holzer LA, Maier R, Holzer G. Parathyroid hormone 1-84 accelerates fracture-healing in pubic bones of elderly osteoporotic women. J Bone Joint Surg Am. 2011;93(17):1583–7.
86. Aspenberg P, Johansson T. Teriparatide improves early callus formation in distal radial fractures. Acta Orthop. 2010;81(2):234–6.
87. Türker M, Aslan A, Çırpar M, Kochai A, Tulmaç ÖB, Balcı M. Histological and biomechanical effects of zoledronate on fracture healing in an osteoporotic rat tibia model. Eklem Hastalik Cerrahisi. 2016;27(1):9–15.
88. Kiely P, Ward K, Bellemore CM, Briody J, Cowell CT, Little DG. Bisphosphonate rescue in distraction osteogenesis: a case series. J Pediatr Orthop. 2007;27(4):467–71.
89. Kuzyk PR, Schemitsch EH. The science of electrical stimulation therapy for fracture healing. Indian J Orthop. 2009;43(2):127–31.
90. Korenstein R, Somjen D, Fischler H, Binderman I. Capacitative pulsed electric stimulation of bone cells. Induction of cyclic-AMP changes and DNA synthesis. Biochim Biophys Acta. 1984;803(4):302–7.
91. Mollon B, da Silva V, Busse JW, Einhorn TA, Bhandari M. Electrical stimulation for long-bone fracture-healing: a meta-analysis of randomized controlled trials. J Bone Joint Surg Am. 2008;90(11):2322–30.
92. Pounder NM, Harrison AJ. Low intensity pulsed ultrasound for fracture healing: a review of the clinical

evidence and the associated biological mechanism of action. Ultrasonics. 2008;48(4):330–8.
93. Schandelmaier S, Kaushal A, Lytvyn L, Heels-Ansdell D, Siemieniuk RA, Agoritsas T, Guyatt GH, Vandvik PO, Couban R, Mollon B, Busse JW. Low intensity pulsed ultrasound for bone healing: systematic review of randomized controlled trials. BMJ. 2017;356:j656.
94. Vulpiani MC, Vetrano M, Conforti F, Minutolo L, Trischitta D, Furia JP, Ferretti A. Effects of extracorporeal shock wave therapy on fracture nonunions. Am J Orthop (Belle Mead NJ). 2012;41(9):E122–7.
95. Zelle BA, Gollwitzer H, Zlowodzki M, Bühren V. Extracorporeal shock wave therapy: current evidence. J Orthop Trauma. 2010;24(Suppl 1):S66–70.

2 Instruments Used in Fracture Reduction

Ippokratis Pountos, K. Newman, and Peter V. Giannoudis

Fracture reduction can be achieved by either direct or indirect means [1, 2]. Direct reduction means that the forces and moments applied when attempting to realign the bony fragments act at the vicinity of the fracture site, while, in indirect reduction, the forces are applied distally to the fracture site [3]. Direct reduction is often performed by direct visualization of the fracture site through surgical exposure. Utilising minimally invasive approaches, fractures can also be reduced percutaneously.

Indirect reduction involves forces along the axis of the limb, which in turn can result in fracture realignment through the action of the surrounding soft tissues (ligamentotaxis) [4, 5]. Indirect reduction can involve manual traction with manipulation or can be combined with tools like traction tables, distractors or external fixators.

In reality, not infrequently, combination of both direct and indirect techniques is often performed. Irrespectively of the reduction technique used, our current armamentarium in fracture reduction aids is ever expanding. The most commonly used instruments are described below. In general terms the instruments can be divided into external devices and internal devices.

External Devices

In this category the most commonly used devices include fracture tables, bumps and bolsters, crutches, skeletal traction, PORD, F-tool, large distractor and external fixator devices, amongst others.

Fracture tables with the capacity for skeletal traction are widely used in fracture management [6]. Fracture tables are radiolucent and designed to achieve and maintain satisfactory reduction of the fracture. The two most commonly used fracture tables are the traction table (Fig. 2.1) and the OSI table (Figs. 2.2 and 2.3).

Most often no further manipulation of the fracture is required once the patient is positioned. Patient positioning on the fracture table is often critical. A thorough preoperative planning with anticipation of potential difficulties and easy access for fluoroscopic imaging is essential [6]. Nowadays, fracture tables are modular, can adjust patient's position with easiness and can take numerous attachments to assist

I. Pountos, M.B., M.D., E.E.C.
Academic Department of Trauma & Orthopaedics, School of Medicine, University of Leeds, Leeds, UK

K. Newman, F.R.C.S.
St Peter's Hospitals NHS Foundation Trust, Chertsey, Surrey, UK

P.V. Giannoudis, M.D., F.R.C.S. (✉)
Academic Department of Trauma & Orthopaedics, School of Medicine, University of Leeds, Leeds, UK
NIHR, Leeds, UK

Musculoskeletal Biomedical Research Center, Chapel Allerton Hospital, Leeds, UK
e-mail: pgiannoudi@aol.com

P.V. Giannoudis (ed.), *Fracture Reduction and Fixation Techniques*,
https://doi.org/10.1007/978-3-319-68628-8_2

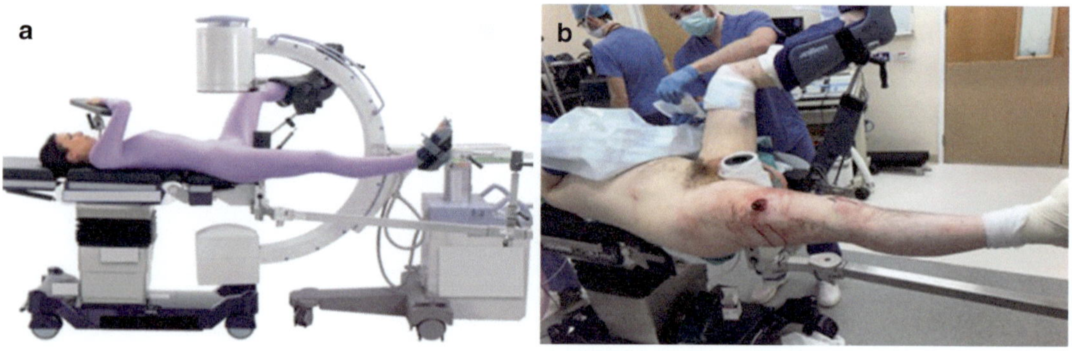

Fig. 2.1 (**a**) Schematic representation of traction applied to right lower leg using a fracture table. (**b**) Patient placed in the supine position on a fracture table with an open right femoral fracture. Traction has been applied on the right hand side to reduce the femoral fracture

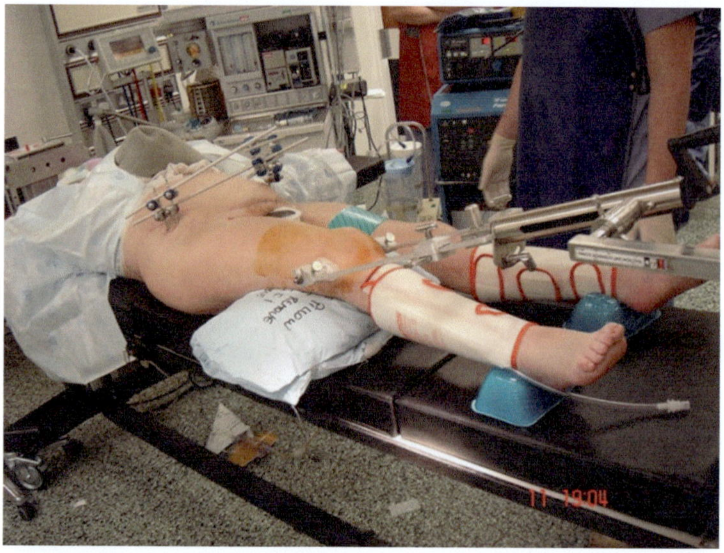

Fig. 2.2 A polytrauma patient with a pelvic external fixator (sustained vertical shear fracture) is placed supine on an OSI table where, with the appropriate attachment device, traction is applied through a right distal femoral pin to reduce the right hemipelvic disruption

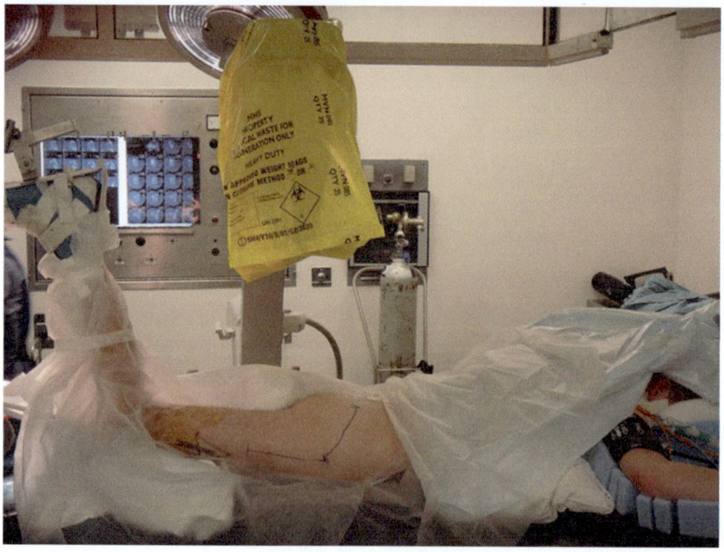

Fig. 2.3 Patient has been positioned prone on the OSI table with skeletal traction (distal femoral pin) applied on the right distal femur to reduce acetabulum fracture

fracture reduction (Fig. 2.4). Setting up the patient can be labour intensive, which increases operative time, and performing multiple surgeries in the same setting is often challenging [7, 8]. Noteworthy, complications from patient positioning can occur and must be minimized. Such complications can range from skin necrosis, nerve palsy and compartment syndrome to iatrogenic fractures [9].

Coexisting injuries and body habitus often preclude the use of the fracture table. In such circumstances the use of the standard radiolucent table is required. Manual traction or the use of skeletal traction (Fig. 2.5) devices can accomplish the same objective with no impact on the final outcome [10]. However, an additional assistant devoted to holding and maintaining traction is required.

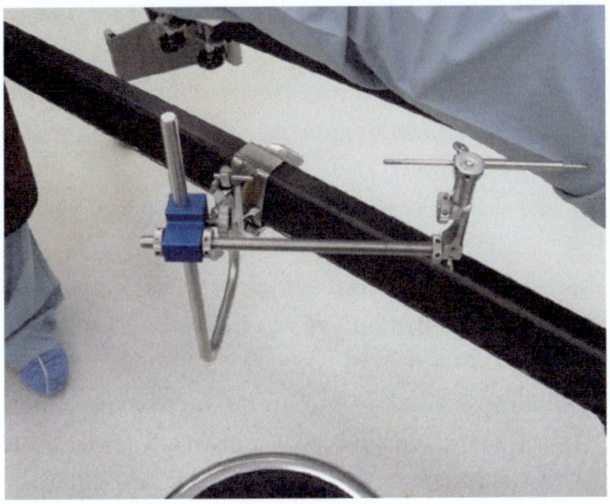

Fig. 2.4 Complementary reduction device attached on the OSI table to assist the reduction of pelvic/acetabulum fractures

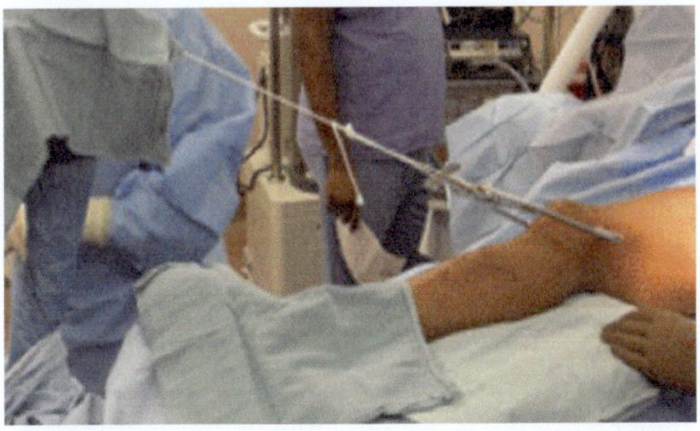

Fig. 2.5 Traction applied using a distal femoral pin intraoperatively

A number of adjuncts can be used during patient positioning on the operating table. Bumps and bolsters can change patient position, maintain the correct orientation of the limb or assist in muscle relaxation during fracture reduction (Figs. 2.6 and 2.7) [11]. Alternatively, special table attachments can be used, for example, the posterior reduction device, (PORD™), which can be used as a fulcrum to relax the gastrocnemius and soleus complexes in femoral or hip fracture fixation (Fig. 2.8) [11, 12].

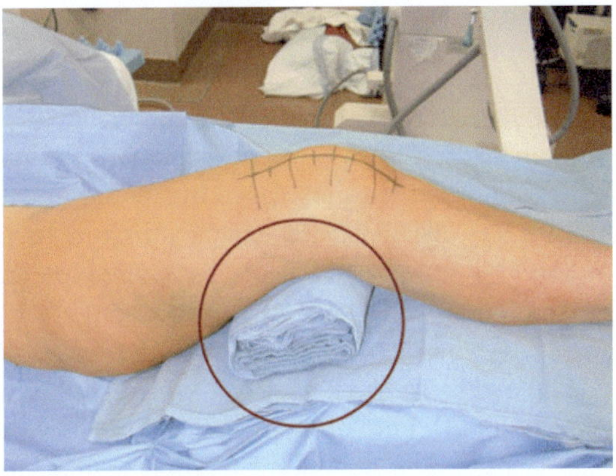

Fig. 2.6 Intraoperative picture showing a bump to control AP sag of knee

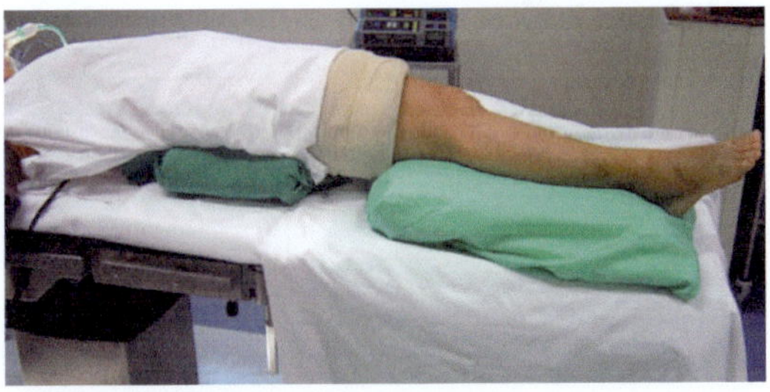

Fig. 2.7 Bolsters to control rotation of leg

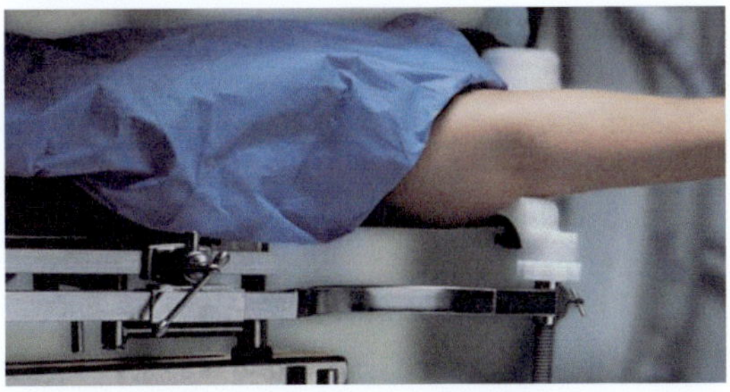

Fig. 2.8 Posterior reduction device (PORD)

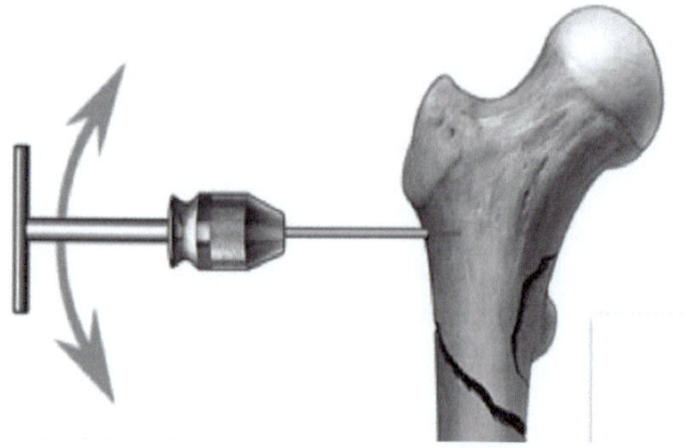

Fig. 2.9 Use of a Schanz screw attached to a T-handed chuck for fracture reduction in sagittal and coronal planes for insertion of nails

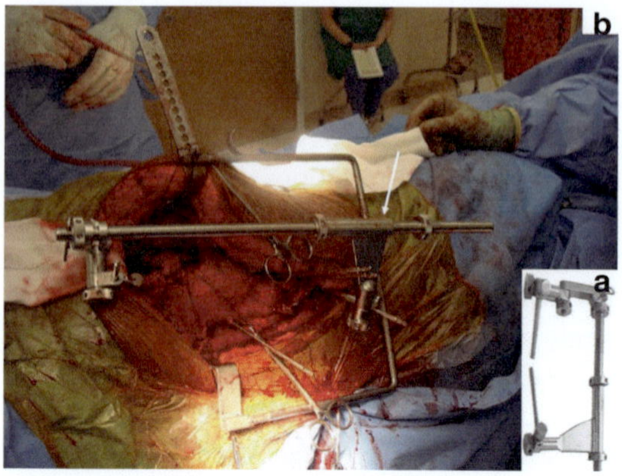

Fig. 2.10 (**a**) Femoral distractor. (**b**) Intraoperative picture of a patient in prone position demonstrating the application of a femoral distractor to reduce a combined acetabulum and proximal femoral fracture

Schanz screws can be inserted percutaneously and can be used as joysticks for manipulation and reduction of the most displaced fracture segment (Fig. 2.9). The T-handed chuck attached to a Schanz pin can be a powerful combination in manipulation and derotating large bony fragments. K-wires applied on the fracture fragments can be used also as joysticks to achieve fracture reduction [13]. Further interfragmentary K-wires can be used as a temporary fixation method to maintain intrafocal reduction. In large bone fragments or when manipulation of the whole limb is required, Schanz pins can be used. Kapandji technique involves the insertion of a K-wire through the fracture gap [14]. Similar to the reduction technique with the use of a Hohmann retractor, manipulation of the distal fragment can occur. Definite stabilization is achieved by passing the K-wire through the distal cortex.

The femoral distractor is composed of a threaded spindle carrying a fixed and a sliding end piece (Fig. 2.10). Schanz screws are fixed through the end pieces, and the distractor is positioned parallel to the axis of the bone. An excursion of about 27 cm is built into the device. More excursion is possible, but angular malposition of the end of the device may occur. Once the bony fragments are adequately reduced, the position is maintained by the secure tightening of the connections. The distractor allows correction of length, rotation and angulation. Also, unlike to the skeletal traction where distraction forces are applied to the whole limb, the femoral distractor applies forces directly to the bone. This makes the distractor readily adaptable in coping with the awkward positioning problems. It also eliminates the risk of nerve injuries, for example, peroneal nerve palsy or pudendal crush syndrome.

The external fixator is a versatile device. Its use can range from the local damage control in cases of compromised soft tissue envelope to the definite management of fractures or bone transport [15]. Not infrequently, the external fixator is a valuable adjunct in fracture reduction and stabilization. With the use of the external fixator, the indirect reduction of the bony fragments can be accomplished under image intensification. Once reduced the position can be maintained while the internal fixation plate is slipped under the soft tissues. In some situations in which the internal fixation does not provide adequate stability, the external fixator can be left in situ for a short period of time, to provide additional support (Fig. 2.11).

The F-tool is a simple device composed of a bar on which different rods can be installed [16]. It allows focused forces to be concentrated at the apex of the deformity. Once longitudinal traction is applied to the limb, the F-tool can be used to correct deformity and angulation along one plane (Fig. 2.12). The F-tool is not radiolucent and should only be used in simple fracture configurations.

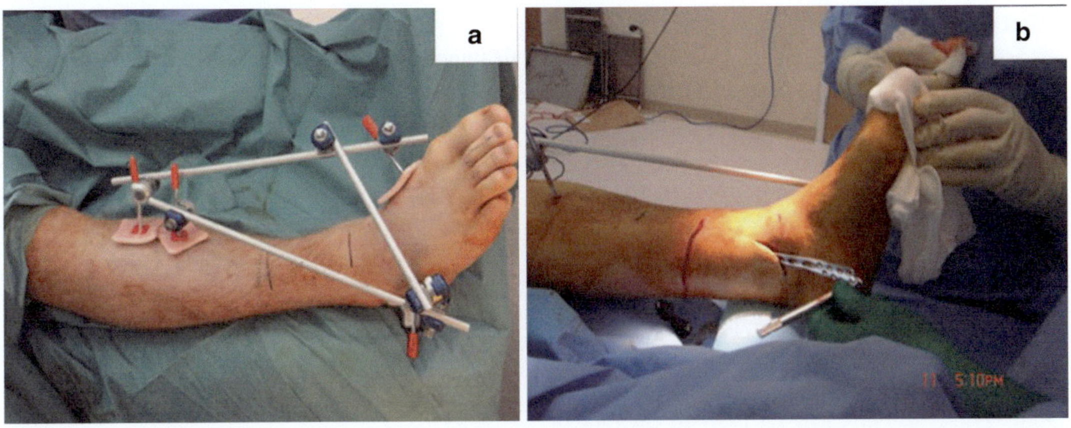

Fig. 2.11 (**a**) Application of an external fixator for a distal tibial fracture. (**b**) Maintaining the lateral component of the external fixator, fracture reduction was possible allowing minimal invasive plating osteosynthesis of the distal tibial fracture

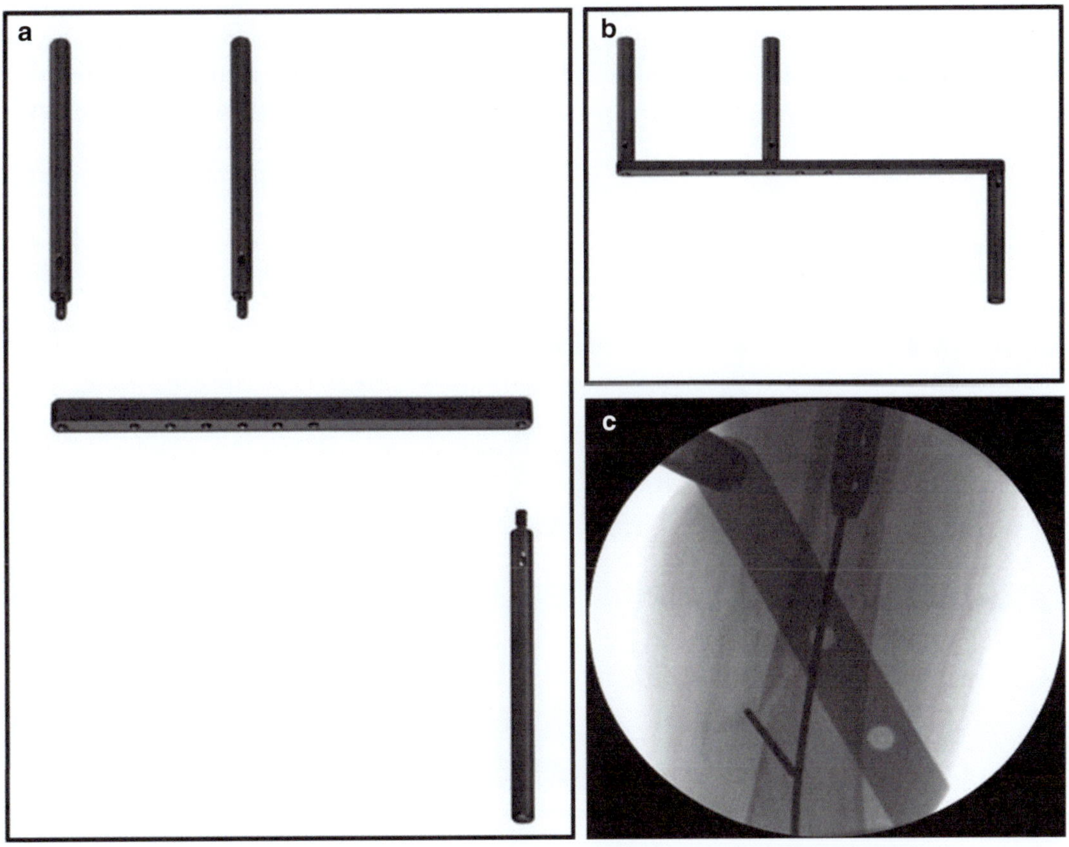

Fig. 2.12 (**a**) F-tool prior to assemblage. (**b**) F-tool connected. (**c**) Fluoroscopic image showing use of the F-tool for reduction of middle one third femoral shaft fracture

Internal Devices

Common reduction tools found in the large and small fracture sets include the following:

(a) Weber forceps (point-to-point forceps)

These forceps have curved sharp pointy tips (Fig. 2.13a). The pointy tips can be applied directly on bones' surface or through drill holes or on screws. They have minimal bone-forceps contact and have minimal impact on the periosteum. These forceps can be used to distract or manipulate fractures when used in two pairs, and when reduction is achieved, they can be used to secure fractures prior to definite fixation. The pointy tips have little interference with other hardware used for fixation like drills, plate and screws. The limitations of the pointy forceps include the easy slippage during fracture manipulation and the potential cortex perforation especially in osteoporotic bone.

(b) Toothed reduction forceps (crocodile forceps, lobster claw)

These forceps have curved serrated jaws designed to have a firm purchase onto the bone (Fig. 2.13b). In contrast to the pointy forceps, these instruments have relatively larger contact area with the bone, and the serrated teeth improve bone-forceps friction. This property, however, comes to a cost, as they can create great periosteal and superficial endosteal damage. They require greater soft tissue dissection around the bone to allow tip placement.

(c) Bone-holding forceps (Verbrugge, ball spike)

The Verbrugge style forceps are self-centring forceps that aim to hold a plate onto the diaphyseal bone (Fig. 2.13c, d). They are comprised of a curved serrated tip that comes in contact with the bone and a sort concave edge that can hold the plate. The hinge mechanism allows the advancement of the forceps tips relative to each other; the forceps centres itself between the plate and the bone. It comes in various sizes from 0 to 3. The use of the appropriate size in relation to the bone fragment is recommended. A modified version of the forceps carrying a ball

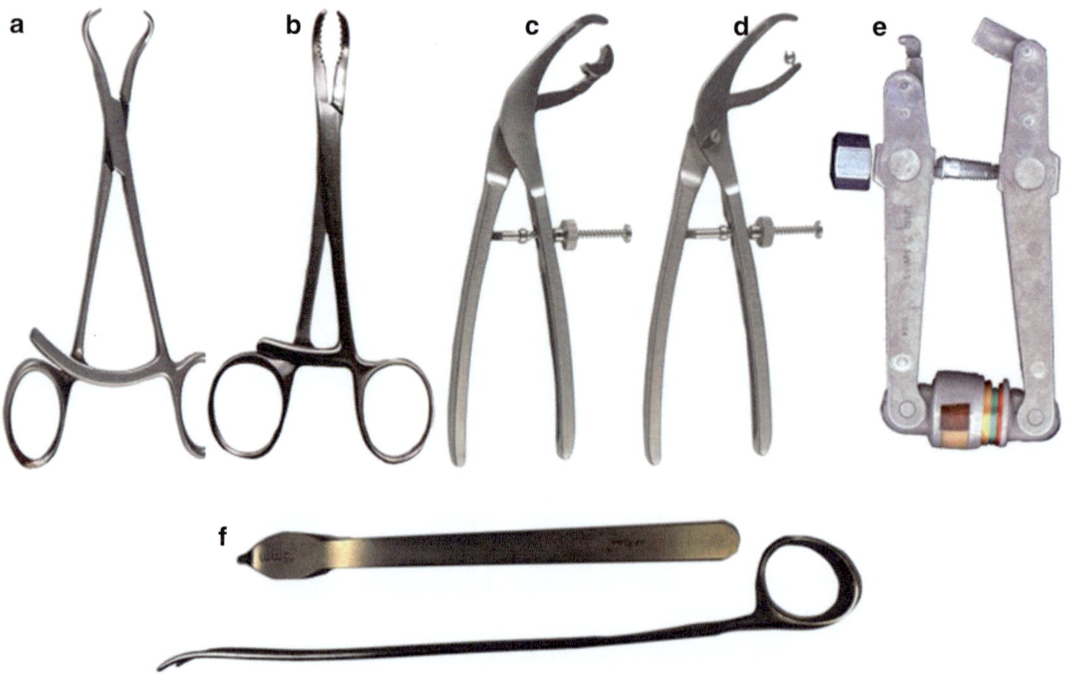

Fig. 2.13 (**a**) Point-to-point forceps. (**b**) Toothed reduction forceps. (**c, d**) Bone-holding forceps. (**e**) The tensioner. (**f**) Hohmann spike retractors

spike, intended to be placed in the hole of the plate, is also available.

(d) Tensioner

The articulating tension device is a device that can exert distraction or compression forces [17, 18] (Fig. 2.13e). It has a built-in strain gauge to indicate the amount of tension applied. It is composed of two legs: a rotatable hook that can fit against plates and a foot that takes a 4.5 mm cortical screw. The standard model has a 40 mm total excursion. Once the tensioner is attached on the bone with the screw, either it can exert a force on the plate to compress the fracture fragments or, in cases of highly comminuted fractures, it can be used to distract and maintain the length of the bone.

(e) Hohmann spike retractors

The Hohmann retractor is often a valuable tool in fracture reduction (Fig. 2.13f). The small tip Hohmann retractor can be inserted in the cortices of diaphyseal bone and used as a lever and pusher to achieve reduction. In diaphyseal fractures, turning and bending of the retractor inside the bone can disengage and reduce the fracture. In translated fractures like the iliac wing fractures, introduction and turning of the retractor inside the bone, followed by a bending force, can reduce the fractures. Often a small area of impaction is created. Due to the fact that the retractor is only inserted into the bone, no soft tissue damage/periosteal stripping is created.

(f) Bone hook and spikes

Bone ball spikes are useful instruments that can temporarily hold and maintain fixation of fragments during fixation (Fig. 2.14a). They are long pointed instruments with a triangular or quadrangular shape in cross-section and with a washer or sphere fixed in distal end. The shape of the ends prevents penetration of the end into the bone during fixation.

Bone hooks are instruments designed to allow the surgeon to grasp, hold and manipulate bony fragments in order to achieve proper alignment and anatomical reduction (Fig. 2.14b).

(g) Push-pull device

The push-pull reduction device is a simple device that aims to temporarily compress a plate to the bone. It acts by pushing the plate and pulling the bone at the same time. It is inserted under

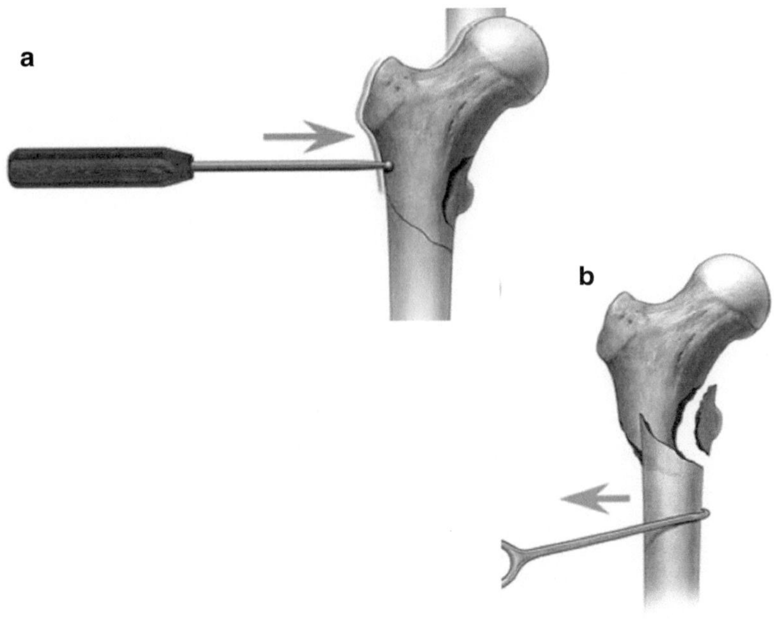

Fig. 2.14 (**a**) Bone ball spike. (**b**) Bone hook

power and requires turning the collet clockwise to start compressing the plate. The device should be inserted in a hole that will be subsequently used for fixation; after removal of the device, a conventional screw can be inserted.

Instruments Found in Specialized Sets

(a) Matta clamps

Joel Matta has initially designed two pairs of clamps, which were subsequently modified in different sizes and configurations (Fig. 2.15a). The original clamps were designed with their handles angling away from critical soft tissues and out of the line of sight. Their tips were of the shape of a ball with sharp points (sharp points provide hold; balls prevent bony penetration of thin cortex).

(b) Farabeuf and Jungbluth forceps

The Farabeuf forceps is an instrument that can be either used directly on the bone or secured on screws through its cut-out jaws (Fig. 2.15b). The Jungbluth forceps on the other hand can be only used in combination to screws. These forceps are designed to be used with 3.5 mm or 4.5 mm screws inserted at the opposite site of the fracture line and away of the site of definite fixation. They allow the application of considerable amount of reduction forces and fracture manipulation in all three planes. They are capable of overcoming the distracting forces without encumbering the plating site avoiding extensive soft tissue striping.

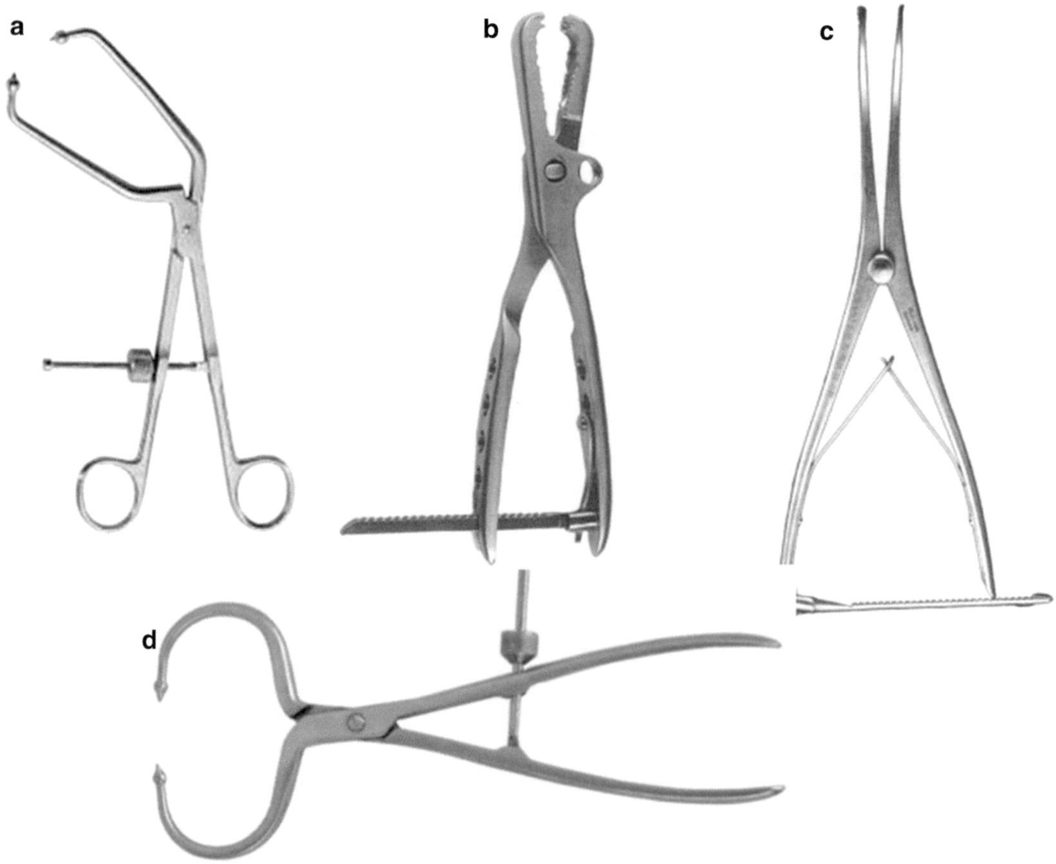

Fig. 2.15 (**a**) Matta clamp. (**b**) Farabeuf forceps. (**c**) Bone spreader. (**d**) Periarticular clamp

(c) Mini-distractor and bone spreaders (laminar spreader)

The mini-distractor belongs to the small fragment instrument set. It connects on 2.5 mm Schanz screws or K-wires and has an overall excursion of 4 cm. These pins should be inserted in 90° angle to the bone in order to maintain the bony axis. Applications of the mini-distractor are limited to smaller bones like fractures of the hand, feet, distal radius, olecranon and distal humerus.

Bone spreaders permit the disimpaction of bony fragments and facilitate the removal of soft tissues trapped interfragmentarily (Fig. 2.15c). It may also be used as a tension device placed off a plate and against a screw to create a distraction force.

A number of bone spreaders that use K-wires are also available and can transmit forces along one axis of the bone. Most commonly they are used to distract small joints in hand and feet but occasionally can be used in fracture management to distract or compress the fracture of small bones.

(d) Periarticular clamp

The periarticular clamp has large bended arms with ball-pointed ends (Fig. 2.15d). This clamp can be applied on previously surgically exposed bone or can be introduced percutaneously through stab incisions. It comes in different sizes, and its most common applications are in distal femoral and proximal tibial fractures. In osteoporotic bone, a spiked disk can be placed onto the tips to prevent bone penetration. A modification of the original design (Vosburg cannulated periarticular clamp) allows the passing of two pins from its two ends. These pins can hold the fragments in place and allow more working space for the application of hardware.

(e) Collinear reduction clamp

The collinear reduction clamp can be used to achieve and maintain fracture reduction through minimally invasive techniques. The device can accept a different attachment arm that makes it versatile allowing the surgeon to create an optimal reduction tool according to the clinical needs. These attachable arms include the percutaneous, pelvic, bone hook-shaped and Hohmann-shaped that can be used in applications in long bone, articular and pelvic fracture types.

(f) Spiked disk

This disk can attach to any ball-pointed instrument. It dispenses the forces applied to the forceps over a greater area; hence, the risk of bone penetration is reduced. The disk has points that prevent slippage and it allows the swivelling of the ball-tip. The spike disk needs to be placed on the bone prior to forceps attachment.

Implants Used as Reduction Tools

(a) Nails

Fracture fixation with the use of an intramedullary device can reduce and stabilize a long bone fracture. Once the guide pin has successfully passed to the distal fragment, the insertion of the nail usually fully reduces the fracture. If coronal or sagittal malalignment is noted, blocking screws (Poller screws) can be placed on the concavity of the deformity [19–21]. These screws serve as pseudocortex guiding the nail in the canal, realigning the bone and increasing the overall construct stiffness. Alternatively, the long reduction tool can be used to guide the guide pin to the centre of the canal (Fig. 2.16a). The positioning of the proximal screws can either aim to fix or compress the fracture. Likewise, in cases where an intramedullary device is used for the management of extracapsular hip fractures, compression of the fracture can be achieved through the axis of the hip screw by a compression attachment (Fig. 2.16b).

(a) Plates

The use of straight plates as antiglide and buttress instruments is an elegant technique that can facilitate fracture reduction. These techniques

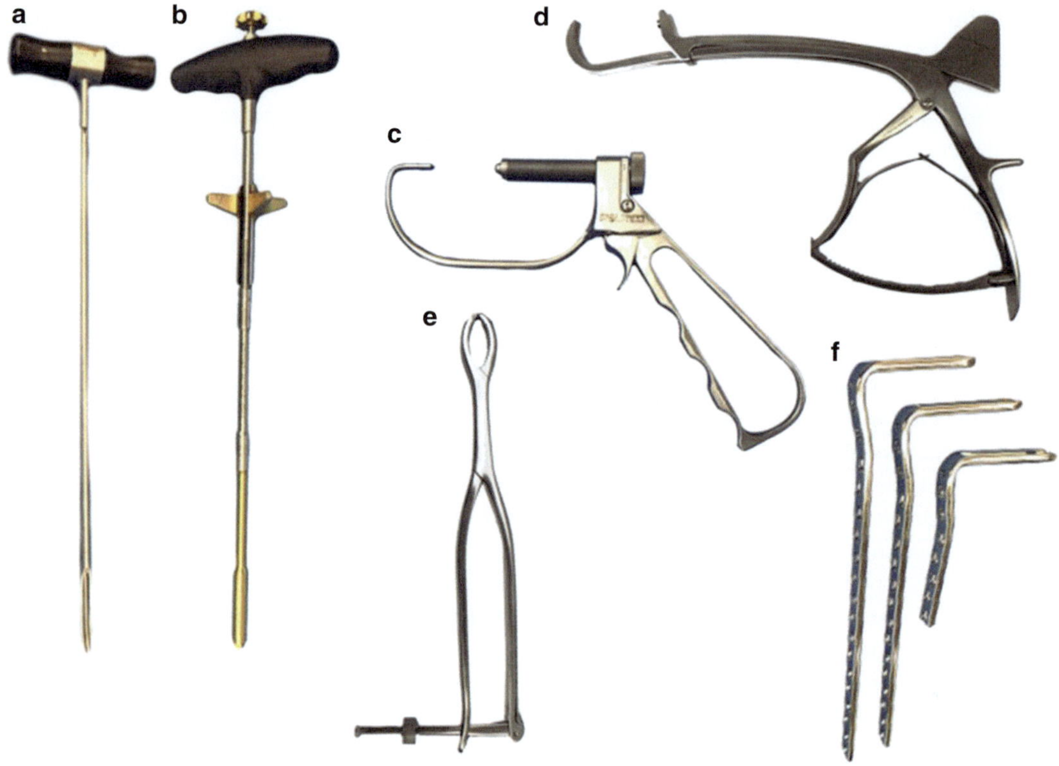

Fig. 2.16 (**a**) Long reduction tool. (**b**) Hip screw handle with compression wheel. (**c, d**) Plate-holding devices. (**e**) Bone-holding forceps. (**f**) Blade plates of different sizes

aim to place the plate in an advantageous position that realigns the bone and could further aid in the axial loading of the fracture with the use of compression screws. In some fracture configurations, the plate can be left in place as a blocking device preventing further displacement. The 'spring plate' used in acetabular fractures and the anterior buttressing plate in distal radial fractures are distinctive examples. In addition to the standard straight plates, our armamentarium includes many specialized plates like the cloverleaf-, 'H'-, 'L'-, 'T'- or 'S'-shaped plates. These plates are mostly intended to fix fracture of the epiphyseal area of long bones. There are specific plate-holding devices to facilitate maintenance of reduction (Fig. 2.16c, d). Bone-holding forceps can also facilitate fracture reduction (Fig. 2.16e).

A condylar blade plate is an alternative hardware that can be used as a reduction tool (Fig. 2.16f). Its use requires a detailed preoperative planning and is most commonly used for comminuted metaphyseal fractures. The principle of its application is the insertion of the blade of the plate in the most distal or proximal fragment, reducing the alignment and splinting the comminuted area by skipping the zone of the fracture. This technique requires minimal soft tissue stripping and does not disturb the fracture site.

(b) Wires and cables

Cerclage with the use of wires and cables can produce interfragmentary compression aiming in the reduction of a fracture [22]. Cerclage is often the only fixation method or can be combined with other devices more often K-wires, screws or Steinmann pins.

Conflict of Interest No benefits in any form have been received or will be received from a commercial party related directly or indirectly to the subject of this chapter.

References

1. Leunig M, Hertel R, Siebenrock KA, Ballmer FT, Mast JW, Ganz R. The evolution of indirect reduction techniques for the treatment of fractures. Clin Orthop Relat Res. 2000;375:7–14.
2. Ruedi T, Sommer C, Leutenegger A. New techniques in indirect reduction of long bone fractures. Clin Orthop Relat Res. 1998;347:27–34.
3. Kurylo JC, Templeman D, Mirick GE. The perfect reduction: approaches and techniques. Injury. 2015;46:441–4.
4. Bindra RR. Biomechanics and biology of external fixation of distal radius fractures. Hand Clin. 2005;21:363–73.
5. Agee JM. External fixation. Technical advances based upon multiplanar ligamentotaxis. Orthop Clin North Am. 1993;24:265–74.
6. Flierl MA, Stahel PF, Hak DJ, Morgan SJ, Smith WR. Traction table-related complications in orthopaedic surgery. J Am Acad Orthop Surg. 2010;18: 668–75.
7. Kumar S, Chadha GN. Dynamic hip screw fixation of intertrochanteric fractures without using traction table. Acta Orthop Belg. 2016;82:346–50.
8. Brumback RJ, Ellison TS, Molligan H, Molligan DJ, Mahaffey S, Schmidhauser C. Pudendal nerve palsy complicating intramedullary nailing of the femur. J Bone Joint Surg Am. 1992;74(10):1450–5.
9. Callanan I, Choudhry V, Smith H. Perineal sloughing as a result of pressure necrosis from the traction post during prolonged bilateral femoral nailing. Injury. 1994;25:472.
10. Lien FC. New tool for applying traction during open reduction and internal fixation of acetabular fractures. Orthopedics. 2012;35:289–91.
11. Trompeter A, Newman K. Femoral shaft fractures in adults. Orthopaedics and Trauma. 2013;27: 322–31.
12. Hammer C, Afolayan J, Trompeter A, Elliott D. A novel approach to closed reduction of distal femur fractures. Ann R Coll Surg Engl. 2014;96:626–8.
13. Dahners LE. Technical notes on a radiolucent distractor for indirect reduction and intramedullary nailing. J Orthop Trauma. 1997;11:374–7.
14. Satish BR, Vinodkumar M, Suresh M, Seetharam PY, Jaikumar K. Closed reduction and K-wiring with the Kapandji technique for completely the displaced pediatric distal radial fractures. Orthopedics. 2014;37:e810–6.
15. Dougherty PJ, Silverton C, Yeni Y, Tashman S, Weir R. Conversion from temporary external fixation to definitive fixation: shaft fractures. J Am Acad Orthop Surg. 2006;14:S124–7.
16. Heffernan MJ, Leclair W, Li X. Use of the F-Tool for the removal of a bent intramedullary femoral nail with a sagittal plane deformity. Orthopedics. 2012;35:e438–41.
17. Gautier E, Perren SM, Ganz R. Principles of internal fixation. Curr Orthop. 1992;6:220–32.
18. Lenz M, Stoffel K, Kielstein H, Mayo K, Hofmann GO, Gueorguiev B. Plate fixation in periprosthetic femur fractures Vancouver type B1-Trochanteric hook plate or subtrochanterical bicortical locking? Injury. 2016;47:2800–4.
19. Krettek C, Stephan C, Schandelmaier P, Richter M, Pape HC, Miclau T. The use of Poller screws as blocking screws in stabilising tibial fractures treated with small diameter intramedullary nails. J Bone Joint Surg Br. 1999;81:963–8.
20. Krettek C, Miclau T, Schandelmaier P, Stephan C, Möhlmann U, Tscherne H. The mechanical effect of blocking screws ("Poller screws") in stabilizing tibia fractures with short proximal or distal fragments after insertion of small-diameter intramedullary nails. J Orthop Trauma. 1999;13:550–3.
21. Ricci WM, O'Boyle M, Borrelli J, Bellabarba C, Sanders R. Fractures of the proximal third of the tibial shaft treated with intramedullary nails and blocking screws. J Orthop Trauma. 2001;15:264–70.
22. Mouhsine E, Garofalo R, Borens O, Blanc CH, Wettstein M, Leyvraz PF. Cable fixation and early total hip arthroplasty in the treatment of acetabular fractures in elderly patients. J Arthroplast. 2004;19:344–8.

3 Direct and Indirect Reduction: Definitions, Indications, and Tips and Tricks

Stuart Aitken and Richard Buckley

Definitions

Fracture reduction can be defined as the restoration of the correct anatomical position of fracture fragments and is a reversal of the process of fracture displacement which occurred at the time of injury. It includes the elevation of impacted cancellous bone and articular fragments in fractures with intra-articular involvement. In extra-articular fractures, reduction includes the restoration of limb length, alignment, and rotation so that the joints above and below the fracture are placed in the correct position. Fracture reduction can be thought of as the recreation of the normal three-dimensional spatial relationship of fracture fragments relative to one another. In clinical practice, this process can be achieved by direct or indirect means and often by a combination of both techniques.

S. Aitken, M.B.Ch.B., M.D., F.R.C.S.Ed.
Department of Surgery, University of Calgary, Calgary, AB, Canada

Department of Orthopaedics, MaineGeneral Medical Center, Augusta, ME, United States

R. Buckley, M.D., F.R.C.S. (✉)
Department of Surgery, University of Calgary, Calgary, AB, Canada
e-mail: buckclin@ucalgary.ca

Direct Reduction

Direct reduction is the act of achieving the above-described objectives when the fracture site has been exposed surgically (or traumatically) thus allowing the surgeon visual access to the fragments. Inherently, it involves some disturbance to the skin, subcutaneous tissues, and vascular supply overlying the fracture. This soft tissue envelope violation can be minimized by placing skin incisions away from areas of superficial abrasion or contusion and keeping deep dissection within muscle and fascial planes. Fracture visualization and subsequent direct reduction afford the surgeon a better chance of anatomical restoration of the fracture but at the expense of conferring some degree of soft tissue stripping and devitalization of fracture fragments. The consequences of this devitalization vary according to the anatomical site involved but include the adverse outcomes of delayed union and nonunion (and potentially implant failure), superficial wound dehiscence, and deep infection of bone and/or adjacent joints.

Indirect Reduction

In contrast, indirect reduction is the act of achieving reduction with the fracture site unexposed and the surrounding soft tissue envelope left intact. Fracture fragments are manipulated by applying corrective forces at a distance from the fracture site which are resisted by tension in the

P.V. Giannoudis (ed.), *Fracture Reduction and Fixation Techniques*,
https://doi.org/10.1007/978-3-319-68628-8_3

intact soft tissues, taking advantage of the general principle of ligamentotaxis. An anatomical reduction is often more difficult to achieve indirectly and requires an understanding of the fracture configuration and the deforming forces acting at the fracture site. However, reduction can be facilitated by the precise placement of reduction clamps or other instruments through strategically located 'stab' incisions, without necessarily imparting the same degree of soft tissue violation involved in a direct approach. Notably, the surgeon does not have the ability to visually inspect the results of indirect reduction, relying instead upon fluoroscopy or other forms of imaging to judge whether bony anatomy has been restored.

Indications

The overarching aim of modern fracture surgery is to obtain an 'acceptable' reduction of the fracture fragments, to maintain that reduction sufficiently while allowing for early range of motion of the injured part, and to achieve this with the least possible disturbance of the soft tissue envelope.

Direct Reduction

In most articular fractures, the aim of reduction is to perfectly restore the joint surface, thereby providing a congruent articular surface and a stable joint which moves normally. Impacted osteochondral fragments are elevated and stabilized in a reduced position (Fig. 3.1). For these reasons, direct inspection of the joint surface via a direct reduction is usually employed. Especially in the lower extremity, reduction of the disrupted joint surfaces and restoration of the normal axial alignment of the limb will reduce the risk of post-traumatic osteoarthrosis. Ideally, no residual joint displacement should be accepted, although different joints with different loading conditions appear to have different tolerances. In general, there is much less malreduction allowed for a constrained weight-bearing joint.

Direct reduction is occasionally used for metaphyseal or diaphyseal fractures. One example is that of a fracture involving the diaphyses of the radius and ulna. Precise restoration of the normal length, alignment, and rotation of both bones is important to prevent limitation of forearm rotation. This can be achieved via careful dissection through tissue planes and the limited soft tissue elevation involved in a direct approach. Simple diaphyseal fractures of other long bones such as the humerus or fibula can also be approached directly, without harmful violation of the soft tissue envelope (Fig. 3.2). Fractures of the tibial or femoral diaphyses can be reduced and treated this way, but the advent of intramedullary fixation has changed the surgical management of even the simplest fracture patterns involving these bones. However, the surgical approach for direct reduction of more complex or comminuted diaphyseal fractures of long bones risks devitalization of segmental fragments and increases the risk of the adverse fracture outcomes previously described. For these reasons, an indirect reduction is often preferred.

Indirect Reduction

In fractures of the diaphysis and metaphysis of long bones, it is the soft tissue envelope that provides vascularity and viability to the underlying fragments. In most circumstances, a method of reduction that preserves this soft tissue envelope but also allows for correction of angular and rotational deformity is preferable. When considering indirect reduction for any fracture, the decision-making process begins with obtaining an accurate history as to the amount of energy involved in the trauma, a detailed examination of the fracture pattern, and a close inspection of the soft tissues at the fracture site. A simple spiral diaphyseal fracture without comminution, sustained from a low-energy fall, with a healthy soft tissue envelope might conceivably be stabilized surgically via an open direct reduction depending upon the surgical strategy and choice of implant. In contrast, direct reduction would be contraindicated in a high-energy meta-diaphyseal injury with marked bony comminution and extensively contused soft tissues due to the risks of further devitalization of already compromised tissues. In these high-energy trauma situations with threatened soft tissues, indirect techniques are preferred.

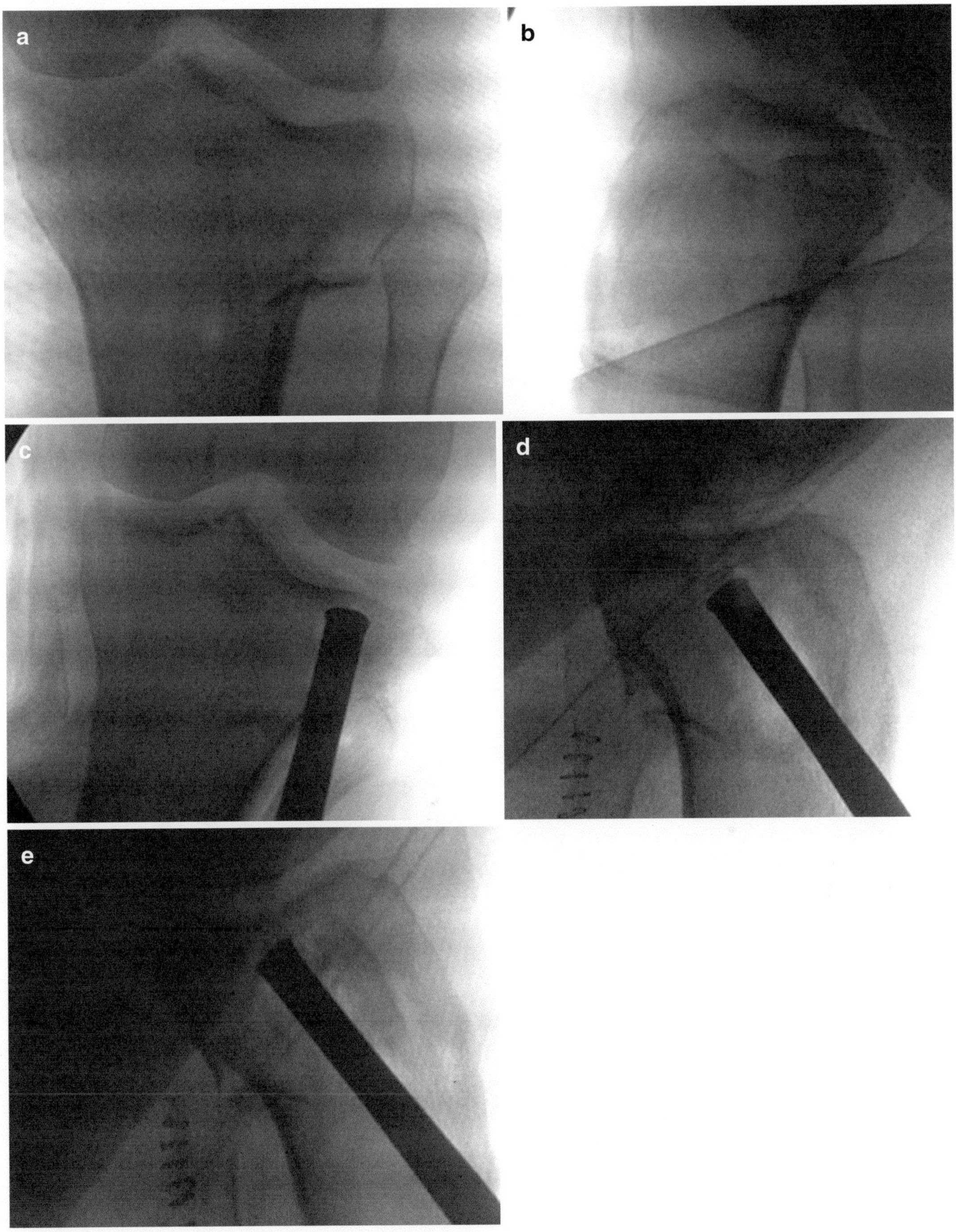

Fig. 3.1 The elevation and reduction of impacted articular osteochondral fragments. Anteroposterior (**a**) and lateral (**b**) fluoroscopic images of a tibial plateau fracture are shown. A bone tamp is introduced and positioned beneath the depressed articular fragments on both views (**c**, **d**) and is then used to elevate the articular fragments back to their anatomic position (**e**)

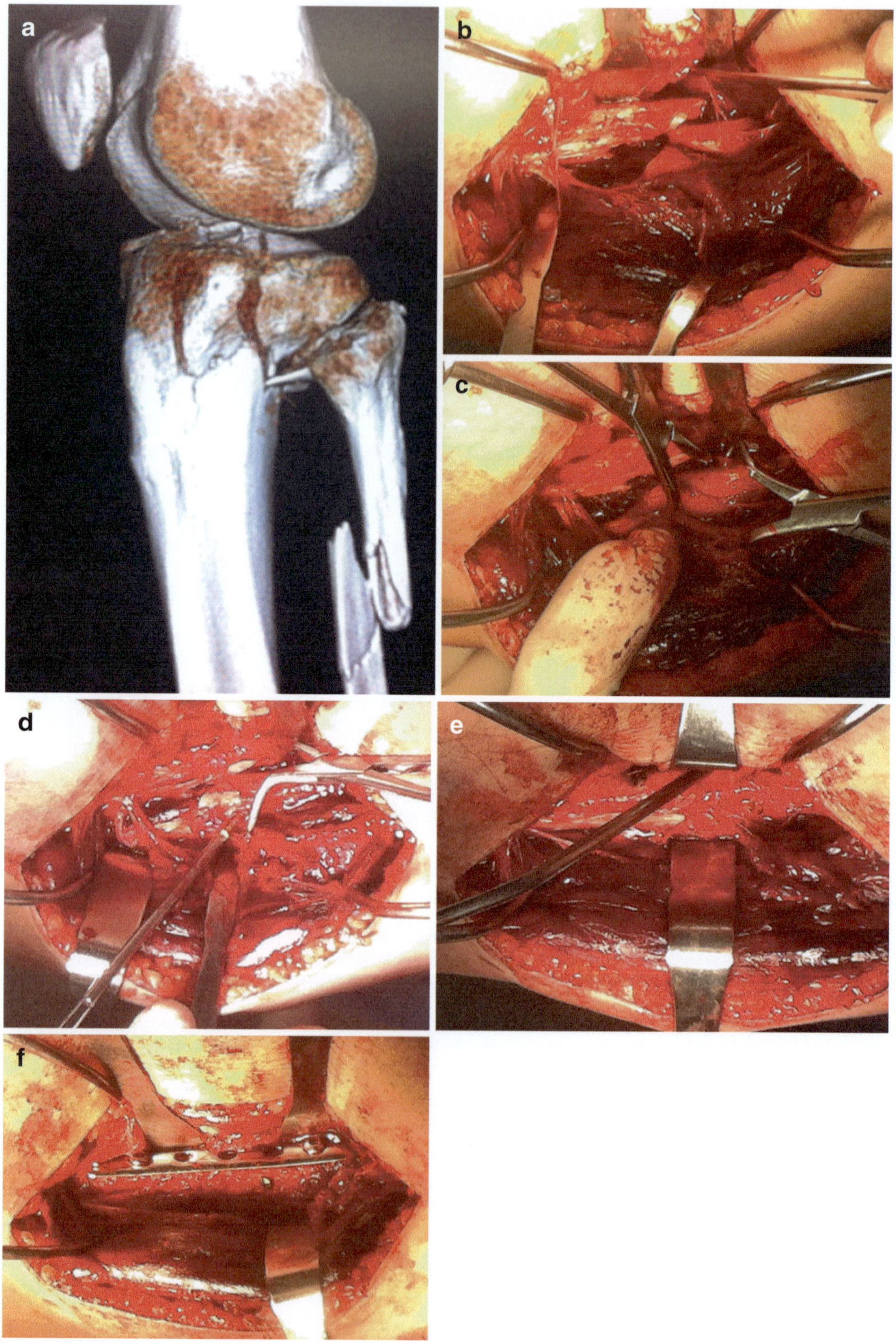

Fig. 3.2 Direct reduction of a fibula shaft fracture. The tibial plateau fracture is associated with a shortened and comminuted fibula fracture (**a**). In order to restore the correct tibial height, the surgeon has chosen to perform an open approach (**b**) and direct anatomic reduction of the fibula. The butterfly fragment is reduced, held with pointed reduction forceps (**c**), and secured with a lag screw (**d**), thereby creating two main fragments. These are reduced and fixed with a second lag screw (**e**). A neutralization plate is then placed to protect the fixation construct (**f**)

With the use of modern fracture implants, indirect reduction techniques are often preferred for *both* low- and high-energy metaphyseal and diaphyseal fracture situations. This highlights the emphasis currently placed on soft tissue envelope preservation in modern fracture surgery.

Tips and Tricks

Table 3.1 provides a list of commonly utilized instruments and techniques for direct and indirect fracture reduction. The subsequent text provides further explanation regarding their application. Of note, some direct techniques may be considered indirect if applied through stab incisions (e.g. Schanz screws, pointed reduction forceps) or if introduced through incisions made at a distance from the fracture site (e.g. pre-contoured plate).

Longitudinal Correction (Traction)

The deforming forces acting on the fracture and preventing reduction result from the combined effects of muscle spasm, ligament and fascial tension, and the effect of gravitational pull. Almost universally, traction applied to the injured segment will create some degree of fracture reduction, as the deforming forces are partially overcome. Traction is most frequently applied indirectly (e.g. by using a traction fracture table, a universal distractor, or external fixation device or by suspending the limb and allowing gravity to create traction), but this is only effective when bone fragments are still connected to soft tissues. The direct application of traction to a fracture overcomes this problem and involves the use of instrumentation at the fracture site (e.g. standard pointed reduction forceps applied with simultaneous rotation of the handles creating distraction between fragments, a retractor placed into the fracture site and used as a lever, a Jungbluth pelvic clamp or laminar spreader creating distraction between two strategically placed cortical screws, or the use of Schanz screws on either side of the fracture as 'joysticks'). In many circumstances, even after the successful application of traction, there will be residual deformity in one or more planes that must be addressed.

Angular Correction

An imbalance of tension in the soft tissues (i.e. muscles or fascia) on either side of a fracture or

Table 3.1 An example of the instrumentation and techniques used to obtain fracture reduction by direct and indirect means [1–6]

Desired correction	Direct reduction	Indirect reduction
Longitudinal	Pointed reduction forceps Bone lever in the fracture Laminar spreader or Jungbluth (between two screws) Schanz screw joysticks Universal AO compression/distraction device	Traction on the fracture table Universal distractor External fixator Gravity
Angular/translational	Schanz screw joysticks Ball spike pusher Bone hook Dental pick Periosteal elevator Cerclage wire Coaxial clamp Pointed reduction forceps	Crutch under the apex Sterile 'bump' Radiolucent triangles F-tool Externally applied mallets
Rotational/multiplanar	Schanz screw joysticks Bone holding clamp External scaffold (Temporary reduction plate) (Pre-contoured plate)	Intramedullary reduction aid Internal scaffold (Intramedullary nail)

a loss of bony integrity affecting one cortex but not the other will cause an angular planar deformity, with or without a rotational deformity, depending on the deforming force vectors. The effect of gravity on a fracture site can also produce angulation. The simplest corrective method is to apply a force at the apex of the deformity. Commonly utilized manoeuvers include placement of a crutch under an apex posterior femoral shaft fracture, placing a sterile 'bump' or radiolucent triangle beneath a distal femoral metaphyseal fracture, or using a Schanz pin placed in the femoral neck to correct the apex anterior deformity in a subtrochanteric fracture.

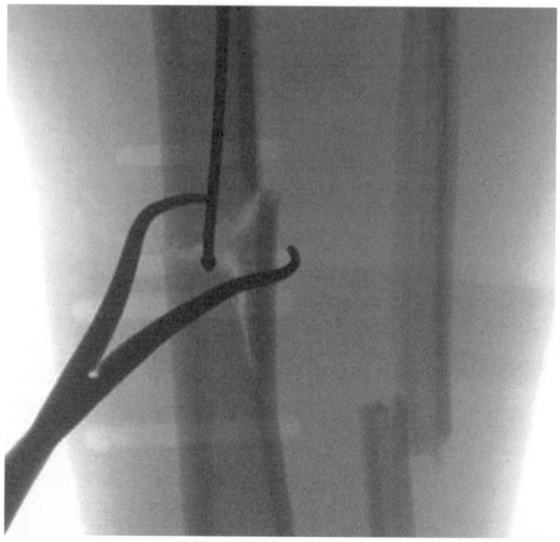

Fig. 3.3 Pointed reduction forceps, placed through stab incisions at the fracture site, are being used to maintain and hold the reduction of the tibial shaft fracture prior to passage of the ball-tipped guide wire and intramedullary reaming

Translational Correction

Any obliquity of fracture orientation will result in tensile forces at a fracture site being converted into translational deformity. The pull of individual musculotendinous units can also create translation dependent upon their site and direction of insertion. Correction of residual translation at a fracture site is often difficult to achieve indirectly, but instruments such as the 'F-tool' or externally applied mallets can be used in some circumstances. More powerful and accurate correction can be achieved by applying instruments at the fracture site via stab incisions (Fig. 3.3) or by utilizing a direct approach. The ball spike pusher, the bone hook, the dental pick, the periosteal elevator, or a cerclage wire can be used to push or pull bone fragments into a reduced position. Depending on the obliquity of the fracture, the application of reduction forceps or a coaxial clamp can be used to directly counteract the translational deforming force.

Rotational and Multiplanar Correction

In most instances, residual deformity exists in multiple planes after traction has been applied to the injured segment. Obtaining control of the bone on one or both sides of a fracture is one way of applying the desired force vector to achieve fracture reduction. This can be achieved by applying one or more 'joystick' devices through the bone (e.g. Kirschner wires or Schanz pins) or by placing some type of forceps around the bone fragments prior to manipulation. With the use of intramedullary fracture implants, a multiplanar reduction can be achieved by using an intramedullary reduction aid (e.g. an undersized nail or a guide wire). However, in contrast to the use of fracture joysticks, these tools are unable to maintain a reduction prior to implantation of the definitive intramedullary device.

Fracture Implants as Reduction Aids

Ideally a fracture implant should contribute to the reduction as well as the stabilization of a fracture. Increasingly, modern fracture implants are 'pre-contoured' and anatomically 'site-specific'. Their shape is designed to closely resemble that of the injured segment to which they are being applied. Perhaps the best example of this is the intramedullary nail. If attention has been paid to its correct site of insertion, then passing the pre-contoured device across the fracture site will confer fracture reduction in the coronal and sagittal planes. The nail acts as an internal scaffold. Alternatively, an external scaffold can be created but serves the same purpose of correcting angular and translational deformity (Fig. 3.4). The use of pre-contoured plates for

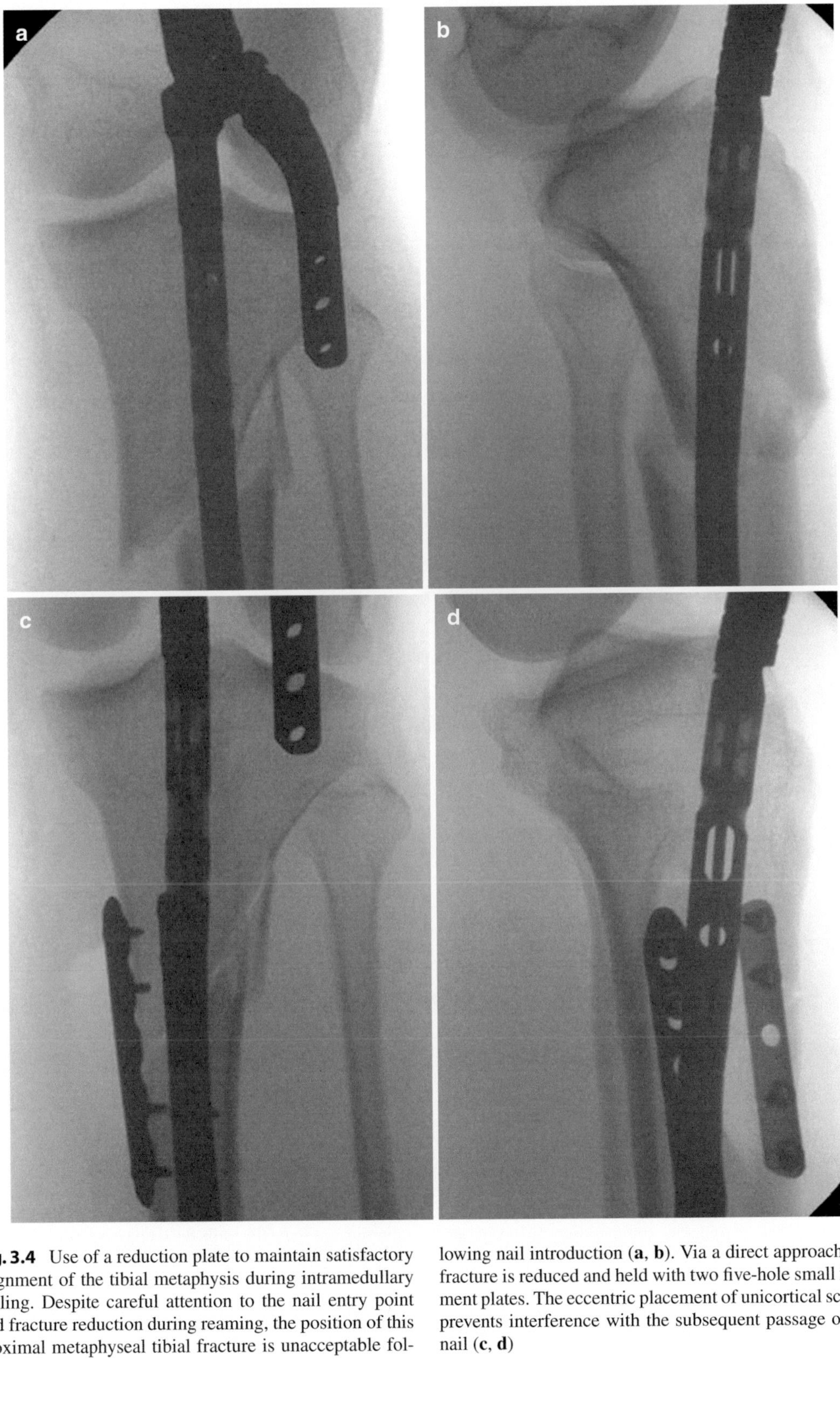

Fig. 3.4 Use of a reduction plate to maintain satisfactory alignment of the tibial metaphysis during intramedullary nailing. Despite careful attention to the nail entry point and fracture reduction during reaming, the position of this proximal metaphyseal tibial fracture is unacceptable following nail introduction (**a**, **b**). Via a direct approach, the fracture is reduced and held with two five-hole small fragment plates. The eccentric placement of unicortical screws prevents interference with the subsequent passage of the nail (**c**, **d**)

stabilization of fractures of the proximal femur, distal femur, or proximal tibia is a good example of the application of this scaffold principle. Provided the plate is applied correctly to the metaphyseal segment and fixed securely, then reduction of the diaphyseal fracture fragment to the plate (or vice versa) will restore coronal and sagittal alignment (Fig. 3.5). The concomitant application of traction will restore length. It is unusual for the application of pre-contoured nails or plates to confer rotational fracture reduction, and it is important to eliminate rotational deformity prior to definitive fixation of the implant to the diaphysis.

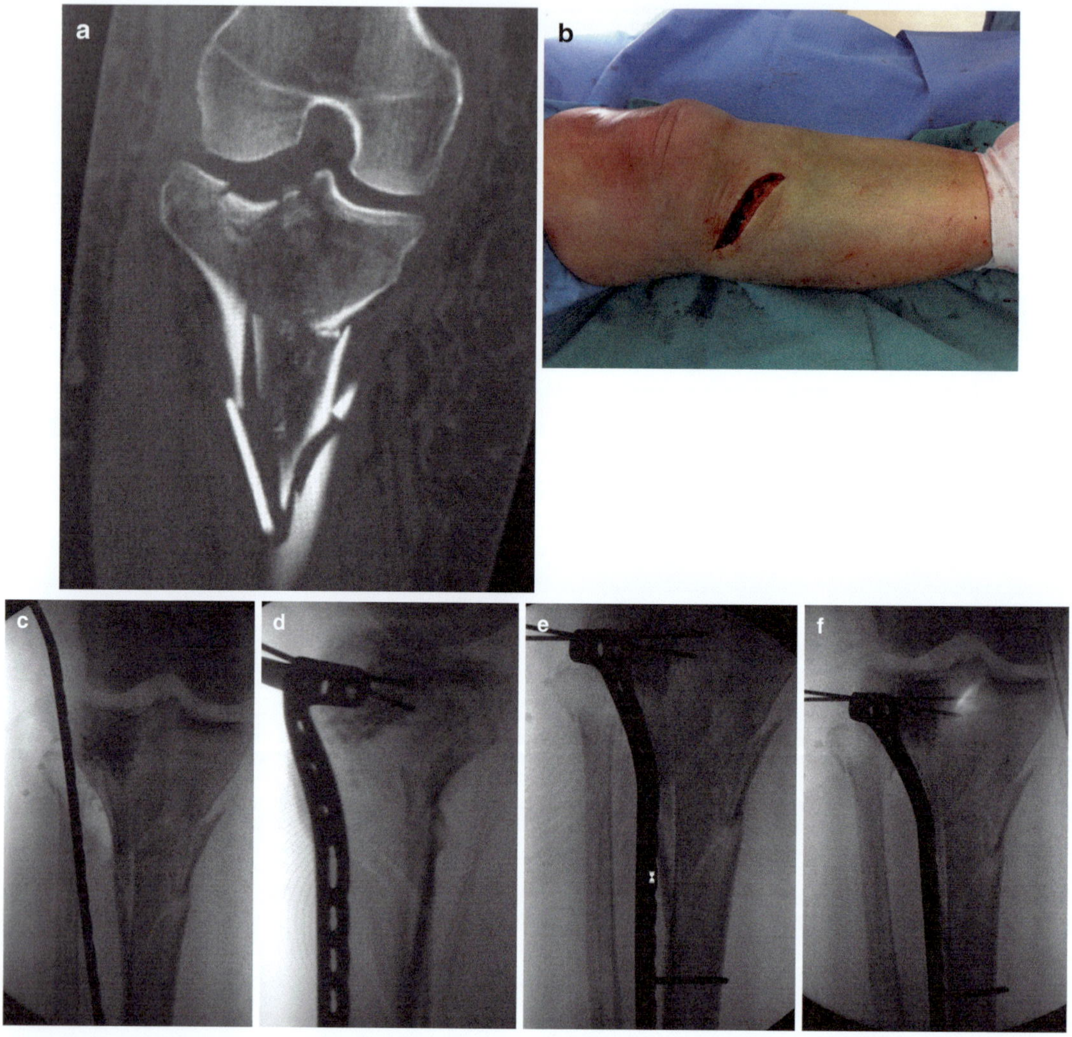

Fig. 3.5 The use of a pre-contoured plate, correctly applied to the proximal fracture segment, restoring coronal and sagittal alignment as the diaphyseal fracture fragment is reduced to it. A tibial plateau fracture with extensive meta-diaphyseal comminution (**a**) is treated using indirect reduction techniques through a proximal skin incision (**b**). Following anatomical reduction of the articular component, a pre-contoured plate is introduced (**c**) and temporarily held proximally and distally with Kirschner wires (**d**). A cortical screw, placed distal to the comminuted segment, pulls the diaphysis to the plate as it is tightened (**e**) thereby restoring limb alignment (**f**)

In summary, a variety of generic techniques exist which can be used to restore the correct anatomical position of fracture fragments. Reduction techniques may be applied directly or indirectly but must always take into consideration the vascularity and viability of the affected bone fragments and surrounding soft tissues. The choice of technique and its particular application will depend largely upon the surgical strategy employed and the anatomical site affected.

Suggested Reading

1. Gautier E, Pesantez RF. Surgical reduction. In: Ruedi TP, Buckley RE, Moran CG, editors. AO Principles of Fracture Management, vol. Volume 1. Stuttgart: Thieme; 2007. p. 165–88. Clin Orthop Relat Res. 2000 Jun;(375):7-14.
2. Perren SM. Trends in internal fixation potential, limits and requirements. Injury. 1999;30(Suppl 2): B2–4.
3. Leunig M, Hertel R, Siebenrock KA, Ballmer FT, Mast JW, Ganz R. The evolution of indirect reduction techniques for the treatment of fractures. Clin Orthop Relat Res. 2000;375:7–14.
4. Wenger R, Oehme F, Winkler J, Perren SM, Babst R, Beeres FJP. Absolute or relative stability in minimal invasive plate osteosynthesis of simple distal meta or diaphyseal tibia fractures? Injury. 2017;48(6): 1217–23.
5. Huang HT, Huang PJ, Su JY, Lin SY. Indirect reduction and bridge plating of supracondylar fractures of the femur. Injury. 2003;34(2):135–40.
6. Krettek C, Müller M, Miclau T. Evolution of minimally invasive plate osteosynthesis (MIPO) in the femur. Injury. 2001;32(Suppl 3):SC14–23.

Part II

Innovations in Fracture Reduction

Innovations in Fracture Reduction Computer-Assisted Surgery

4

Rami Mosheiff and Amal Khoury

Computer-Assisted Surgery in Trauma

Computer-Assisted Surgery (CAS) systems provide the surgeon with a precise, more complete, and up-to-date view of the intraoperative situation. By incorporating real-time tracking of the location of instruments and anatomy, and their precise relation to preoperative and intraoperative images, the systems create a new modality akin to continuous imaging [1]. In this sense, CAS systems are like navigators based on global positioning systems (GPSs), currently found in cars which help drivers find their way to a desired destination. During driving, the system shows the exact location of the car at all times on a computerized map and provides turn-by-turn directions ahead of time. Today, a variety of image-free and image-based systems exist for planning and executing a variety of orthopedic procedures, including primary and revision total hip and total knee replacement, anterior cruciate ligament reconstruction, spinal pedicle screw insertion, and trauma. CAS has already become an integral part of the orthopedic trauma surgery setup [2]. The rapid development in the use of computers in this field provides many feasible options at all stages of treatment of the orthopedic trauma patient, from preoperative planning to postoperative evaluation. The role of computerization in the treatment of trauma patients is not only to enhance the surgical options in the preplanning stage but also to shorten surgery, an advantage that could be crucial for patient morbidity in a trauma setup. This integrates well with the current tendency toward minimal invasive surgery [3]. CAS technology brings important digitized information into the operating room, enabling the accomplishment of two main goals: minimal invasive surgery and maximal accuracy. Moreover, both surgeon and patient enjoy a significant reduction in the amount of radiation exposure usually associated with orthopedic trauma surgery. Computerized navigation has made a breakthrough in expanding the use of CAS from the preplanning to the postoperative stage, yet the crucial stage of fracture reduction is a dynamic stage which makes the intraoperative integration of this new technology more difficult [4].

Computer-Assisted Surgery for Closed Reduction of Long Bone Fractures

Open reduction of a long bone fracture can result in higher rates of infection and non-union. Several techniques have been suggested to accomplish closed reduction, such as the use of a femoral dis-

R. Mosheiff, M.D. (✉) • A. Khoury, M.D.
Department of Orthopedic Surgery,
Hadassah Medical Center, Jerusalem, Israel
e-mail: ramim@hadassah.org.il

P.V. Giannoudis (ed.), *Fracture Reduction and Fixation Techniques*,
https://doi.org/10.1007/978-3-319-68628-8_4

tractor, percutaneous Schanz screws to manipulate the fragments, and traction. These solutions rely exclusively on fluoroscopy, thus exposing both the patient and the surgeons to a significant amount of radiation [5].

From the different computer-assisted surgery (CAS) systems, the main modality which has been adapted to trauma surgery is fluoroscopy-based navigation. While this technology might be viewed by some as only improved fluoroscopy, it is undoubtedly this feature that has allowed computer-based navigation systems to become a pioneer in the process of CAS integration in the orthopedic trauma operating room. The use of a fluoroscopy-based computerized navigation system can improve the nailing technique by locating the entry point of the nail, inserting locking and Poller screws, and providing accurate nail and screw measurements. These tasks then can be performed with markedly reduced radiation exposure. However, fracture reduction in vivo has not been achieved by computerized navigation systems without difficulties, since it requires simultaneous dynamic imaging of two separate anatomic sites, such as fracture fragments [6].

The first innovative technique for closed reduction in intramedullary nailing utilizing a fluoroscopy-based computerized navigation system was published in 2005 [7]. A modular infrared-emitting active instrument tracker is mounted on a cannulated intramedullary fracture-aligning device which is inserted into the medullary canal of the proximal fragment, advanced to the fracture site, and will at a later stage be used as a "joystick" for fracture reduction. A bone tracker is inserted into the distal segment of the fracture. Two fluoroscopic images (AP and lateral) of the distal fragment are taken and stored in the computer. The fluoroscope is now removed from the surgical field and will not be used throughout the reduction process. At the same time, the position sensor (infrared camera) is tracking the intramedullary fracture alignment device by locating the instrument tracker on it and the distal fragment using the bone tracker. Since the intramedullary device is located inside the proximal fragment, its image represents both the device and the proximal fragment as a single unit. The image seen on the computer screen displays the tracked instrument only, but actually represents the proximal fragment surrounding it. This eliminates the need to fix a reference frame to the proximal fragment. The actual fracture reduction is then carried out by manipulating the proximal fragment, using the tracked intramedullary alignment device, and directing its virtual image on the computer screen toward the medullary canal of the distal fragment. While navigating, the images seen on the computer screen during the reduction process are the virtual image of the device and the distal fragment itself. The fracture is reduced when both images are aligned on both previously taken AP and lateral views. The procedure is entirely performed without the use of fluoroscopy.

Computer-Assisted Surgery to Control Length and Rotation of Long Bone Fractures

Femoral fracture nailing is considered to be a highly successful procedure, with healing rates approaching 98–99%. However, the procedure is not devoid of complications [8]. As more high-energy shaft fractures with excessive comminution and metaphyseal involvement are being treated, malunions can occur, with malrotation deformity being the most common. The incidence of clinically significant rotational deformity (more than15°) is found in 10–22% of cases [9]. Several solutions and radiographic techniques aimed at reducing malrotation during femoral shaft fixation have been proposed, such as the cortical step sign, the lesser trochanter profile, and radiographic comparisons of both extremities in the lateral view. However, despite the use of these techniques, there is no clear evidence that the incidence of femoral malrotation has decreased.

A significant breakthrough of fluoroscopy-based navigation in trauma surgery is the ability to simultaneously track more than one bone fragment during navigated fracture reduction surgery, enabling a real-time tracking and manipulation of the two main bone fragments. The fracture reduction navigation software includes both single-bone tracking and the ability to follow in real time two bone-attached trackers, one for each bone fragment [10]. This software application allows for performing femoral fracture fixation using fluoroscopy-based navigation with different modules, including navigation of nail entry point, segmentation of the fracture fragments and virtual reduction without the use of live fluoroscopy, virtual implant insertion, and nail locking. Most importantly, it is possible to determine the length and rotation of the fixed bone by comparing it with the intact contralateral femur. By using images obtained from both proximal and distal ends of both the intact and the injured femurs, the length and rotational profile of each bone can be calculated. As a result, before nail locking, the fractured femur can be matched in length and rotation to the healthy limb (Fig. 4.1).

At the start of each surgical procedure after anesthesia, a noninvasive optical tracker is placed on the uninjured thigh. Four images of the intact femur are taken as follows: an anteroposterior (AP), a lateral view of the proximal femur, an AP, and a true lateral of the distal femur. The software automatically calculates the axial rotation angle between the acquired proximal and distal femoral landmarks, as well as the femoral length. All images and data are stored in a computerized database. After nail insertion and before nail interlocking, trackers are placed in both proximal and distal ends of the injured femur. The process of image acquisition and marking is similar to the one described above for the uninjured extremity. The same four images are taken while tracking with both a handheld fluoroscopic tracker (X-spot)

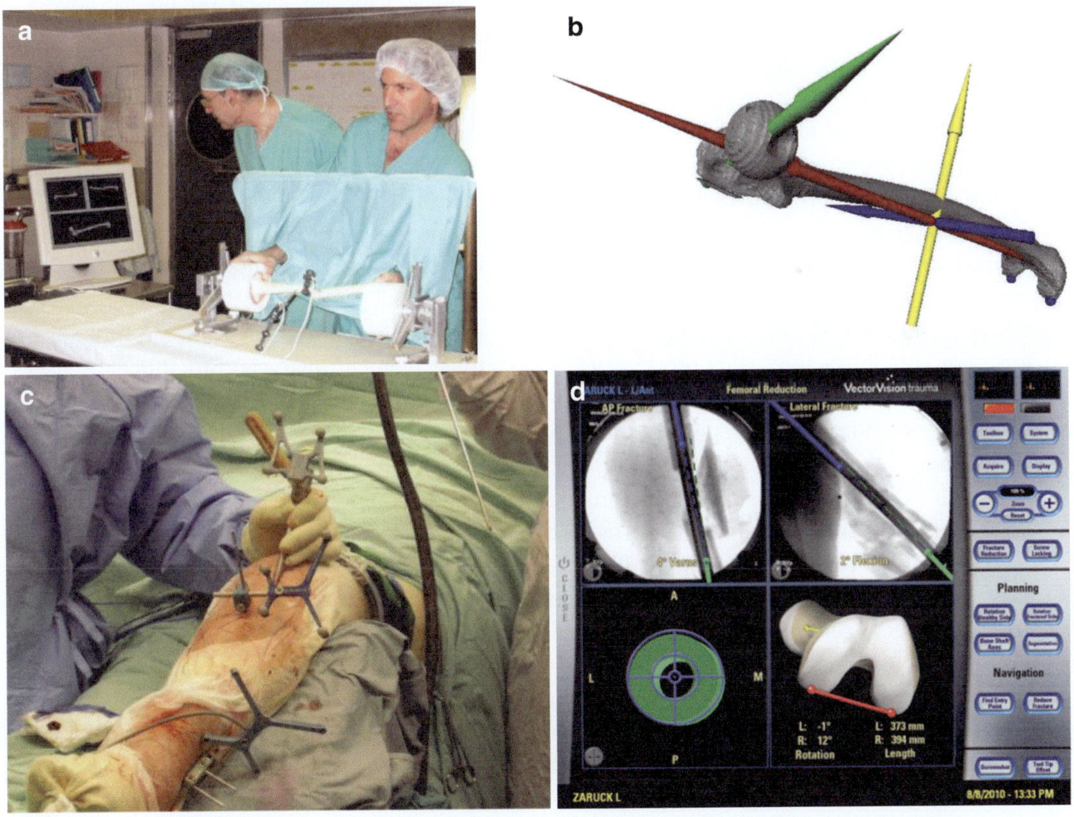

Fig. 4.1 A significant breakthrough is the ability to simultaneously track more than one bone fragment during navigated fracture reduction surgery. The fracture reduction navigation software has the ability to follow in real time two bone-attached trackers, one for each bone fragment. In vitro experiments in our lab (**a** and **b**) followed by real-time intramedullary nailing of a tibial fracture (**c** and **d**)

and bone trackers placed in the proximal and distal ends of the femur. The images are marked for the center of the femoral heads, the tip of the greater trochanter, the posterior condyles, and the intercondylar line. At this point, the tracking camera of the navigation system is recording the length and rotation of the injured nailed extremity. The computer screen displayed the length in millimeters and rotation of both the intact and broken femurs. After obtaining a satisfactory alignment, interlocking screws are placed in both proximal and distal fracture ends.

Computerized Virtual Fracture Reduction Methods

The current standard of care starts with the acquisition of X-ray images and the evaluation of the fractures. Next, the surgery is planned to determine the surgical approach, the bone fracture reduction, and the type, number, and locations of the fixation hardware. Surgeons can plan the fracture reduction and fixation with commercial software packages, based on 2D digital overlay templates of the fixation hardware on the X-ray images. In more complex cases, the planning is performed on CT scan 3D bone fragment models. During surgery, the surgeon reproduces the preoperative plan based on new fluoroscopic X-ray images. For simple fractures, this process yields adequate results in most cases. However, a higher incidence of complications is reported for complex fractures.

Although 3D CT has considerably improved imaging, complete understanding of the fracture lines and fragments can, at times, still be difficult. One of the most discussed difficulties is the choice of a correct operative approach. Taking all of this into account, it is obvious that strict preoperative planning is a crucial step especially in percutaneous surgical treatment. It is not surprising that new technologies have been introduced to help the surgeon plan the operative procedures more precisely. Computer programs that have been developed during recent years have enabled the performance of a virtual operation of the injured skeleton. The purpose of this preoperative stage is to virtually perform all steps of the real surgical procedure. This method might improve surgery in general, but could make a colossal advance in percutaneous surgery of this area. The ability to exercise a virtual surgical procedure marking the safe zones allows for precise planning of fragment reduction, screw dimensions, and pathways and enables the pre-checking of the percutaneous option as an alternative to the open approach. Moreover, since the information is based on specific imaging of the fracture, it can be used intraoperatively. The highly detailed information that is acquired in the preoperative stage may be transferred to the execution stage and thus direct the navigation accordingly. Nowadays, all computerized preoperative planning softwares, available either experimentally or in clinical use, are based on preoperative CT scans [11]:

1. 3D imaging allowing for the performance of the different stages of a virtual surgical procedure, including segmentation, reduction, and fixation [12]
2. 3D imaging in which the virtual reduction is based on a mirror image of the healthy side as a template [13]
3. 3D imaging allowing for the performance of finite element analysis, providing the necessary information for choosing the most preferred biomechanical composition of fixation [14]
4. Haptic computer-assisted patient-specific preoperative planning [15].

Computerized Intra-articular Fracture Fixation

C-arm radiographs are commonly used for intraoperative image guidance in surgical interventions. Fluoroscopy is a cost-effective real-time modality, although image quality can vary greatly depending on the target anatomy. Intra-articular fracture fixation presents unique technical difficulties. In many cases, the fracture is comminuted and has complex geometry that is difficult to evaluate on conventional CT slices or fluoroscopic radiography images. For more than a decade, 3D intraoperative imaging was introduced, such as Siremobil Iso-C 3D (Siemens Medical Solutions); it has been positively investigated to improve intraoperative understanding for fracture reduction and tool placement. However, this tool has its limitations: It can be used only once or twice during surgery because of radiation exposure, and it has a static and limited field of view. Other obstacles include tracking of small bone fragments and possible fragment motion during fixation. Modifications of the isocentric C-arm have recently been introduced, offering superior image quality, increased field of view, higher spatial resolution, and soft tissue visibility, as well as the elimination of the need to rotate around a fixed point (isocentricity).

In addition, newly developed patented software modules have recently been developed which allow for intraoperative 3D assessment, with decreased cost and less radiation, using conventional fluoroscope techniques.

Advanced 3D Intraoperative Imaging for the Judgment of Fracture Reduction

A relatively new technology in 3D intraoperative imaging is offered by the application of flat-panel detectors (developed for radiographic/fluoroscopic imaging) to cone-beam CT. Cone-beam CT (CBCT) provides volumetric image reconstructions from 2D projections acquired across a given source-detector trajectory about the patient (e.g., a circular orbit). Cone-beam computed tomography (CBCT) scans are sometimes available, so 2D-3D registration is needed for intra-procedural guidance. This technology is an important advancement over existing intraoperative imaging (e.g., Iso-C 3D), offering superior image quality, increased field of view, higher spatial resolution, and soft tissue visibility. CBCT imaging provides exquisite visualization of articular details, subtle fragment detection and localization, and confirmation of fracture reduction and implant placement. CBCT imaging revealed areas of malalignment and displaced fragments in intra-articular fracture reduction surgeries. CBCT facilitated fragment localization and improved anatomic reduction. CBCT image noise increased gradually with reduced dose; it has been proved in tibial plateau fracture reduction and fixation surgery [16]. Moreover, CBCT can provide intraoperative high-resolution images with a large field of view. This quality of imaging enables surface matching algorithms to be utilized even with large areas of comminution. This was proved to be useful in judging precisely the femoral shaft rotation in femoral fracture surgery using surface mapping algorithms [17].

In the former decade, challenges in improving intraoperative quality have led to the combination of robotic, floor-based 3D flat-panel CBCT C-arm, known as Artis zeego (Siemens). In recent years hybrid operating rooms were established over the world. In our setting we combined a 3D flat-panel C-arm (Artis zeego) with a navigation system (Brainlab Curve, Brainlab). This unique combination enables the surgeon to visualize an entire pelvis in CT-like image quality with a single 3D scan (figure). This way a surgeon is able to control fracture reduction and to alternate his plan accordingly (Fig. 4.2). The Ulm group has shown superior results in terms of precision in the placement of sacroiliac screws using the abovementioned modality [18].

The use of the Artis zeego system allows for the validation of fracture reduction and intraoperative hardware placement in different intra-articular fracture surgeries. It is routinely used in our institution in Pilon, calcaneus, tibial plateau, and some pelvic and acetabular fracture surgeries (figure). The need for a revision of fracture reduction is evaluated before final hardware placement. If a further reduction is needed, the provisional fixation is removed, and the reduction is improved.

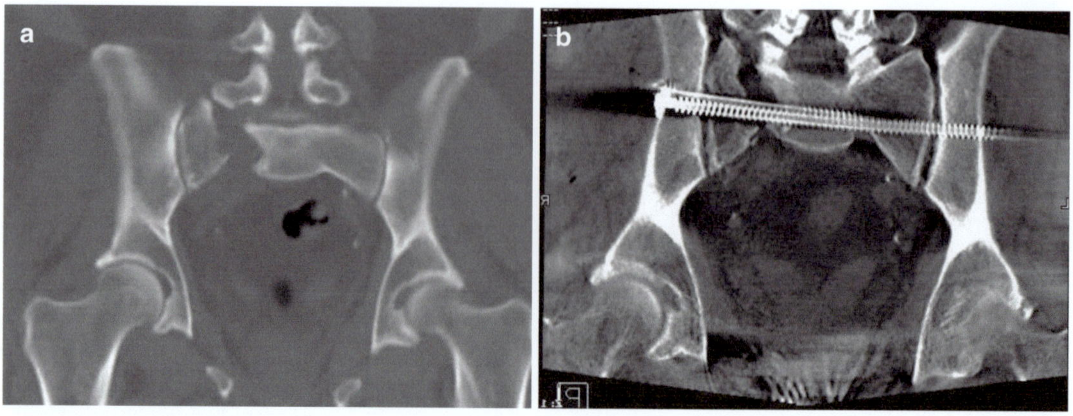

Fig. 4.2 Advanced intraoperative 3D imaging assists in the judgment of the quality of the fracture reduction and implant placement. A coronal reformat of a pelvic CT scan shows posterior pelvic non-union before surgery (**a**). An intraoperative coronal reformat of a CT, acquired by the Artis zeego system, shows the status of the reduction and fixation of the pelvis (**b**)

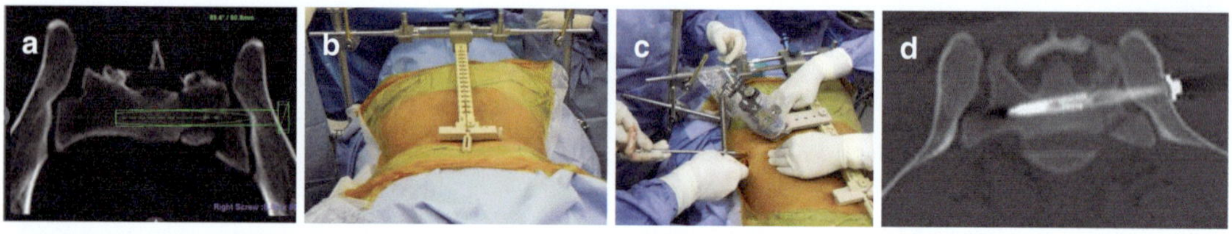

Fig. 4.3 On the basis of combined CT scan and fluoroscopic data (**a**), the miniature robot (SpineAssist; Mazor Surgical Technologies, Caesarea, Israel) aligns itself to the desired entry point and trajectory, as dictated by the surgeon's preoperative plan (**b** and **c**). We use the same for the placement of sacroiliac screws (**d**)

Future Directions

One of the promising developments of computer-assisted surgery is the robotic execution of the preoperative plans (Fig. 4.3). Today tool placement is well guided by different means of navigation, but not the fracture reduction. A decade ago a new miniature robot (SpineAssist; Mazor Surgical Technologies, Caesarea, Israel), which has been developed as a surgical assistant for accurate percutaneous placement of pedicle screws and translaminar facet screws, was introduced. On the basis of combined CT scan and fluoroscopic data, the robot aligns itself to the desired entry point and trajectory, as dictated by the surgeon's preoperative plan. A vast experience has been gained during this time, and recently we use the same system with minor modifications for the placement of sacroiliac screws. This enables 3D environment navigation, based on the preoperative plan, for the placement of screws in narrow safe zones [19, 20].

This is an example of a computerized coupling between preplanning and execution of fixation. Direct computerized control of fracture reduction based on the digital preplanning doesn't exist yet. In the near future, we hope to be able to integrate this crucial stage of fracture care in the existing sequence of technologies of preoperative planning and intraoperative guided navigation (Fig. 4.4).

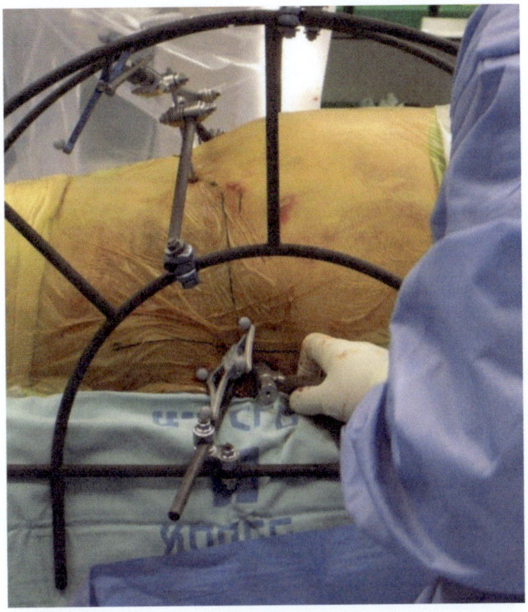

Fig. 4.4 Integration of the reduction stage in the sequence of technologies of preoperative planning and intraoperative guided navigation is desired. Part of our in vivo trials is based on table-skeletal pelvic fixation frame which secures the normal side of the pelvis to the table and enables maneuvering the other hemipelvis. This pelvic frame has increased our ability to obtain a closed reduction of the pelvic ring and is coupled to the navigation system

References

1. Nolte L, Beutler T. Basic principles of CAOS. Injury. 2004;35(suppl 1):6–16.
2. Liebergall M, Ben-David D, Weil Y, et al. Computerized navigation for the internal fixation of femoral neck fractures. J Bone Joint Surg Am. 2006;88A:1748–54. Reddix RN, Webb LX. Computed-assisted preoperative planning in the surgical treatment of acetabular fractures. J Surg Orthop Adv. 2007;16:138–143.
3. Mosheiff R, Khoury A, Weil Y, et al. First generation of fluoroscopic navigation in percutaneous pelvic surgery. J Orthop Trauma. 2004;18:106–11.
4. Weil YA, Liebergall M, Mosheiff R, et al. Assessment of two 3-D fluoroscopic systems for articular fracture reduction: a cadaver study. Int J Comput Assist Radiol Surg. 2011;6(5):685–92.
5. Kahler DM. Virtual fluoroscopy: a tool for decreasing radiation exposure during femoral intramedullary nailing. Stud Health Technol Inform. 2001;81:225–8.
6. Weil YA, Liebergall M, Mosheiff R, et al. Long bone fracture reduction using a fluoroscopy-based navigation system: a feasibility and accuracy study. Comput Aided Surg. 2007;12:295–302.
7. Mosheiff R, Weil Y, Peleg E, et al. Computerised navigation for closed reduction during femoral intramedullary nailing. Injury. 2005;36:866–70.
8. Tornetta P III, Ritz G, Kantor A. Femoral torsion after interlocked nailing of unstable femoral fractures. J Trauma. 1995;38:213–9.
9. Jaarsma RL, Pakvis DF, Verdonschot N, et al. Rotational malalignment after intramedullary nailing of femoral fractures. J Orthop Trauma. 2004;18:403–9.
10. Weil Y, Gardner MJ, Helfet DL, et al. Accuracy of navigated femoral fracture reduction–a laboratory study. Clin Orthop Rel Res. 2007;460:185–91.
11. Attias N, Lindsey RW, Starr AJ, Borer D, Bridges K, Hipp JA. The use of a virtual three-dimensional model to evaluate the intraosseous space available for percutaneous screw fixation of acetabular fractures. J Bone Joint Surg Br. 2005;87(11):1520–3.
12. Cimerman M, Kristan A. Pre-operative planning in pelvic and acetabular surgery: the value of advanced computerised planning modules. Injury. 2007;38(4):442–9.
13. Noser H, Heldstab T, Schmutz B, Kamer L. Typical Accuracy and Quality Control of a Process for Creating CT-Based Virtual Bone Models. J Digit Imaging. 2011;24(3):437–45.
14. Varga E, Erdőhelyi B. Severe Pelvic Bleeding: The Role of Primary Internal Fixation. Eur J Trauma Emerg Surg. 2010;36(2):107–16.
15. Kovler I, Joskowicz L, Weil Y, Khoury A, Kronman A, Mosheiff R,·Liebergall M, Salavarrieta J. Haptic computer-assisted patient-specific preoperative planning for orthopedic fractures surgery. Int J CARS. 2015: 10: 1535–1546.
16. Khoury A, Siewerdsen JH, Whyne CM, Daly MJ, Kreder HJ, Moseley DJ, Jaffray DA. Intraoperative cone-beam CT for image-guided tibial plateau fracture reduction. Comput Aided Surg. 2007;12(4):195–207.
17. Khoury A, Whyne CM, Daly M, Moseley D, Bootsma G, Skrinskas T, Siewerdsen J, Jaffray D. Intraoperative cone-beam CT for correction of periaxial malrotation of the femoral shaft: a surface-matching approach. Med Phys. 2007;34(4):1380–7.
18. Richter PH, Gebhard F, Dehner C, Scola A. Accuracy of computer-assisted iliosacral screw placement using a hybrid operating room. Injury. 2016;47(2):402–7. https://doi.org/10.1016/j.injury.2015.11.023. Epub 2015 Dec 12.
19. Lieberman IH, Togawa D, Kayanja MM, Reinhardt MK, Friedlander A, Knoller N, Benzel EC. Bone-mounted miniature robotic guidance for pedicle screw and translaminar facet screw placement: Part I-Technical development and a test case result. Neurosurgery. 2006;59(3):641–50. discussion 641-50
20. Stüer C, Ringel F, Stoffel M, Reinke A, Behr M, Meyer B. Robotic technology in spine surgery: current applications and future developments. Acta Neurochir Suppl. 2011;109:241–5. https://doi.org/10.1007/978-3-211-99651-5_38.

5 Inflatable Bone Tamp (Osteoplasty) for Reduction of Intra-articular Fractures

Peter V. Giannoudis and Theodoros Tosounidis

Introduction

Extra-vertebral balloon osteoplasty (the so-called inflatable bone tamp) has lately gained a lot of popularity being used as a tool for reduction of fractures. This technique has been applied successfully for reduction of depressed distal radius, humeral head and calcaneal and tibia plateau fractures amongst others [1–4]. In this chapter the technique will be demonstrated for the management of tibial plateau Schatzker type II and III depressed intra-articular fractures.

Anatomical Fracture Location: Radiograph of Fracture Pattern

A tibial plateau fracture with intra-articular involvement occurs following an axial force exerted from the femoral condyles against the articular surface of the tibia.

P.V. Giannoudis, M.D., F.R.C.S. (✉)
Academic Department of Trauma and Orthopaedics, School of Medicine, University of Leeds, Leeds, UK
NIHR, Leeds, UK

Musculoskeletal Biomedical Research Center, Chapel Allerton Hospital, Leeds, UK
e-mail: pgiannoudi@aol.com

T. Tosounidis, M.D., Ph.D.
Academic Department of Trauma and Orthopaedics, School of Medicine, University of Leeds, Leeds, UK

The Schatzker et al. classification of tibial plateau fractures continues to be the most commonly used classification for these injuries [5] (Fig. 5.1). For the type II and III fracture patterns, like any other intra-articular fracture, the goals of treatment remain: anatomical fracture reduction, stable fixation and early range of motion.

Currently, the most commonly reduction technique used involves a bone punch using a cortical window that allows access to the depressed fragment.

Recently however, borrowing from the successful vertebral kyphoplasty technique, an inflatable balloon acting as a tamp can reduce the depressed tibial plateau fracture. This technique gives the advantage of reducing the bone window to a drill hole while simultaneously increasing the area of force transmission, resulting in easy and satisfactory fracture reduction and minimal trauma.

Brief Preoperative Planning

Initial clinical examination of the affected extremity is vital to assess the state of the soft tissues and the neurovascular status and to exclude the presence of compartment syndrome. In polytrauma patients initial ATLS assessment is mandatory as well as secondary and tertiary surveys to exclude injuries to other anatomical locations. Radiological examination consists of AP and lateral knee (Fig. 5.2) and tibia radiographs. Acquisition of

P.V. Giannoudis (ed.), *Fracture Reduction and Fixation Techniques*,
https://doi.org/10.1007/978-3-319-68628-8_5

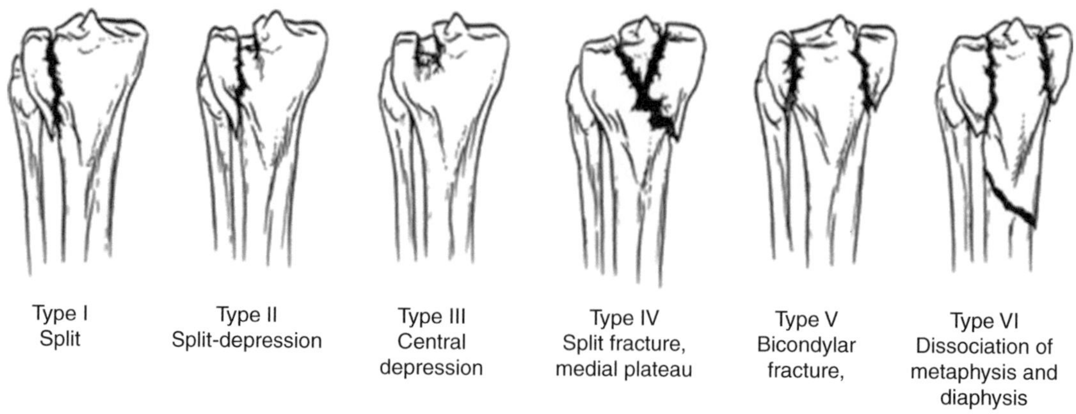

Fig. 5.1 The Schatzker classification of tibial plateau fractures

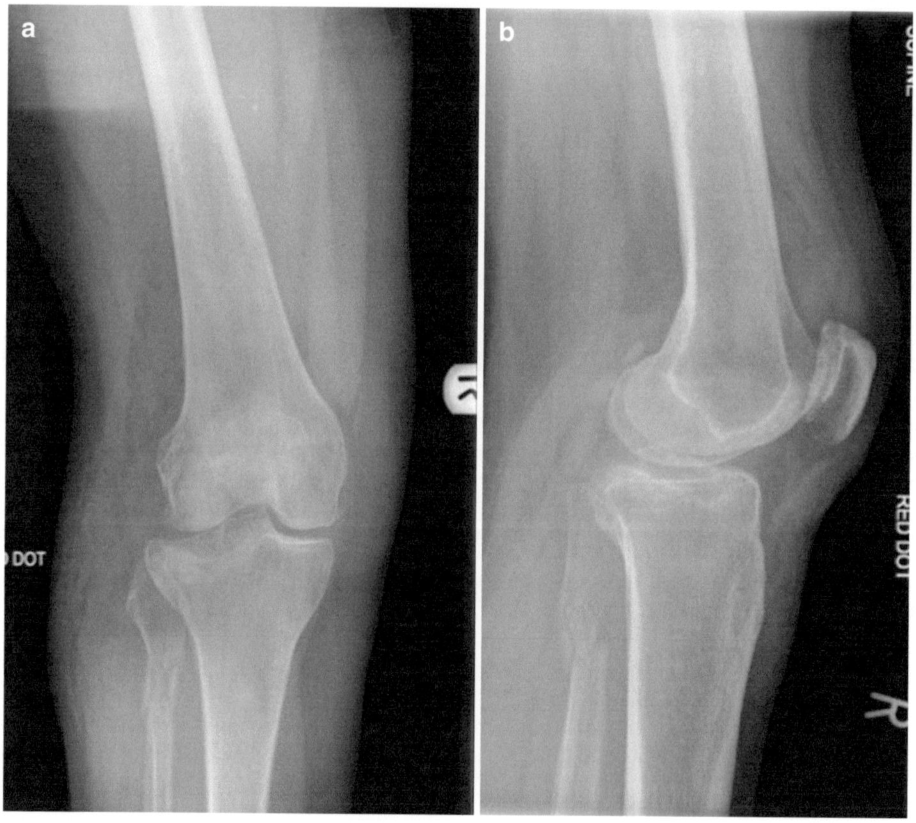

Fig. 5.2 (**a**) AP and (**b**) lateral radiograph of a right type II lateral tibial plateau fracture

computed tomography (CT) scan (Fig. 5.3) is crucial to appreciate in more detail the extent of depression, comminution and the existence of other fracture lines that may affect the placement of the metal work for achieving optimum stability.

Patient Set-Up in Theatre

In the operating room, the patient is placed in the supine position on a radiolucent table (Fig. 5.4).

The image intensifier is positioned to the opposite side of the surgeon who will be standing

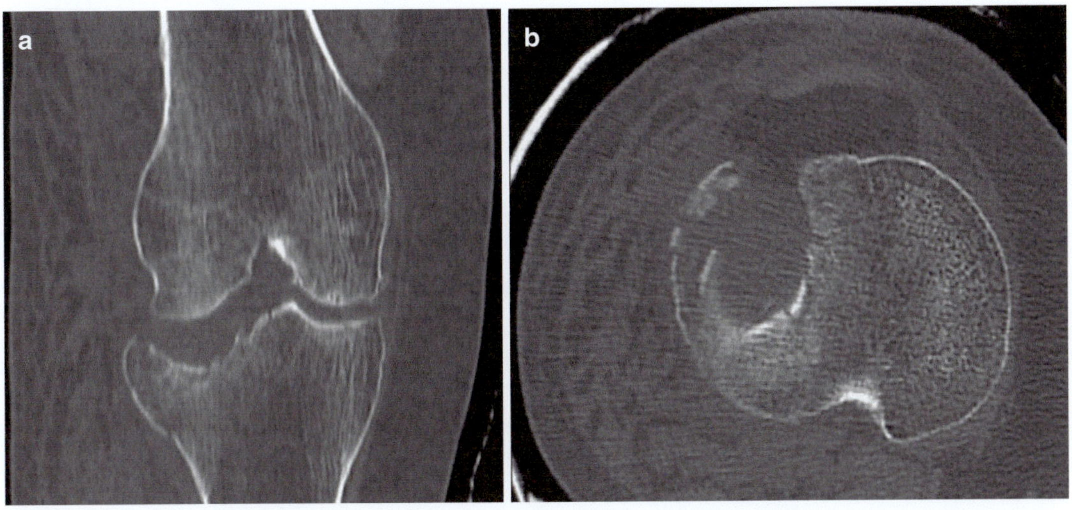

Fig. 5.3 (**a**, **b**) CT images of right lateral tibial plateau fracture

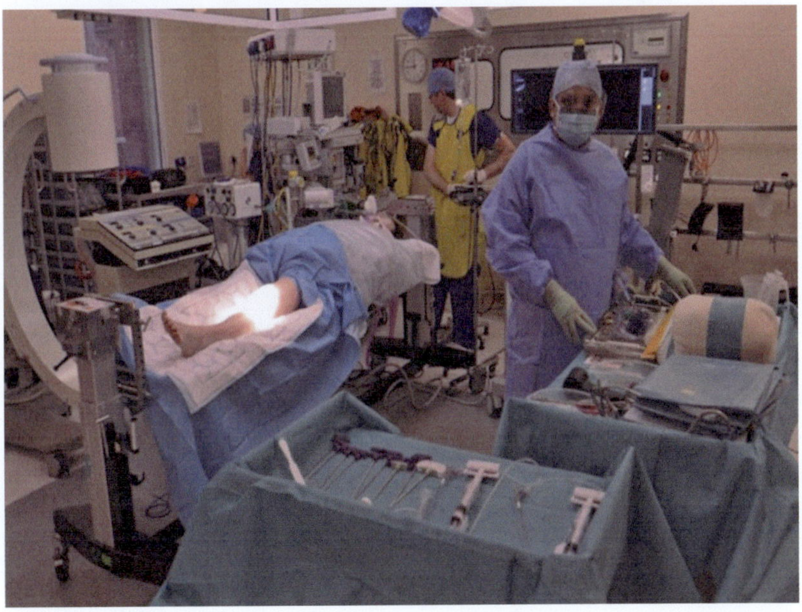

Fig. 5.4 Patient is placed in the supine position on a radiolucent table

at the side of the injured limb. The opposite leg can be flexed and supported with a leg-holding attachment device to allow easy acquisition of lateral knee radiographs (Fig. 5.5).

Closed Reduction Manoeuvres

Closed reduction is difficult to achieve in such fractures. However, placing the knee in slight flexion over the triangle or a bolster to allow 15° of flexion will facilitate relaxation of the gastrocnemius muscle (Fig. 5.5).

Reduction Instruments

Instrumentation that is required consists of Osteo Introducer, precision drill, Kyphon inflation syringe, inflatable balloon (IBT) of appropriate size, contrast liquid, bone filler device, bone void filler, k-wires, reduction forceps, plates and screws (Fig. 5.6).

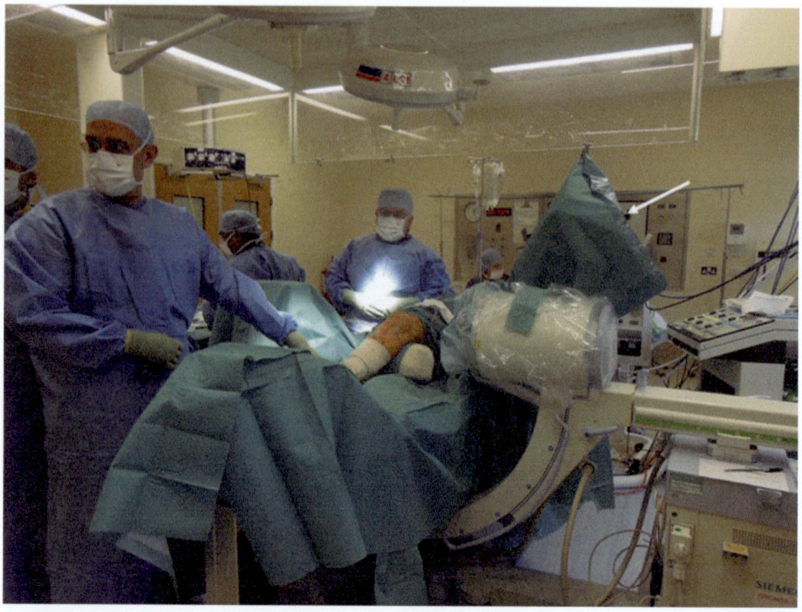

Fig. 5.5 Image intensifier is positioned to the opposite side of the surgeon. The uninjured leg is flexed and supported with a leg-holding attachment device to allow easy acquisition of lateral radiographs. Note that the injured leg is supported with a bolster

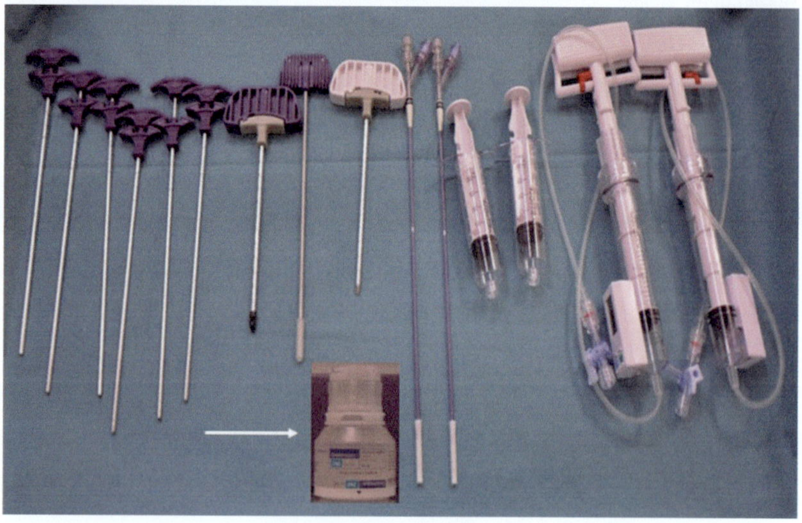

Fig. 5.6 Kyphon inflatable balloon set

Surgical Approach: Identification of the Area of Articular Depression

This technique is used through a minimal invasive approach. A thigh tourniquet is applied.

Under fluoroscopic guidance, the tip of a k-wire or a metal marker is placed on the medial aspect of the tibial plateau, approximately 2–3 mm below the depression, in the anteroposterior and lateral planes of the fluoroscopic acquisition images (Fig. 5.7).

When the right level is identified, a small percutaneous skin incision on the medial side is made, and the trocar for the inflatable bone tamp is advanced from the medial to the lateral direction, underneath the impaction area (Fig. 5.8).

To avoid subsidence of the inflatable balloon tamp away from the depressed fragment into the cancellous metaphyseal bone, the authors have recommended placing two or three rafting 2 mm k-wires just below the balloon. However, a special cannula is currently available that prevents expansion of the balloon inferiorly, thus eliminating the need for inserting k-wires.

A carved incision is carried out posterior to the lateral joint line. A tunnel is created to elevate

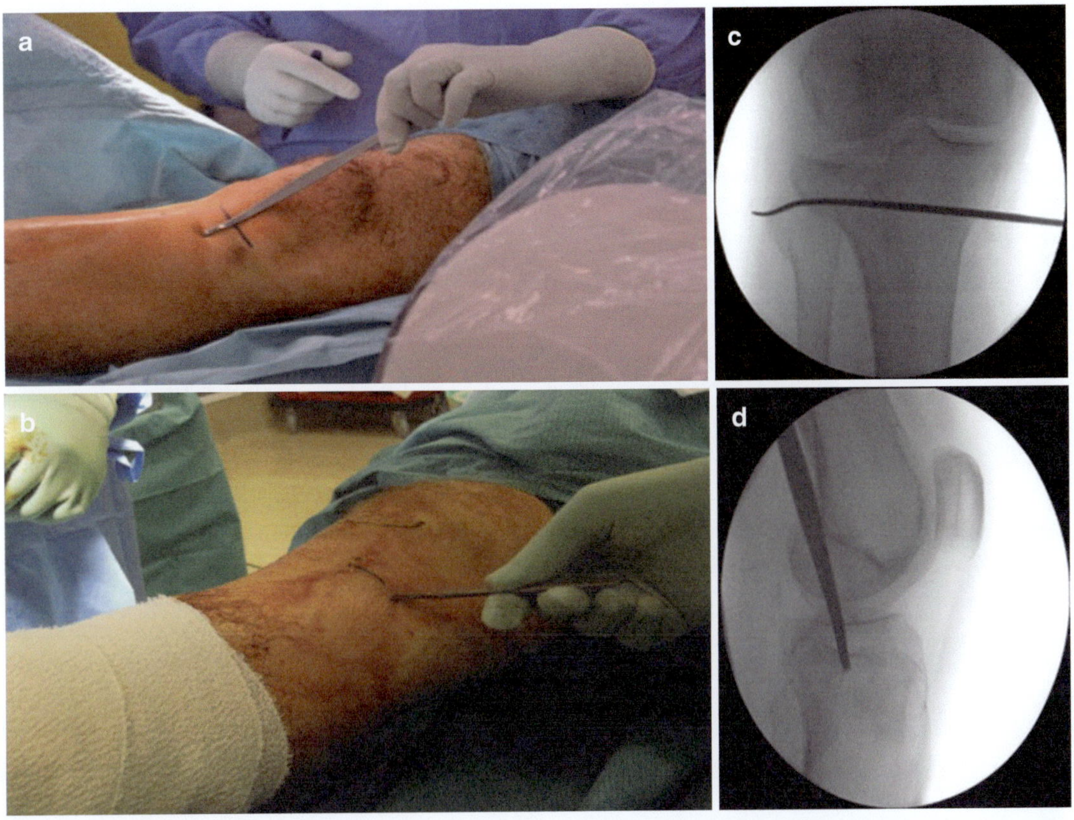

Fig. 5.7 (**a–d**) Under fluoroscopic guidance, the tip of the metal marker is placed on the medial aspect of the tibial plateau, approximately 2–3 mm below the depression, in the anteroposterior and lateral planes of the fluoroscopic acquisition images

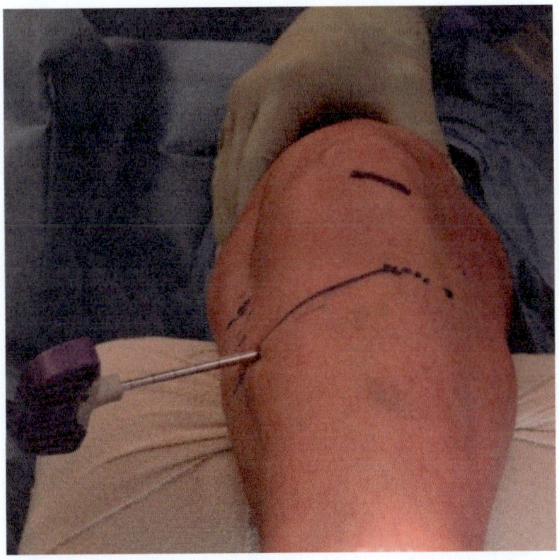

Fig. 5.8 Following a small percutaneous skin incision on the medial side, the trocar is advanced from the medial to the lateral direction, underneath the impaction area

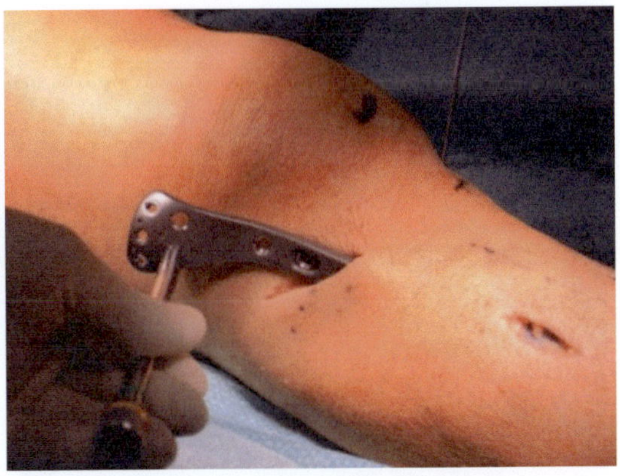

Fig. 5.9 Following a carved incision, a locking plate is advanced and inserted over the lateral wall fragment

the proximal structures of the anterior compartment of the leg. A plate to buttress the latter wall and to prevent displacement of the lateral wall is inserted (Fig. 5.9).

Structure at risk during this step is in the common peroneal nerve around the neck of the fibula. If the surgeon feels that it is necessary to inspect the articular surface, a submeniscal arthrotomy is made through the coronary ligament to expose the lateral plateau fracture.

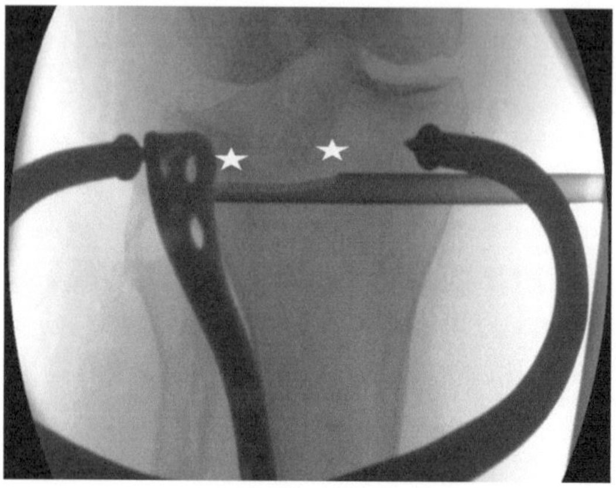

Fig. 5.10 A large, pointed reduction clamp has been applied percutaneously in order to prevent displacement of the lateral split fracture fragment during inflation of the balloon

Reduction Manoeuvres

A large, pointed reduction clamp is applied in a percutaneous fashion holding the plate and the medial tibial plateau in order to prevent displacement of the lateral split fracture fragment during inflation of the balloon (Fig. 5.10).

The precision drill then is inserted through the cannula to prepare the path for the ITB. After removal of the precision drill, the IBT is inserted in the cannula and is advanced under the area of depression to allow a targetted expansion of the balloon. The balloon is gradually inflated, and reduction is progressively achieved to anatomical level by taking the necessary fluoroscopic acquisition images (Fig. 5.11).

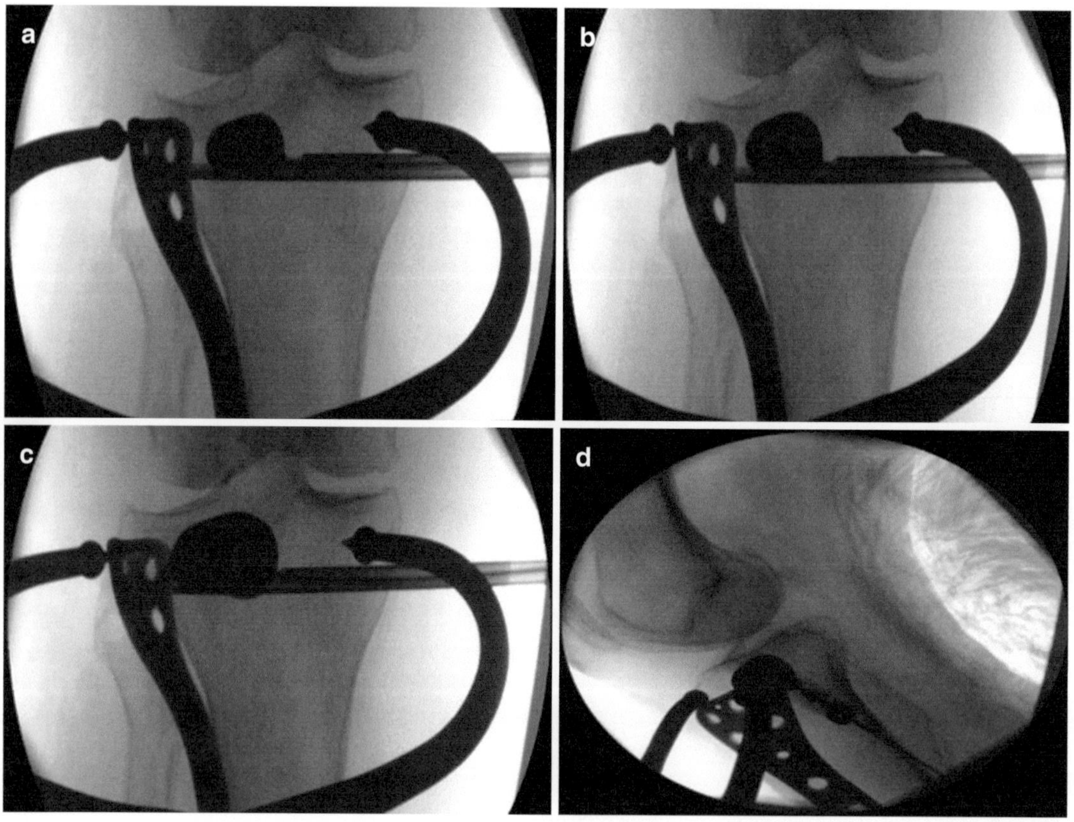

Fig. 5.11 (**a–d**) The IBT is inserted in the cannula and the balloon is gradually inflated and reduction is progressively achieved to anatomical level by taking the necessary fluoroscopic acquisition images

When reduction is achieved and prior to the deflation of the balloon, a k-wire is inserted from the latter side in order to secure maintenance of the reduction (Fig. 5.12a).

Following removal of the IBT, a bone filler device is inserted to facilitate delivery of the bone substitute at the area where the void has been created. Prior to delivery of the bone substitute, the suction tip can be placed at the entry hole of the bone filler device to remove blood from the void (create a dry void area) for optimum interdigitation of the cement filler (Fig. 5.12b, c). Following filling of the void with the bone graft substitute (tricalcium phosphate), the bone filler device is removed.

Osteosynthesis then can be carried out by inserting the proximal and distal screws through the selected plate (Fig. 5.12d, e). Occasionally, if indicated, and following reduction of the depressed articular segment, the lateral tibial plateau can be stabilised with 1–2 cannulated screws prior to the plate application for neutralisation of the fixation.

Post-operatively, the patient can initiate early range of motion of the affected knee joint. Mobilisation is toe-touch weight bearing for 4 weeks followed by partial weight bearing for another 4 weeks, and then full weight bearing is advised. Thromboprophylaxis is recommended for a period of 6 weeks.

Summary of Tips and Tricks: Pitfalls

- Accurate targeting of the depressed intra-articular segment with the trocar is essential for subsequent optimum positioning of the ITB.
- Attention must be paid not to overcompress the lateral condyle because this may lead to entrapment of the depressed fragment

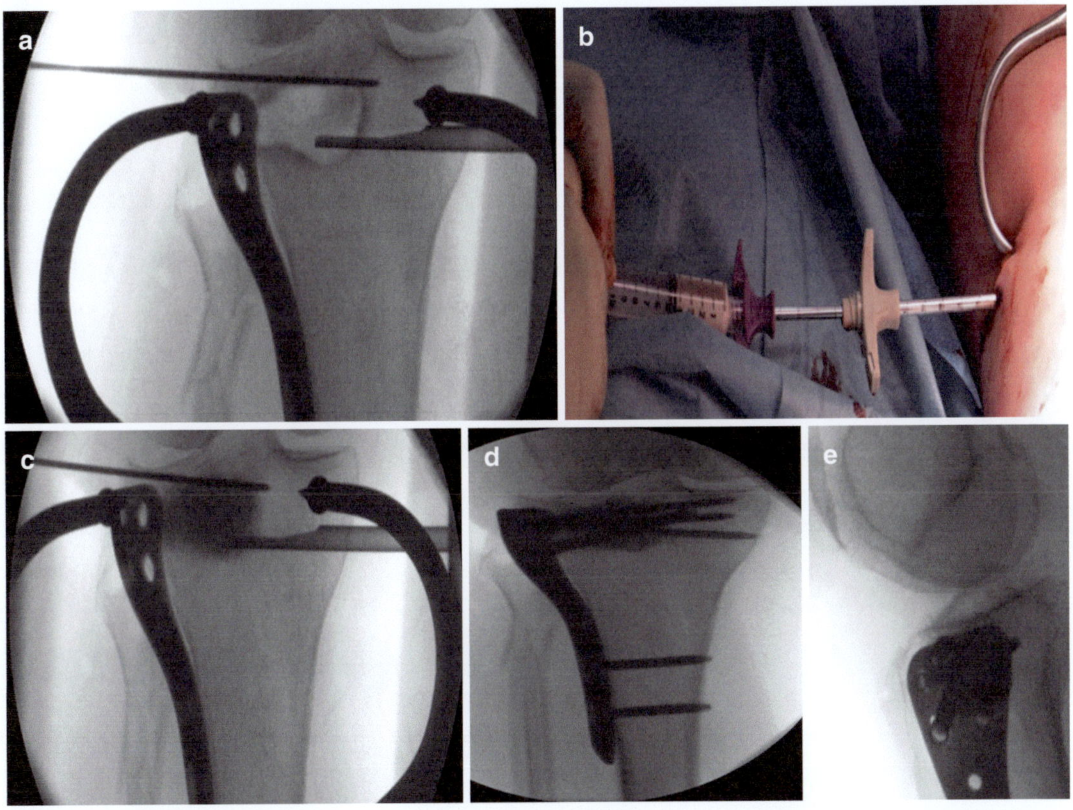

Fig. 5.12 (**a**) After successful reduction and prior to deflation of the balloon, a k-wire is inserted from the lateral side in order to secure maintenance of the reduction. (**b, c**) Delivery of bone substitute to fill the void for structural support. (**d, e**) Definitive osteosynthesis with insertion of proximal and distal screws through the plate

and the inability to achieve an anatomic articular congruence (so-called trapdoor effect).

- When there is extensive articular surface collapse, consider the implantation of a second ITB and the simultaneous inflation of both balloons.
- Follow the manufacturer's instructions not to go beyond the maximum recommended pressure for the balloon inflation in order to minimise the risk of bursting of the balloon.
- Adequate quantity of the bone substitute must be delivered within the void for reducing the risk of secondary fracture collapse.

Conflict of Interest No benefits in any form have been received or will be received from a commercial party related directly or indirectly to the subject of this chapter.

References

1. Sandmann GH, Siebenlist S, Imhoff FB, Ahrens P, Neumaier M, Freude T, Biberthaler P. Balloon-guided inflation osteoplasty in the treatment of Hill-Sachs lesions of the humeral head: case report of a new technique. Patient Saf Surg. 2016;10(1):4.
2. Ollivier M, Turati M, Munier M, Lunebourg A, Argenson JN, Parratte S. Balloon tibioplasty for reduction of depressed tibial plateau fractures: Preliminary radiographic and clinical results. Int Orthop. 2016;40(9):1961–6.
3. Broome B, Mauffrey C, Statton J, Voor M, Seligson D. Inflation osteoplasty: in vitro evaluation of a new technique for reducing depressed intra-articular fractures of the tibial plateau and distal radius. J Orthop Traumatol. 2012;13(2):89–95.
4. Hahnhaussen J, Hak DJ, Weckbach S, Heiney JP, Stahel PF. Percutaneous inflation osteoplasty for indirect reduction of depressed tibial plateau fractures. Orthopedics. 2012;35(9):768–72.
5. Schatzker J, McBroom R, Bruce D. The tibial plateau fracture. The Toronto experience 1968-1975. Clin Orthop Relat Res. 1979;138:94–104.

Innovations in Fracture Reduction: Poller Screws

6

Theodoros H. Tosounidis and Peter V. Giannoudis

Rationale of the Clinical Use of Poller Screw

The use of "Poller" or "blocking" screws is a minimally invasive reduction technique used in intramedullary nailing of long bones. Its clinical use was first described in English literature by Krettek et al. in 1995 [1], and since then it has been widely accepted as a safe and efficient truly percutaneous technique. Their original indication, which was the reduction and supplemental stabilisation of long bone metaphyseal fractures, has been recently expanded and is currently used in the management of nonunions and in intramedullary limb lengthening. The basic logic behind the use of Poller screws is to reduce the width of the medullary canal, block the nail and increase the mechanical stiffness of bone-implant construct [2, 3].

Poller screws are predominantly used in nailing of metaphyseal fractures. In such cases the short or flared segment is difficult to be aligned to the long one, and even if this is achieved by other means (unicortical plating, multiplanar traction, percutaneous clamps), the reduction is difficult to be maintained until the secure proximal and distal interlocking screw application. Poller screws were initially recommended to be applied at the short segment on the concave side of the deformity. Other descriptions of the correct position include "place the screw were you don't want the nail to go" or to the "deficient cortex". Nevertheless, these descriptions can be quite confusing and difficult to translate in the clinical setting especially for the less experienced surgeon.

Various fine-tuning methods of the original technique have been described, with common denominator being the meticulous preoperative planning and the careful intraoperative technique. We have found the method presented by Hannah et al. [4] very useful and accurate, when only one Poller screw is used or in the case of the first screw application when multiple Poller screws are used. This method is based on the fact that most of the metaphyseal long bone fractures have an oblique configuration. Initially the long axes of the short and long fragments are drawn. The fracture line is then drawn. This divides the short and long fragments in four quarters: two with an acute angle facing the facture and two with an obtuse angle facing the fracture. The Poller screws are placed in the acute angle close to the midline and close to the fracture line (Fig. 6.1 illustrates the use of Poller screws in a distal tibial fracture).

T.H. Tosounidis, M.D., Ph.D. (✉)
P.V. Giannoudis, M.D., F.A.C.S., F.R.C.S.
Academic Department of Trauma and Orthopaedic Surgery, University of Leeds, Leeds, UK

NIHR Leeds Biomedical Research Unit,
Chapel Allerton Hospital, Leeds, West Yorkshire, UK
e-mail: ttosounidis@yahoo.com

P.V. Giannoudis (ed.), *Fracture Reduction and Fixation Techniques*,
https://doi.org/10.1007/978-3-319-68628-8_6

For the application for multiple screws, we consider the method recently described by Muthusamy et al. [5] very effective. According to this, the deformity is reduced by simultaneously pushing the apex and the peripheries of the deformity towards the midline. This can be conceptualised by applying a pushing moment to the apex and bending moment to the peripheries using the surgeon's fingers (thumbs and indexes) as reduction tools. In the so-called "reverse rule of thumb" technique, the subsequent blocking screws are inserted on the side of the nail opposite to where the thumbs and the fingers are placed on the bone. Figure 6.2 illustrates the application of Poller screws with this technique.

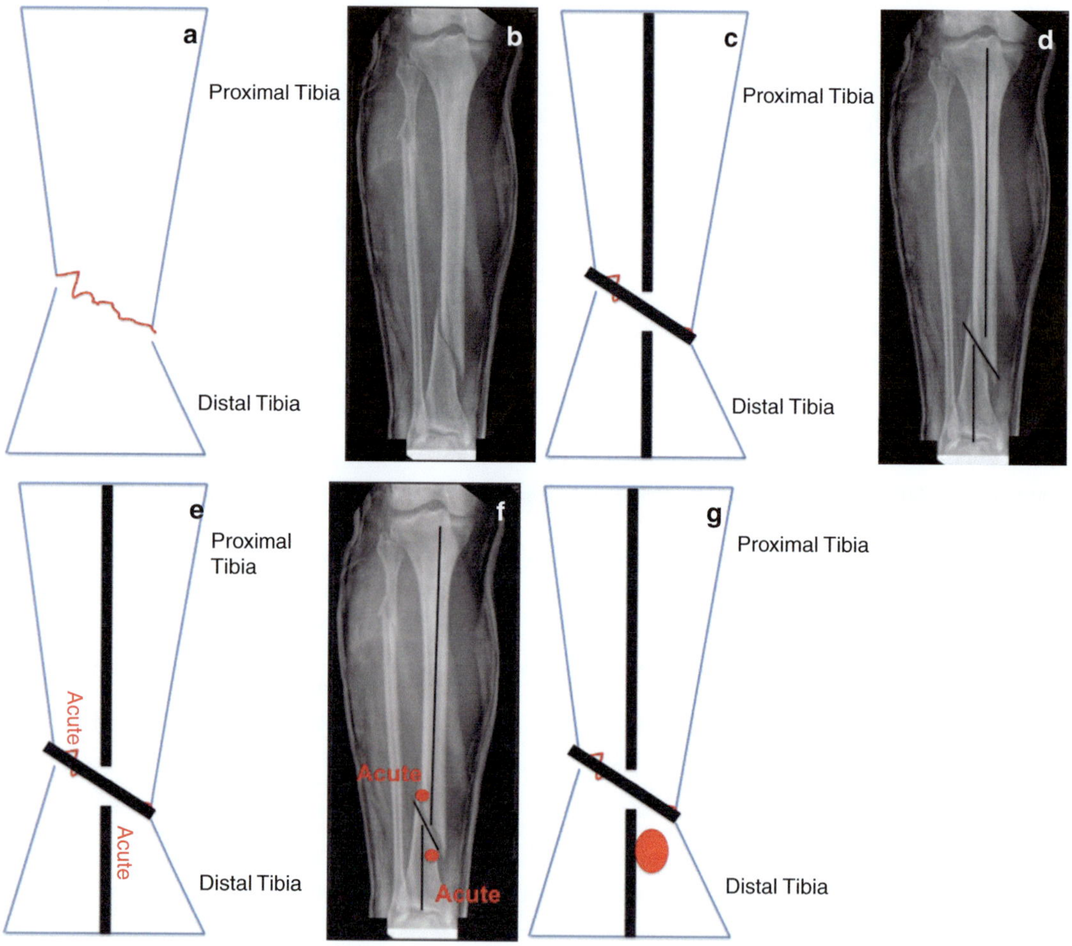

Fig. 6.1 The use of Poller screws in intramedullary nailing of a distal tibia. (**a, b**) Schematic and anteroposterior radiograph of a right distal tibia fracture. (**c, d**) The fracture line and the lines of the long axes of the short and long fragments are drawn. (**e, f**) The fracture line on each segment and the corresponding long axis produce two angles, one acute and one obtuse. (**g, h**) The first Poller screw is inserted to the acute angle area of the short segment. (**i, j**) The ball-tipped guide wire and the reamer are inserted. (**k**) The nail is inserted. Note that the deformity is corrected when the nail is touching the Poller screws and is directed towards the opposite side. (**l**) Final intraoperative anteroposterior and lateral fluoroscopic views showing the central position of the nail. (**m**) Anteroposterior and lateral radiographs showing the healed fracture 5 months post-operatively

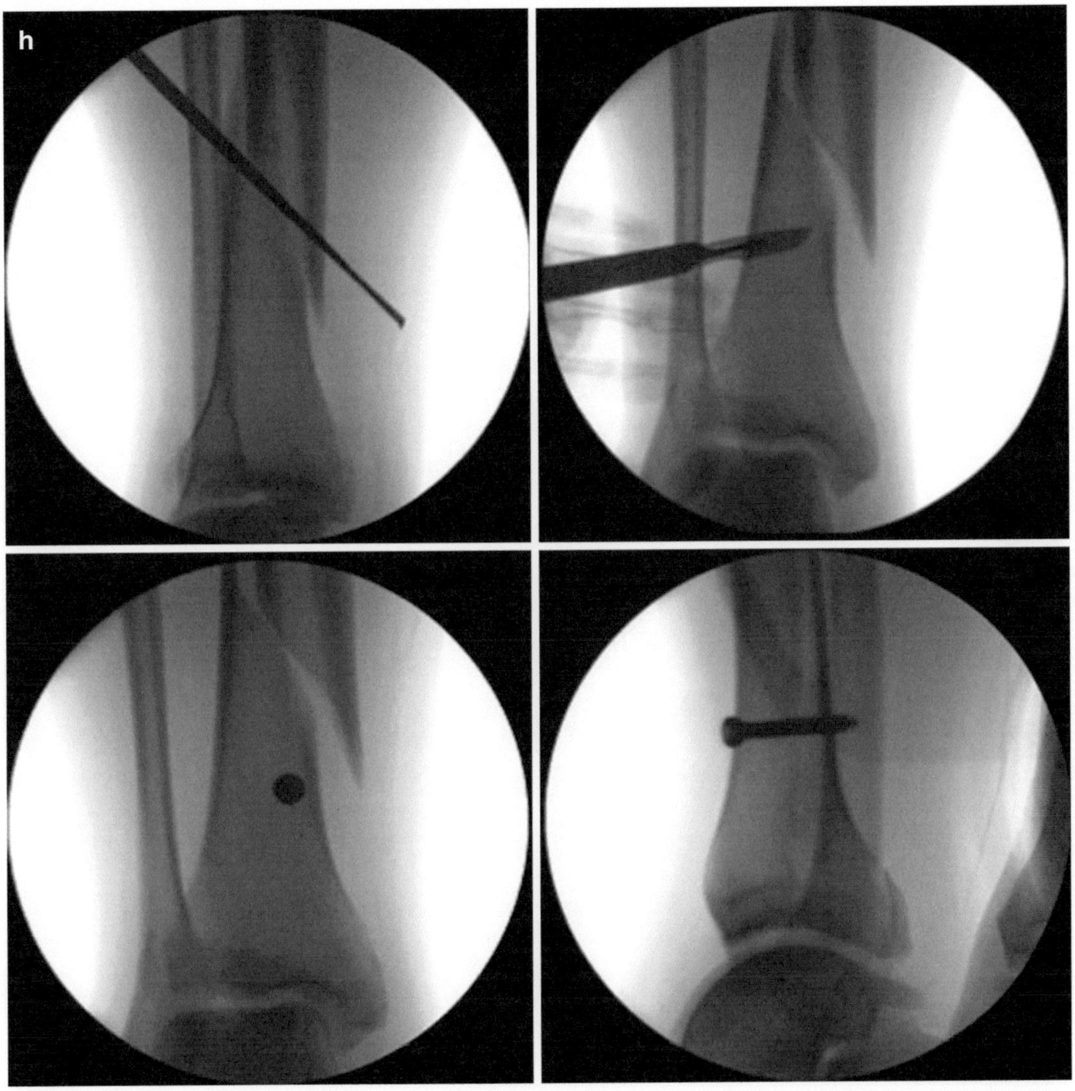

Fig. 6.1 (continued)

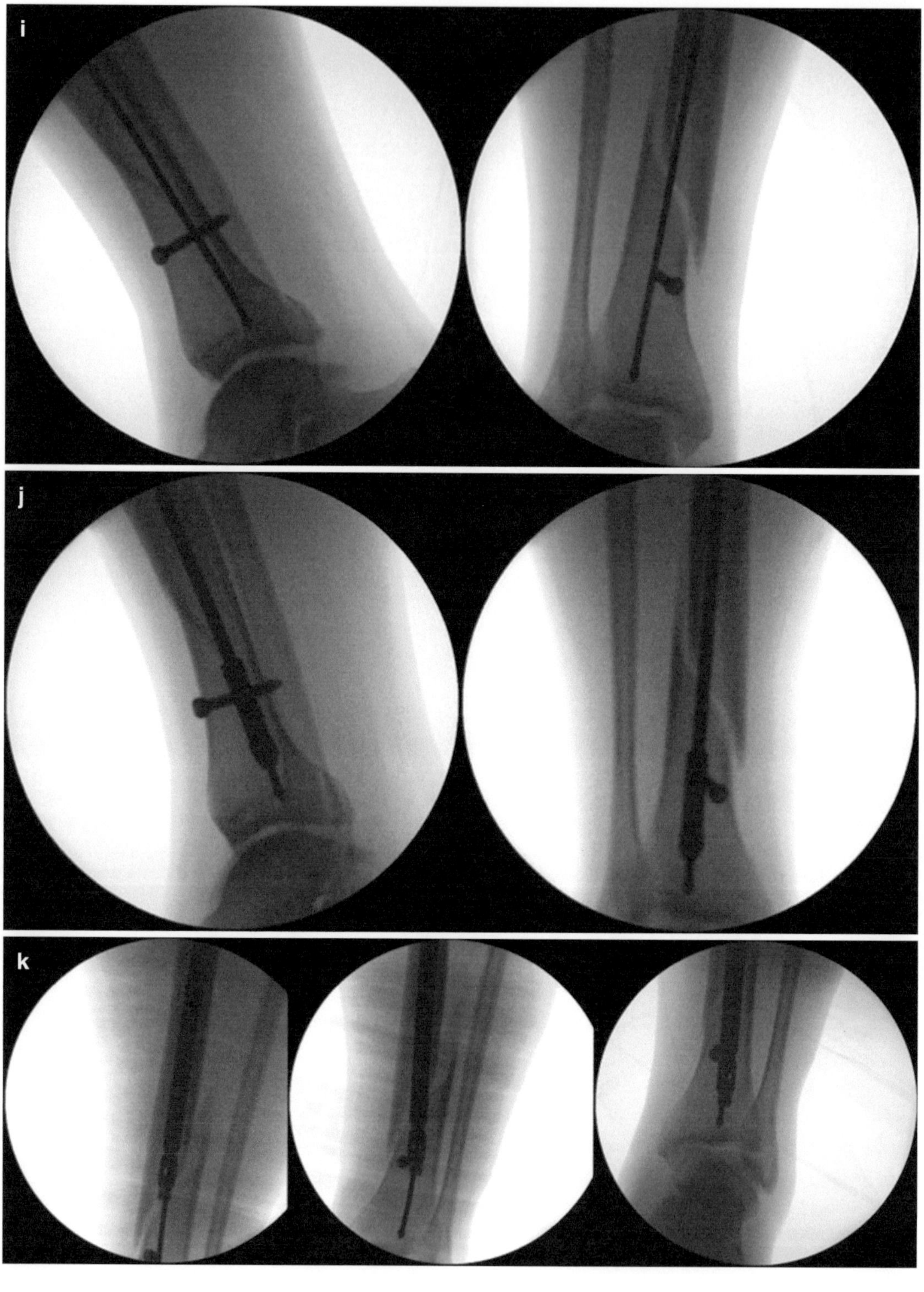

Fig. 6.1 (continued)

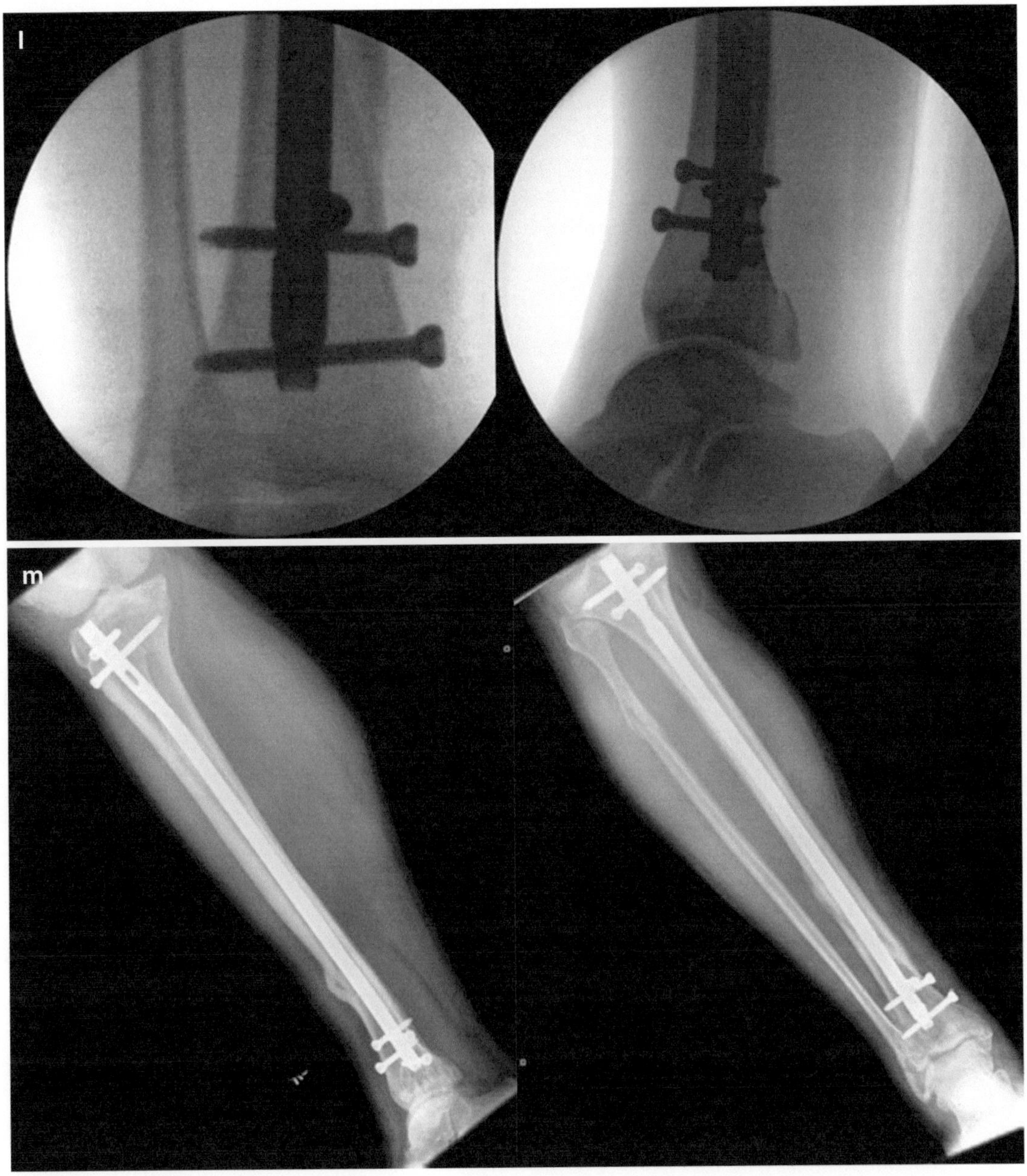

Fig. 6.1 (continued)

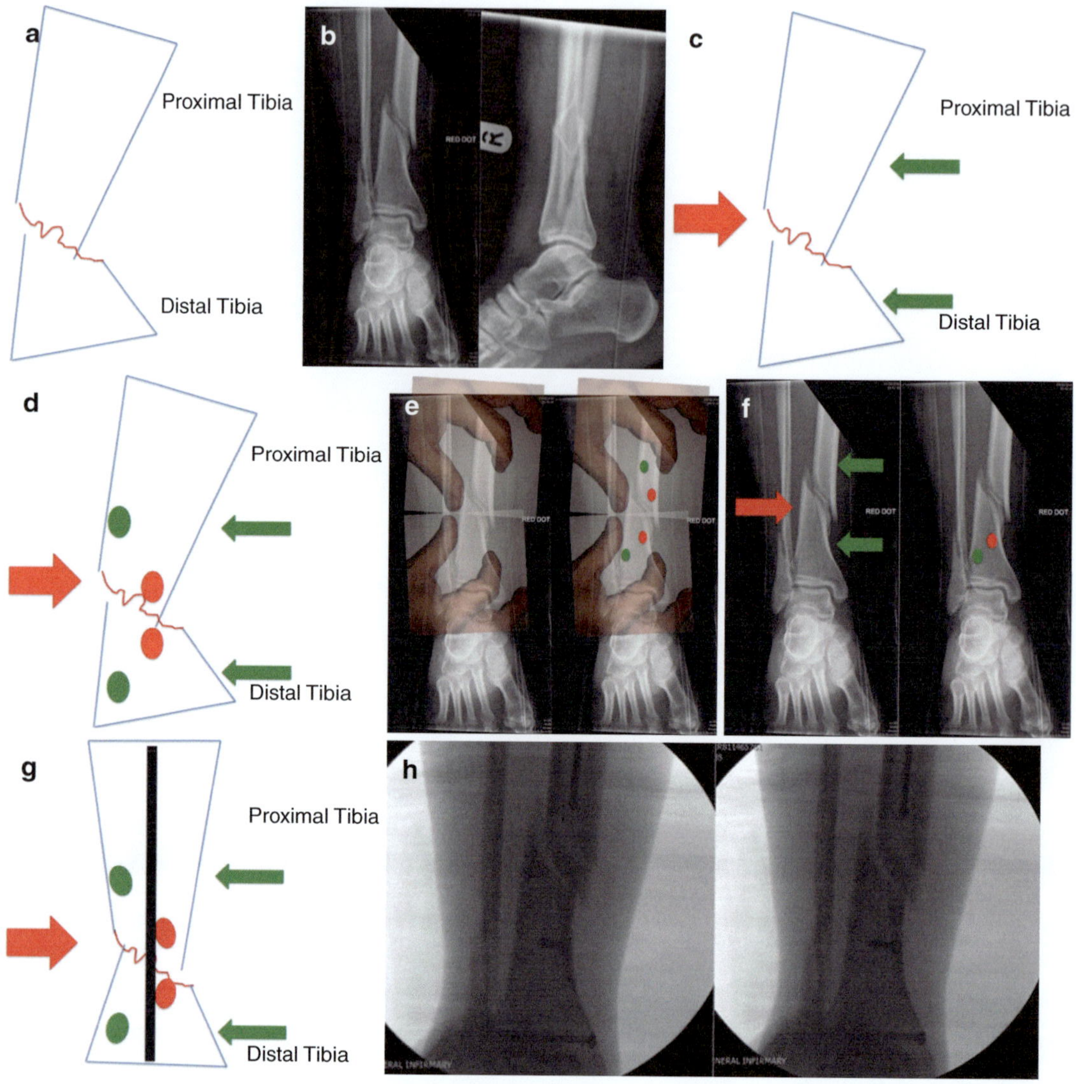

Fig. 6.2 Demonstration of the use of the "reverse rule of thumb" technique in a distal tibia fracture. (**a, b**) Schematic and plain radiographs showing the fracture with apex lateral angulation (varus deformity). (**c, d**) In order to correct the deformity, the apex has to be pushed medially, whilst the ends of the deformity have to be displaced laterally. The Poller screws are inserted opposite to the side of the application of correcting force, i.e. opposite to the apex of the deformity and to the same of the apex side at the periphery. (**e**) The "reverse rule of thumb" shows the position of the screws opposite to thumbs and indexes. (**f, g, h, i, j, k**) In this case Poller screws were placed only at the distal short fragment. Initially the most proximal to the fracture, distal Poller screw was applied. This was not enough to correct the deformity, and subsequently an additional distal screw was applied to the opposite distal cortex on the same (i.e. short) fragment. (**l, m**) Final intraoperative and immediate post-operative radiographs showing the final reduction and position of the nail in relation to the Poller screws

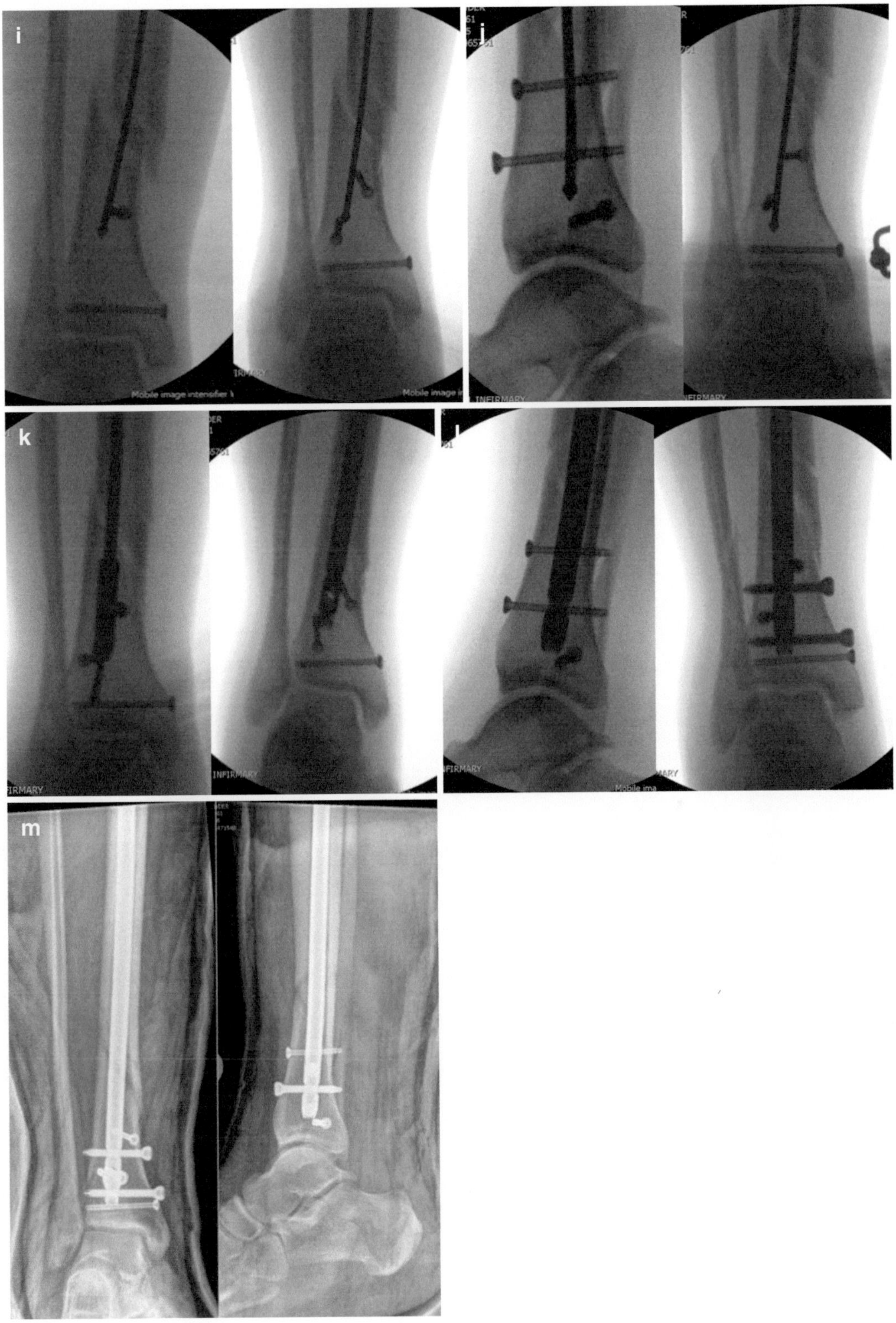

Fig. 6.2 (continued)

Tips and Tricks

Technical points that deserve special consideration include the following:

- Poller screws can be used either before or after the nail insertion. When they are used after the nail insertion, only minor corrections can be performed. The critical point is that Poller screw insertion must be performed before the application of the proximal and distal interlocking screws.
- The exact distance of Poller screws from the midline and from the fracture line is not well defined with suggestions being from 1 to 3 cm [6, 7] away from the fracture line and as close to midline as safe as it could be (6–7 mm) [6]. The above depends on the fracture configuration and the diameter of the nails used. Application of the Poller screw very close to the fracture line can result in propagation of the fracture; on the other hand, application very close to the midline can potentially block the screw insertion. Figure 6.3 illustrates the application of "ineffective Poller screws".
- Other "Poller devices" that can be used include K-wires and Steinmann pins. K-wires have a minimal footprint and offer versatility in their applications allowing for "trial placement". The Steinmann pin can also be used as a joystick for fracture manipulation and reduction [6].
- The use of cannulated screws should be performed with caution since they can deform

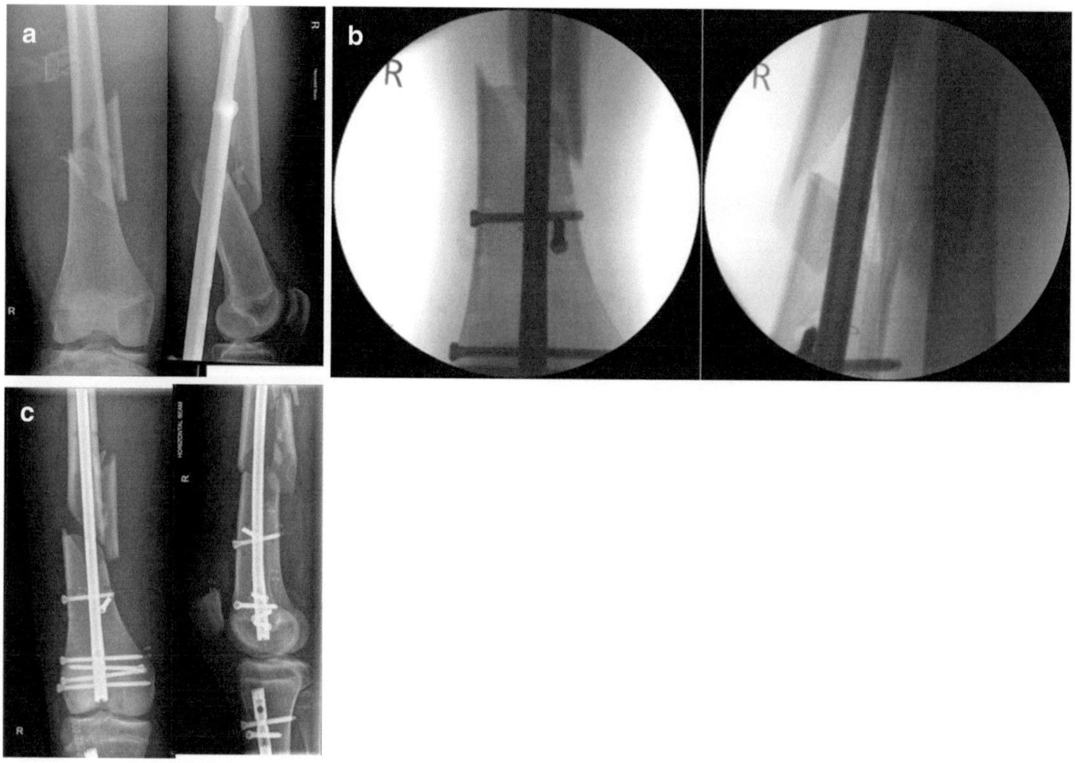

Fig. 6.3 The application of ineffective Poller screws to the distal femur. (**a**) Anteroposterior and lateral radiographs showing a comminuted distal femoral fracture. (**b**) Intraoperative fluoroscopic views showing the application of two Poller screws, one anterior to posterior and one lateral to medial. It is obvious that the Poller screw at the sagittal plane is not abutting on the nail, and thus it exerts no effect in reduction and stabilisation of the fracture. The remaining translation of the proximal fragment in relation to the distal is apparent. (**c**) Post-operative radiographs showing that distal femur in malreduced position (varus malreduction)

intra- or post-operatively making their removal problematic.

- Reaming of the canal adjacent to the Poller screw should be done with great caution or even avoided.
- A second Poller screw can be used on the opposite site of the short fragment. This technique can be used in short oblique or very distal metaphyseal fractures. By placing a second Poller screw on the opposite site of the short fragment and closest to the articular surface, a "goalpost" for insertion of the nail is created.
- Poller screws can be used in either sagittal or frontal planes. They can also be used in both of these planes simultaneously. Their position depends on the displacement/deformity, and they should be positioned perpendicular to this plane. This means that if the displacement exists on the frontal plane (varus/valgus), the Poller screws should be inserted on the sagittal plane (anterior to posterior). Similarly, if the displacement exists on the sagittal plane (procurvatum or recurvatum), then the Poller screw should be inserted on the frontal/coronal plane.
- Poller screws can be left in place in order to augment the stability of the construct. This is particularly helpful in very distal fractures where the insertion of three interlocking screws to the distal fragment is not always feasible. The principle of implant stability augmentation with Poller screws is used in the management of nonunions [8].
- When a Poller screw is overcorrecting the deformity, disengagement of the screw from the far cortex makes it less "efficient" and allows nail to correct to a more central position [9].
- Metaphyseal long bone fractures and especially those involving the distal tibia often have an additional intra-articular component not always visible on plain radiographs. We strongly recommend additional CT imaging of the joint adjacent to the short fragment so that the use of the Poller screw can carefully be planned and avoid any propagation of fracture lines and further comminution of the fragment. Apparently, the intra-articular component should be addressed prior to the metaphyseal fracture.

References

1. Krettek C, Schandelmaier P, Tscherne H. Nonreamed interlocking nailing of closed tibial fractures with severe soft tissue injury. Clin Orthop Relat Res. 1995;315:34–47.
2. Krettek C, Miclau T, Schandelmaier P, et al. The mechanical effect of blocking screws ("Poller screws") in stabilizing tibia fractures with short proximal or distal fragments after insertion of small-diameter intramedullary nails. J Orthop Trauma. 1999;13:550–3.
3. Krettek C, Stephan C, Schandelmaier P, et al. The use of Poller screws as blocking screws in stabilising tibial fractures treated with small diameter intramedullary nails. J Bone Joint Surg Br. 1999;81:963–8.
4. Hannah A, Aboelmagd T, Yip G, et al. A novel technique for accurate Poller (blocking) screw placement. Injury. 2014;45:1011–4.
5. Muthusamy S, Rozbruch SR, Fragomen AT. The use of blocking screws with internal lengthening nail and reverse rule of thumb for blocking screws in limb lengthening and deformity correction surgery. Strategies Trauma Limb Reconstr. 2016;11:199–205.
6. Shahulhameed A, Roberts CS, Ojike NI. Technique for precise placement of poller screws with intramedullary nailing of metaphyseal fractures of the femur and the tibia. Injury. 2011;42:136–9.
7. Seyhan M, Cakmak S, Donmez F, et al. Blocking screws for the treatment of distal femur fractures. Orthopedics. 2013;36:e936–41.
8. Eom TW, Kim JJ, Oh HK, et al. Challenge to treat hypertrophic nonunion of the femoral shaft: the Poller screw augmentation technique. Eur J Orthop Surg Traumatol. 2016;26:559–63.
9. Guthrie HC, Bellringer SF, Nicol S. Fine-tuning of blocking screws in long bone nailing. Ann R Coll Surg Engl. 2015;97:240–1.

7 Assessment of Reduction

David J. Hak

Using a direct reduction method, the fracture site is visualized greatly increasing the likelihood of an anatomic reduction in simple fracture patterns. In contrast, the fracture site is commonly not visualized during indirect reductions, and the surgeon relies on various methods to ensure restoration of accurate length, alignment, and rotation. The benefits of indirect reduction methods include decreased soft tissue dissection and less stripping of periosteal blood supply, with the goal of improving fracture healing and decreasing soft tissue wound complications. Because indirect reduction methods are being increasingly used, methods to assess fracture reduction have become vitally important.

Direct Vision

Direct visual inspection of the fracture reduction can easily assess the accuracy of the reduction but often requires significant soft tissue exposure. Usually only one side of the reduction can be visually inspected, and it is important to note that while the visualized cortex may be well aligned, there can occasionally be a cortical gap along the far cortex that cannot be directly visualized.

D.J. Hak, M.D., M.B.A., F.A.C.S.
Denver Health Medical Center, University of Colorado School of Medicine, Aurora, CO, USA
e-mail: david.hak@dhha.org

Palpation

Palpation of the fracture reduction can be performed either with your finger or an instrument such as a Freer elevator. It allows assessment of areas that may not be seen with direct vision, but soft tissues may not allow full access to the entire area of reduction, and the ability to assess the degree of step-off or malrotation may be limited.

Intraoperative Fluoroscopy

Intraoperative fluoroscopy is used to assess fracture reduction and implant position during minimally invasive procedures. Limitations of fluoroscopy include a limited field of view, difficulty in obtaining certain views, and degradation of image quality in obese patients. The ability to manipulate the fluoroscopic angles allows the surgeon to find and save the best-looking image, which may not always reflect accuracy of the reduction. In addition, fluoroscopy exposes the operative team to radiation and requires the use of protective equipment that may increase surgeon fatigue.

The accuracy of fluoroscopic assessment of articular reduction may be limited. Investigators studied a simulated intra-articular lateral tibial plateau fracture cadaveric model. Anterior-posterior (AP), lateral, and joint line fluoroscopic views were obtained of each specimen with anatomic reduction, 2 mm of articular dis-

P.V. Giannoudis (ed.), *Fracture Reduction and Fixation Techniques*,
https://doi.org/10.1007/978-3-319-68628-8_7

placement, and 5 mm of articular displacements. Assessment of whether the articular surface was reduced was performed by eight orthopedic traumatologists. For 5 mm of displacement, using both the AP and lateral views yielded the highest accuracy for detecting reduction at 90% (95% confidence interval, 83–94%), but for the other conditions, agreement was poor to moderate, and accuracy ranged from 37 to 83%. The authors concluded that applying these findings clinically suggests that direct visualization of the articular surface may be necessary to ensure malreduction less than 5 mm [1].

Intraoperative fluoroscopy can be used to assess lower extremity alignment by using an electrocautery cord as a radiopaque "plumb" line. Center one end of the cord over the femoral head and the other over the ankle joint to represent the mechanical axis. Pull the cord taut and assess the location where the cord crosses the knee joint (Fig. 7.1). Compare this with the preoperative plans or with the contralateral leg mechanical axis. The average normal mechanical axis crosses the knee 10 mm medial to the center of the knee joint (normal range 3–17 mm) [2, 3].

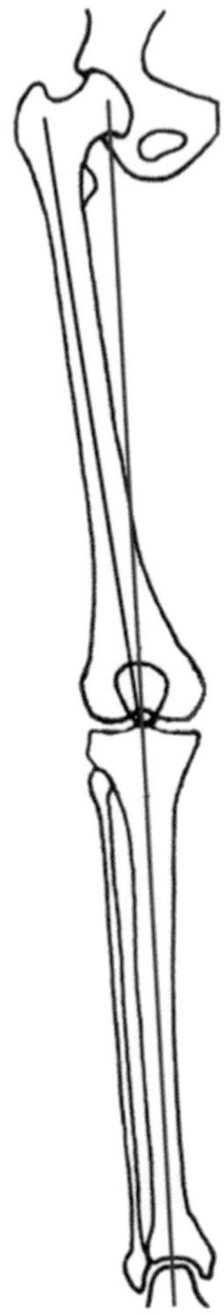

Fig. 7.1 An electrocautery cord can be used as a radiopaque "plumb" line. Center one end of the cord over the femoral head and the other end over the ankle joint, and then pull taut to represent the mechanical axis. The varus/valgus alignment of the limb can be assessed by the position that the "plumb" line crosses the knee joint

Intraoperative Plain Radiographs

While the quality of fluoroscopic imaging has increased with improved technology, the resolution of plain radiographs is still superior. Plain radiographs were found to be superior to fluoroscopy in the assessment of articular gap, step-off, and displacement in a cadaveric model of closed reduction and percutaneous pinning of simulated Bennett's fractures [4]. Another benefit of plain radiographs is the ability to image a larger field of view, which can be advantageous in assessing angular alignment such as in a tibial osteotomy [5]. Disadvantages of intraoperative plain radiographs are that it is time-consuming and may represent a sterility concern. While a fluoroscopic machine is typically covered with a sterile drape, such precautions are not typically followed with a standard the portable radiograph unit.

Arthroscopic Assessment

Arthroscopic assessment of articular reduction has primarily been promoted for fractures of the distal radius and tibial plateau. Its use in fracture reduction and assessment has been described in almost every joint in which arthroscopic assessment is feasible including the hip, shoulder, ankle, and other smaller joints. It provides the benefit of direct visualization of the articular surface. It can also identify additional soft tissue injuries. The disadvantages include the need for additional equipment and potential risks of fluid extravasation [6].

A retrospective case-matched study compared 15 comminuted intra-articular distal radius fractures treated with arthroscopically assisted reduction with

15 that were treated with fluoroscopic-assisted reduction. Investigators reported that those who underwent arthroscopically assisted reduction had significantly improved supination, wrist extension, and wrist flexion. The authors concluded that arthroscopically assisted reduction permits a more thorough inspection of the ulnar-sided components of the injury [7].

Investigators performed arthroscopic assessment of 17 consecutive tibial plateau fractures following reduction under fluoroscopic visualization. Persistent fracture depression (≥2 mm) was seen on arthroscopic assessment in 10 of the cases necessitating intraoperative correction. The authors concluded that arthroscopic assessment significantly improved visualization of articular displacement, particularly in the posterolateral central region of the tibial plateau [8]. In contrast, a study that compared ten consecutive unicondylar tibial plateau fractures treated by arthroscopically assisted control of reduction were compared with 23 consecutive unicondylar tibial plateau fractures treated by fluoroscopic control. The investigators in this study concluded that they were not able to demonstrate any significant benefit from arthroscopy compared with fluoroscopic reduction [9].

Computed Tomography

Fracture reduction and fixation using computed tomography was initially popularized in the early 1990s for placement of iliosacral screws [10, 11]. The major advantage of computed tomography-guided sacral fixation is direct visualization of the course of the guidewire and screw placement, avoiding significant complications from misplaced implants. Because of limitations of access during the procedure, typically only percutaneous procedures can be performed in real time.

Computed tomography has been shown superior to conventional radiographs in detecting articular steps and gaps following open reduction and internal fixation of fractures of the distal radius and the acetabulum [12–14]. Because these CT findings are only discovered following the procedure, additional surgery may be required if the findings indicate revision is indicated.

3D Fluoroscopy

Several 3D intraoperative imaging systems that use CT technology are available for verifying anatomic relationships. They can also be used in conjunction with intraoperative navigation. Three-dimensional (3D) fluoroscopic imaging uses a mobile C-arm unit that is modified to provide a motorized rotational movement and combined with a computer workstation. These allow real-time intraoperative assessment and correction of reduction and implant position. The use of 3D fluoroscopy provides increased understanding of fracture patterns and implant position during fracture surgery.

The ARCADIS Orbic 3D devices (Siemens, Malvern, Pennsylvania, USA) are a high-end C-arm with an isocentric design and 190° orbital movement that provide 3D functionality. In contrast to the standard C-arm used in two-dimensional fluoroscopy, the C-arm rotates around an isocentric point such that the distance between the X-ray tube and targeted region remains constant. The device acquires a series of approximately 100 fluoroscopic two-dimensional images at equidistant angles, which are then reconstructed into a three-dimensional image at a volume of 120 mm. The images have comparable resolution and similar clinical value compared with standard CT images [15].

The O-arm imaging system (Medtronic, Louisville, Colorado, USA) provides surgeons with real-time, 3D images, as well as multiplane, 2D, and fluoroscopic imaging. The unique design allows a 360° orbital movement. It can be used with navigation for image-guided surgery. While it is used primarily for navigated spinal and neurosurgery, it can also be used to assess fracture reduction [16]. Both 2D and 3D volumetric imaging can be obtained within seconds, yielding high-quality imaging comparable to fixed CT systems.

Investigators reported that three-dimensional fluoroscopy exhibited higher precision in reduction assessment in a cadaveric tibial plateau fracture model compared to standard fluoroscopy [17]. Intraoperative 3D imaging has been studied in fractures of the distal radius, scaphoid, calcaneus, pelvis, and acetabulum [18–22]. The use of this advanced intraoperative imaging may provide improved articular reduction and optimal implant position [23].

Leg Length Measurement

Leg length discrepancy can occur when treating comminuted fractures. The contralateral leg, if uninjured, can serve as a guide for restoration of normal length. Leg lengths should be clinically assessed at the conclusion of any operation involving a comminuted femur or tibia. To measure leg lengths in the supine position, the torso and pelvis should be aligned straight, and the patients' feet brought together until their ankles touch. Knee or hip flexion deformities can affect this measurement. Another method to assess leg length is measure the distance from anterior superior iliac spine to the medial malleolus with a tape measure. Additional quantification of leg length inequality can be obtained with a CT scanogram.

In a study of 91 comminuted femoral shaft fractures treated with intramedullary nailing, investigators found a mean leg length discrepancy of 0.58 cm in 98% of the patients, but only six (7%) patients had a leg length discrepancy greater than 1.25 cm [24].

Various radiographic methods are also available for assessment of leg lengths. There is general consensus that radiographic methods are more accurate and reliable than clinical examination for assessment of leg length discrepancy [25].

For the orthoroentgenogram radiographic technique, the patient lies supine next to a calibrated ruler. Three distinct exposures centered over the hip, knee, and ankle are obtained using a long cassette that accommodates all three images. It was developed to minimize measurement error secondary to magnification. The scanogram radiographic technique also utilizes three distinct exposures centered over the hip, knee, and ankle in order to minimize magnification error. The patient lies supine next to a calibrated ruler, and unlike the orthoroentgenogram, the standard length radiographic cassette is moved for the three exposures.

CT scanogram can also be obtained to measure leg lengths. CT scout images of the joints are obtained, and measurements are obtained with the CT cursor. Measurements from the CT scanogram are more consistently reproducible, and it requires lower radiation doses than conventional imaging techniques. Typically the leg lengths are measured using an anterior-posterior (AP) scout view of the bilateral femurs and tibias. Assessment of leg lengths on the lateral scout view is especially useful for patients with flexion contractures of the knee, in whom measurements on standard anterior-posterior views may be underestimated [26].

Rotational Assessment

Assessment of rotational alignment is very challenging during indirect reductions. Malrotation abnormalities have been reported following intramedullary nailing of both femoral and tibial fractures. Twenty-eight percent (21 of 76) of patients that had undergone IM femoral nailing on a fracture table had a rotational deformity of 15° or greater as assessed by postoperative CT scans. Twelve of these were external rotation deformities, and nine were internal rotation deformities [27]. Malrotation greater than 10° was found in 22% of tibial fractures treated with intramedullary nailing [28].

Krettek popularized several useful techniques that can be used to judge the proper rotation of femoral shaft fractures during either IM nailing or minimally invasive plate fixation [29]. These techniques include assessment of cortical thickness, internal and external cortical diameters, and profile of the lesser trochanter.

Comparison of the cortical thickness may be used to evaluate rotational alignment of simple transverse and short oblique fractures. In the absence of comminution or eccentric reaming, the cortical thickness of the proximal fragment should match the cortical thickness of the distal fragment (Fig. 7.2). Comparison of the outer cortical diameter may be used to evaluate rotational

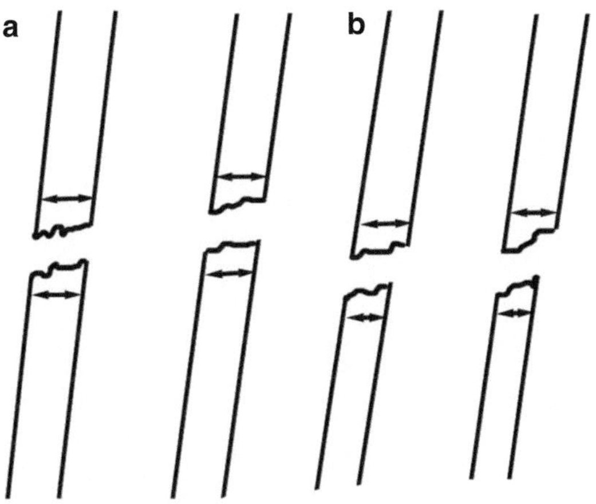

Fig. 7.2 Evaluation of cortical thickness at the fracture site to assess accuracy of rotational reduction. The cortical thickness of the proximal fragment is equivalent to the distal fragment, suggesting correct rotational alignment (**a**). The cortical thickness of the proximal fragment is not equivalent to the distal fragment indicating that the rotational alignment is off (**b**)

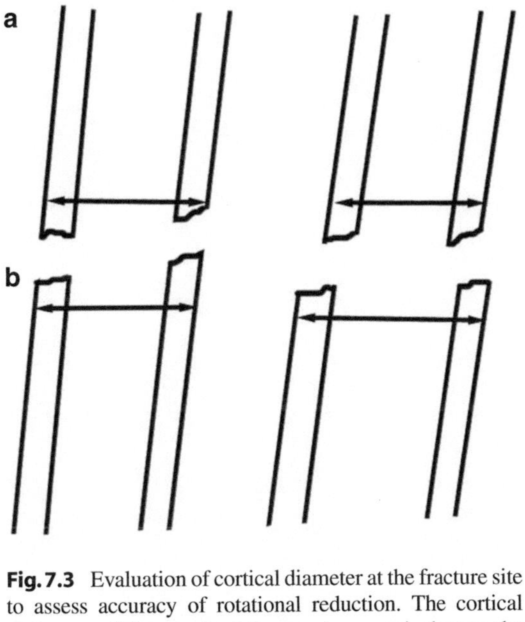

Fig. 7.3 Evaluation of cortical diameter at the fracture site to assess accuracy of rotational reduction. The cortical diameters of the proximal fragment are equivalent to the distal fragment suggesting correct rotational alignment if the fracture is at a level where the femoral cross section is oval rather than round (**a**). The cortical diameters of the proximal fragment are not equivalent to the distal fragment indicating that the rotational alignment is not correct (**b**)

alignment because at many levels the femur is oval in shape, rather than round (Fig. 7.3). If the cortical diameters are different, it suggests malrotation. However, if the cortical diameters are equal, it may not necessarily indicate malreduction, since if the femoral shaft cross section is round at the level of the fracture, the diameters will be equal even with marked rotational malalignment.

The most accurate fluoroscopic method for assessing the accuracy of rotation during IM femoral nailing is assessment of the profile of the lesser trochanter, with comparison to the uninjured side. Since the lesser trochanter is a posteromedial structure, its profile changes depending on the rotation of the proximal femoral segment. Since there is some variation from patient to patient, the profile of the lesser trochanter on the uninjured side should be obtained and saved. Begin by first obtaining a true AP knee image. With the uninjured leg held stationary, move the fluoroscope to the hip, and save an image of the lesser trochanter profile.

The fluoroscopic process is repeated on the injured side. Again a true AP image of the knee is obtained. The fluoroscope is moved to the hip and an image obtained. If the profile of the lesser trochanter matches that seen on the uninjured side, then the rotational alignment is correct (Fig. 7.4). If the profile of the lesser trochanter is smaller than the uninjured side, it indicates that the proximal segment is internally rotated compared to the AP image of the knee (an external rotational deformity of the distal segment). If the profile of the lesser trochanter is larger than the uninjured side, it indicates that the proximal segment is externally rotated compared to the AP image of the knee (an internal rotational deformity of the distal segment).

Jeanmart et al. have described a technique for evaluating femoral malrotation using limited CT cuts through the proximal and distal femur [30]. A line is drawn along the posterior border of the femoral condyles and another line drawn through the femoral neck. The angle between these two lines is measured, and any difference between the injured and uninjured sides is compared (Fig. 7.5). A decrease in angle of the fractured side indicates increased external rotation of the distal fragment, while an increase of this angle indicates an increased internal rotation of the distal femoral fragment.

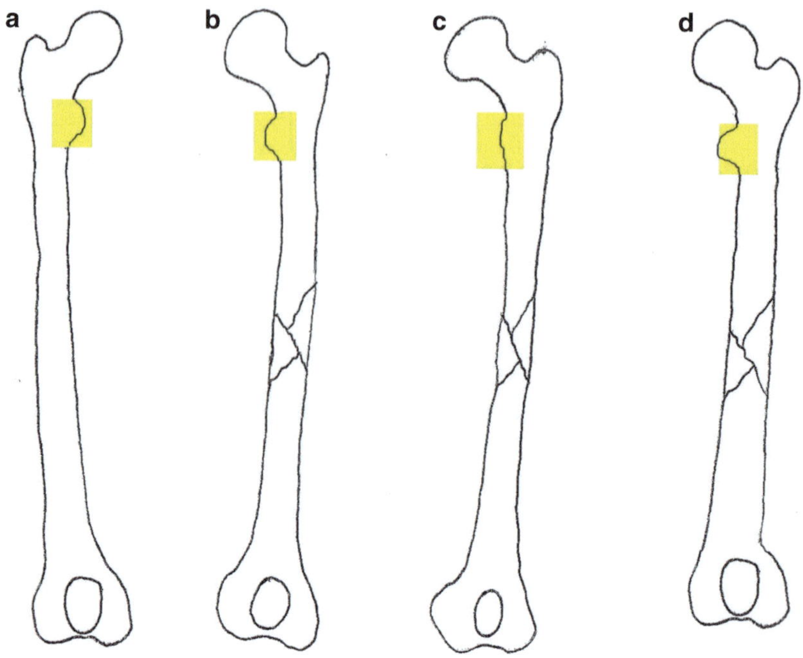

Fig. 7.4 Assessment of the lesser trochanter profile. Assessment of the lesser trochanter profile on the uninjured side with the leg in neutral rotation (AP image of the knee) (**a**). Matching profile of the lesser trochanter on the injured side indicates correct rotation (**b**). A smaller profile of the lesser trochanter indicates that the proximal segment is internally rotated (an external rotational deformity of the distal segment) (**c**). A larger profile of the lesser trochanter indicates that the proximal segment is externally rotated compared to the AP image of the knee (an internal rotational deformity of the distal segment) (**d**)

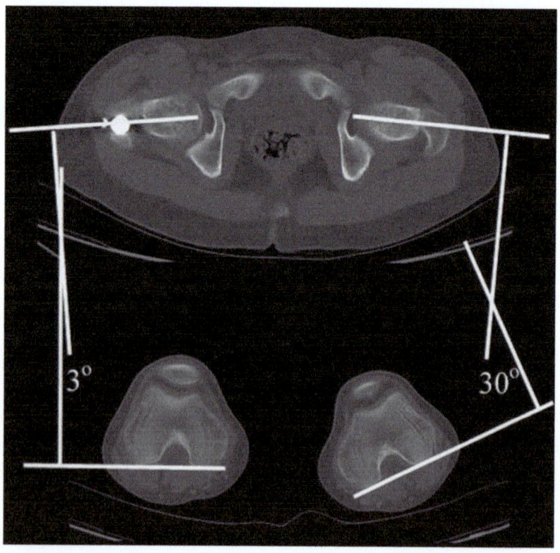

Fig. 7.5 Computerized tomographic evaluation of femoral malrotation. Right-angle lines are drawn from the axis of the femoral neck and from the posterior border of the femoral condyles. The angle of the intersection of these lines is measured as shown. Rotational malalignment is determined by differences between the fractured and uninjured side. A decrease in angle of the fractured side indicates increased external rotation of the distal fragment, while an increase in angle indicates increased internal rotation of the distal femoral fragment. The angle on the uninjured side measures 30°, while the malrotated fractured side measures only 3°, indicating a 27° external rotation deformity

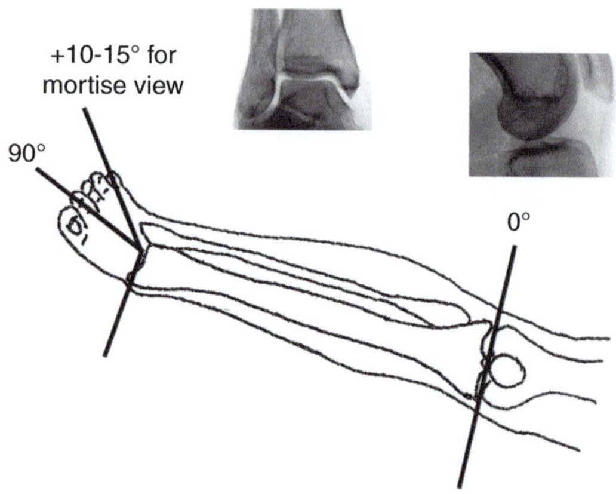

Fig. 7.6 Fluoroscopic technique to evaluate tibial rotation. First, a true lateral of the knee is obtained by superimposing the medial and lateral femoral condyles. With the leg held stable, the fluoroscopic unit is rotated 90°, which provides a true AP view. If the tibial fracture is accurately reduced, rotation of an additional 10–15° should provide an accurate mortise view of the ankle

Tibial torsion can be assessed by measuring the rotational difference between a true AP of the knee and a true mortise view of the ankle (Fig. 7.6). A true lateral of the knee can be obtained by superimposing the medial and lateral femoral condyles. With the leg held stationary, the fluoroscope is rotated 90° obtaining a true AP of the knee. The fluoroscopic unit is then moved down to the ankle, and further rotation is added until a true mortise of the ankle is obtained. In general an additional 10–15° of rotation from the true AP should produce an accurate mortise view [31]. A more precise degree of rotation can be obtained by imaging the uninjured extremity to determine the patient's normal tibial torsion. However, in a study of 100 normal patients, the difference in tibial torsion between legs reached up to 15°. The mean difference between sides was 2.1° with a standard deviation of 5.2° [32].

References

1. Haller JM, O'Toole R, Graves M, Barei D, Gardner M, Kubiak E, Nascone J, Nork S, Presson AP, Higgins TF. How much articular displacement can be detected using fluoroscopy for tibial plateau fractures? Injury. 2015;46(11):2243–7.
2. Paley D, Tetsworth K. Mechanical axis deviation of the lower limbs: Preoperative planning of uniapical angular deformities of the tibia or femur. Clin Orthop. 1992;280:48–64.
3. Paley D, Herzenberg JE, Tetsworth K, McKie J, Bhave A. Deformity planning for frontal and sagittal plane corrective osteotomies. Orthop Clin North Am. 1994;25(3):425–65.
4. Capo JT, Kinchelow T, Orillaza NS, Rossy W. Accuracy of fluoroscopy in closed reduction and percutaneous fixation of simulated Bennett's fracture. J Hand Surg Am. 2009;34(4):637–41.
5. Probe RA. Lower extremity angular malunion: evaluation and surgical correction. J Am Acad Orthop Surg. 2003;11(5):302–11.
6. Belanger M, Fadale P. Compartment syndrome of the leg after arthroscopic examination of a tibial plateau fracture. Case report and review of the literature. Arthroscopy. 1997;13(5):646–51.
7. Ruch DS, Vallee J, Poehling GG, Smith BP, Kuzma GR. Arthroscopic reduction versus fluoroscopic reduction in the management of intra-articular distal radius fractures. Arthroscopy. 2004;20(3):225–30.
8. Krause M, Preiss A, Meenen NM, Madert J, Frosch KH. 'Fracturoscopy' is superior to fluoroscopy in the articular reconstruction of complex tibial plateau fractures – an arthroscopic assisted fracture reduction technique. J Orthop Trauma. 2016;30(8):437–44.
9. Lobenhoffer P, Schulze M, Gerich T, Lattermann C, Tscherne H. Closed reduction/percutaneous fixation of tibial plateau fractures: arthroscopic versus fluoroscopic control of reduction. J Orthop Trauma. 1999;13(6):426–31.
10. Nelson DW, Duwelius PJ. CT-guided fixation of sacral fractures and sacroiliac joint disruptions. Radiology. 1991;180:527–32.
11. Duwelius PJ, Van Allen M, Bray TJ, Nelson D. Computed tomography-guided fixation of unstable posterior pelvic ring disruptions. J Orthop Trauma. 1992;6(4):420–6.
12. Cole RJ, Bindra RR, Evanoff BA, Gilula LA, Yamaguchi K, Gelberman RH. Radiographic evaluation of osseous displacement following intra-articular fractures of the distal radius: reliability of plain radiography versus computed tomography. J Hand Surg [Am]. 1997;22:792–800.
13. Borrelli J Jr, Goldfarb C, Catalano L, Evanoff BA. Assessment of articular fragment displacement in acetabular fractures: a comparison of computerized tomography and plain radiographs. J Orthop Trauma. 2002;16:449–56.
14. Moed BR, Carr SE, Gruson KI, Watson JT, Craig JG. Computed tomographic assessment of fractures of the posterior wall of the acetabulum after operative treatment. J Bone Jt Surg Am. 2003;85-A:512–22.
15. Hott JS, Papadopoulos SM, Theodore N, Dickman CA, Sonntag VK. Intraoperative Iso-C C-arm navigation in cervical spinal surgery: Review of the first 52 cases. Spine. 2004;29(24):2856–60.
16. Hsu AR, Gross CE, Lee S. Intraoperative O-arm computed tomography evaluation of syndesmotic reduction: case report. Foot Ankle Int. 2013;34(5):753–9.
17. Gösling T, Klingler K, Geerling J, Shin H, Fehr M, Krettek C, Hüfner T. Improved intra-operative reduction control using a three-dimensional mobile image intensifier – a proximal tibia cadaver study. Knee. 2009;16(1):58–63.
18. Mehling I, Rittstieg P, Mehling AP, Küchle R, Müller LP, Rommens PM. Intraoperative C-arm CT imaging in angular stable plate osteosynthesis of distal radius fractures. J Hand Surg Eur Vol. 2013;38(7):751–7.
19. Eckardt H, Lind M. Effect of intraoperative three-dimensional imaging during the reduction and fixation of displaced calcaneal fractures on articular congruence and implant fixation. Foot Ankle Int. 2015;36(7):764–73.
20. Grossterlinden L, Nuechtern J, Begemann PG, Fuhrhop I, Petersen JP, Ruecker A, Rupprecht M, Lehmann W, Schumacher U, Rueger JM, Briem D. Computer-assisted surgery and intraoperative three-dimensional imaging for screw placement in different pelvic regions. J Trauma. 2011;71(4):926–32.
21. Luria S, Safran O, Zinger G, Mosheiff R, Liebergall M. Intraoperative 3-dimensional imaging of scaphoid fracture reduction and fixation. Orthop Traumatol Surg Res. 2015;101(3):353–7.
22. Eckardt H, Lind D, Toendevold E. Open reduction and internal fixation aided by intraoperative 3-dimensional imaging improved the articular reduction in 72 displaced acetabular fractures. Acta Orthop. 2015;86(6):684–9.
23. Weil YA, Liebergall M, Mosheiff R, Singer SB, Joskowicz L, Khoury A. Assessment of two 3-D

fluoroscopic systems for articular fracture reduction: a cadaver study. Int J Comput Assist Radiol Surg. 2011;6(5):685–92.
24. Herscovici D Jr, Scaduto JM. Assessing leg length after fixation of comminuted femur fractures. Clin Orthop Relat Res. 2014;472(9):2745–50.
25. Terry MA, Winell JJ, Green DW, Schneider R, Peterson M, Marx RG, Widmann RF. Measurement variance in limb length discrepancy: Clinical and radiographic assessment of interobserver and intraobserver variability. J Pediatr Orthop. 2005;25:197–201.
26. Sabharwal S, Kumar A. Methods for assessing leg length discrepancy. Clin Orthop Relat Res. 2008;466(12): 2910–22.
27. Jaarsma RL, Pakviz DFM, Verdonschot N, et al. Rotational malalignment after intramedullary nailing of femoral fractures. J Orthop Trauma. 2004;18:403–9.
28. Puloski S, Romano C, Buckley R, Powell J. Rotational malalignment of the tibia following reamed intramedullary nail fixation. J Orthop Trauma. 2004;18: 397–402.
29. Krettek C, Miclau T, Grun O, et al. Intraoperative control of axes, rotation and length in femoral and tibial fractures. Technical note. Injury. 1998;29(Suppl 3): C29–39.
30. Jeanmart L, Baert AL, Wackenheim A. Computer tomography of neck, chest, spine and limbs. Atlas of pathologic computer tomography, vol. 3. New York, NY: Springer-Verlag; 1983. p. 171–7.
31. Clementz BG. Assessment of tibial torsion and rotational deformity with a new fluoroscopic technique. Clin Orthop Rel Res. 1989;245:199–209.
32. Clementz BG. Tibial torsion measured in normal adults. Acta Orthop Scand. 1988;59(4):441–2.

8 General Principles of Preoperative Planning

Charalampos G. Zalavras

Definition

Planning is the process of thinking about and organizing the activities required to achieve a desired goal. It involves the creation and maintenance of a plan, which is defined by the American Heritage Dictionary of the English Language as "a systematic arrangement of elements or important parts," "a proposed or intended course of action," and "an orderly or step-by-step conception or proposal for accomplishing an objective" [1].

Planning consists of the following key components:

1. Analysis of the current situation, definition of the problem at hand, and determination of the desired goal.
2. Evaluation of potential solutions and determination of the optimal course of action in order to achieve the goal (tactic). Tactic (from the ancient Greek "τακτική" meaning "art of arrangement") is a conceptual action aiming at the achievement of a goal.
3. Implementation of the plan (logistics). Logistics (from the ancient Greek "λόγος" meaning reason or speech; "λογιστικός" meaning accountant or responsible for counting) is the detailed organization and implementation of a complex operation.

Similarly, in fracture surgery, preoperative planning involves the careful evaluation of various variables (fracture characteristics, extremity condition, patient status) in order to define the current problem, determine the goal of management, and develop and implement an individualized management plan that will optimize outcome for a patient with a fracture.

Importance of Preoperative Planning

Preoperative planning is very important for several reasons [2, 3]. Most importantly, preoperative planning improves patient outcomes. Without careful analysis in a systematic fashion of the specific characteristics of the fracture, the extremity, and the patient and without detailed evaluation of all available treatment options, the best treatment plan may be overlooked, and the final outcome may be compromised. For example, a fracture pattern that is relatively uncommon may not be readily recognized, and the fixation method selected may not be the optimal one, thereby leading to failure. Such failure could have been prevented by careful planning.

C.G. Zalavras, M.D., Ph.D., F.A.C.S.
Department of Orthopaedics, Keck School of Medicine, University of Southern California, Los Angeles, CA, USA
e-mail: zalavras@usc.edu

P.V. Giannoudis (ed.), *Fracture Reduction and Fixation Techniques*,
https://doi.org/10.1007/978-3-319-68628-8_8

Preoperative planning optimizes efficiency and operative performance of the surgeon. The mental exercise of developing a plan and rehearsing each step of the procedure will prepare the surgeon and will lead to less time thinking and debating between options during the procedure. As a result, unnecessary delays on the part of the surgeon will be minimized, and he/she will be free to dedicate his/her mental resources to the task at hand without having to think about the next step for the first time. The procedure will flow better, and any stress will be minimized. Potential problems can be anticipated, and in addition to the surgical tactic, alternative plans can be developed in advance in case intraoperative difficulties arise. A well-defined plan will also improve communication between members of the operative team.

Attention to the logistics will ensure that implementation of the plan is not compromised because of a preventable lack of resources. For example, some of the necessary implants and equipment may not be readily available and may have to be requested in advance.

Finally, the process of preoperative planning is of unique educational value for the surgeon him/herself and for the residents and medical students participating in the care of the patient. The careful assessment of each specific fracture patient and the detailed analysis of potential treatment options stimulate critical thinking and improved decision-making ability of everyone involved.

Antoine de Saint-Exupéry's statement that a goal without a plan is just a wish and Benjamin Franklin's warning that by failing to prepare you are preparing to fail, both apply to fracture surgery as well. Prior to an operation, the time that a surgeon devotes to a careful preoperative plan is of critical importance and often determines the success or failure of the procedure [4]. The author of the current chapter believes that the decision-making process and the preoperative plan are a component of patient's care that is as, or even more, important than technical execution of the procedure.

Unfortunately preoperative planning is not routinely practiced, although almost all surgeons understand how important this is. A study by Wade et al. reported that 94% of consultants and 100% of residents considered preoperative planning important in orthopedic trauma; however, only half routinely planned fracture surgery [5]. Time constraints may be a potential explanation. However, time invested in planning and preparation is time well spent. As Abraham Lincoln exclaimed "Give me six hours to chop down a tree and I will spend the first four sharpening the axe."

Methodology of Preoperative Planning

Preoperative planning involves the careful evaluation of various variables in order to develop and implement an individualized management plan that will optimize outcome for a patient with a fracture. More specifically, preoperative planning consists of the following elements:

1. *Analysis of the current situation, definition of the problem, and determination of the desired goal*

Preoperative planning starts with the analysis of fracture characteristics, extremity condition, and patient status. Based on this analysis, the surgeon needs to define the current problem and determine what the goal of treatment should be. In an ideal situation, the goal should be union of the fracture without any complications and restoration of preexisting function of the extremity and the patient. However, this goal may not always be attainable.

The treating surgeon needs to obtain as much information as possible from a detailed history and clinical exam, from assessment of relevant imaging studies, and from review of all available records in case of a preexisting injury or surgery, for example, in case of a new peri-implant fracture at the end of the plate used to fix a previous fracture.

Fracture characteristics need to be carefully evaluated. In addition to the anatomic location of the fracture (specific bone) and the diaphyseal, metaphyseal, or intra-articular location of the fracture, the surgeon needs to determine the exact fracture pattern and the presence of associated fractures, since this will have implications for selection of the optimal fixation method. Good-quality orthogonal radiographs should be obtained and scrutinized. Further imaging studies, such as computed tomography (CT) scan, CT scan with 3-D reconstructions, or magnetic resonance imaging (MRI), may assist the surgeon understand the exact fracture pattern and/or detect presence of an associated fracture with important implications for management, for example, a femoral neck fracture associated with a diaphyseal femoral fracture.

The presence of osteoporosis, for example, in elderly patients, may compromise stability of the fixation construct, and this needs to be considered when selecting fixation implants, for example, by using locking implants when plate fixation would be the preferred fixation method.

Previous trauma and/or surgery in the involved bone may create unique challenges for fixation of a fracture. A deformity may be present and the medullary canal may be obliterated, which will make intramedullary nailing difficult to perform. Implants may be present at the location of the fracture (such as in peri-implant fractures at the end of an existing plate or in periprosthetic fractures associated with an arthroplasty), which will necessitate a decision and plan for maintaining or removing the existing implants and for selecting implants for fixation of the new fracture. The existing implants should be identified by careful evaluation of radiographs and by obtaining previous medical records.

The soft tissue envelope should be carefully assessed. Small punctate wounds indicating an open fracture may be overlooked. Intraarticular fractures, such as tibial plateau or pilon fractures, are usually associated with a considerable amount of soft tissue swelling and development of fracture blisters. Resolution of the swelling will help reduce soft tissue complications and timing of surgery needs to be adjusted accordingly.

The neurovascular and functional status of the extremity should be taken into account. Presence of an associated vascular injury compromising perfusion of the extremity requires not only emergent intervention but also a specific plan for the order of vascular repair versus fracture fixation and for provisional versus definitive fixation. Decisions on the management of an associated peripheral nerve injury need to be incorporated in the overall a management plan, for example, timing of repair and primary repair versus nerve grafting. Functional deficits due to existing conditions, such as adjacent joint stiffness, previous injuries, or neurologic problems, may compromise the final outcome and may not allow restoration of function following healing of the fracture.

Associated injuries need to be carefully considered. For example, respiratory compromise may necessitate a damage control approach with provisional external fixation of a femoral fracture instead of intramedullary nailing to avoid further insult to the lungs. A spine injury may preclude lateral positioning of a patient and may necessitate intramedullary nailing in a supine position for fixation of a femoral fracture. An associated injury, such as an ipsilateral fracture of the patella or tibia, may make retrograde intramedullary nailing preferable to the antegrade technique.

The health status of the patient is an important factor that affects the healing potential as well as the surgical risk. Patient's condition needs to be optimized before surgery and specific measures taken postoperatively to minimize complications and improve outcome.

2. *Evaluation of potential solutions and determination of the optimal course of action (tactic)*

Starting with the goal in mind, which should be union of the fracture without any complications and restoration of preexisting function, the surgeon then evaluates different courses of action to achieve this goal and various potential solutions to the current problem.

The surgeon assesses the potential advantages and disadvantages, risks and benefits, and feasibility for each course of action. The surgeon needs to evaluate whether a specific fracture would benefit from absolute or relative stability, which surgical techniques and approaches may achieve that, and how stability can be optimized, while at the same time minimizing soft tissue damage. Often more than one courses of action may be reasonable with unique advantages and disadvantages. These need to be discussed with the patient, and he/she should participate in the decision-making.

The optimal course of action is decided upon, and all its individual components are determined, thereby developing the surgical tactic, which is a step-by-step guide to the procedure. Preoperative and postoperative considerations are also included in the plan.

During the mental exercise of planning, it is also important that the surgeon develops alternative plans to accommodate possible intraoperative findings or a change in the patient's condition. Having a plan A and a plan B (or even a plan C) beforehand will optimize the flow of the procedure (Fig. 8.1).

Preoperative Considerations

If emergent management of the fracture is not necessary, the patient's condition needs to be evaluated and optimized before surgery in consultation with appropriate specialties and with the anesthesiologist, for example, by correcting coagulopathies or electrolyte imbalances. The type of anesthesia and need for advanced intraoperative monitoring or blood products are discussed and decided upon in advance.

Operative Considerations and Surgical Tactic

Assuming that surgical management is indicated, the first decision involves the optimal **timing of surgery.** A fracture with an associated vascular injury requires emergent management, whereas an intra-articular fracture with soft tissue swelling may require a delay of 2 weeks or more until the swelling resolves.

An associated decision involves the **provisional versus definitive fixation** of the fracture. An associated vascular injury may require expedient provisional fixation with an external fixator prior to vascular repair. Presence of soft tissue swelling over an intra-articular fracture may require provisional fixation with a joint-spanning external fixator, followed by definitive fixation when the swelling has resolved. When provisional fixation is employed, it is useful to think about the definitive fixation and avoid compromising it in any way. For example, external fixator pins should be preferably inserted outside of the area that would be occupied by a plate for definitive fixation of the fracture. The operative setup details and the steps of the surgical procedure (tactic) are then decided upon.

The operative setup includes preparation of the operative room and preparation of the patient. The **operative room setup** includes having the

Fig. 8.1 A 55-year-old female patient sustained a dislocation of the left elbow after a fall. Anteroposterior and lateral radiographs of the elbow demonstrate associated fracture of the radial head and fracture of the coronoid process constituting the terrible triad injury (**a**, **b**). The largest part of the radial head appears to be intact, and the treating surgeon may plan to fix this radial head fracture to help restore stability of the elbow joint. Careful evaluation of the CT scan coronal cuts demonstrates that in that addition to the displaced fragment of the radial head, there is impaction of the remainder of the radial head (**c**). This impaction is also evident in the sagittal cuts (**d**). Understanding the complexity of the fracture pattern warns the surgeon about the difficulty of achieving stable fixation of the radial head fracture and allows the surgeon to plan accordingly. Radial head replacement implants and trays should be available in terrible triads of the elbow in order to be able to proceed with radial head replacement if needed. Depending on fracture characteristics, the surgeon may elect to proceed directly with radial head replacement or to attempt fixation of the radial head fracture. If fixation of the radial head is the chosen course of action (plan A), the surgeon should be prepared to proceed with the alternative plan of replacement (plan B) in case stable fixation of the radial head fracture cannot be achieved. In addition, the surgeon should be prepared to address residual instability of the elbow after fixation or replacement of the radial head (plan C). Options include fixation of the coronoid process fracture, repair of the lateral collateral ligament, repair of the medial collateral ligament, application of a hinged external fixator, or combinations of the above. Preoperative planning allows the surgeon to be prepared and have the necessary equipment for different courses of action according to the specific demands of each procedure. In this patient the author elected to proceed directly with radial head replacement, which successfully restored stability of the elbow as seen in intraoperative fluoroscopic view (**e**). The lateral collateral ligament was also repaired (**f**), but fixation of the coronoid fracture or any additional interventions was not deemed necessary

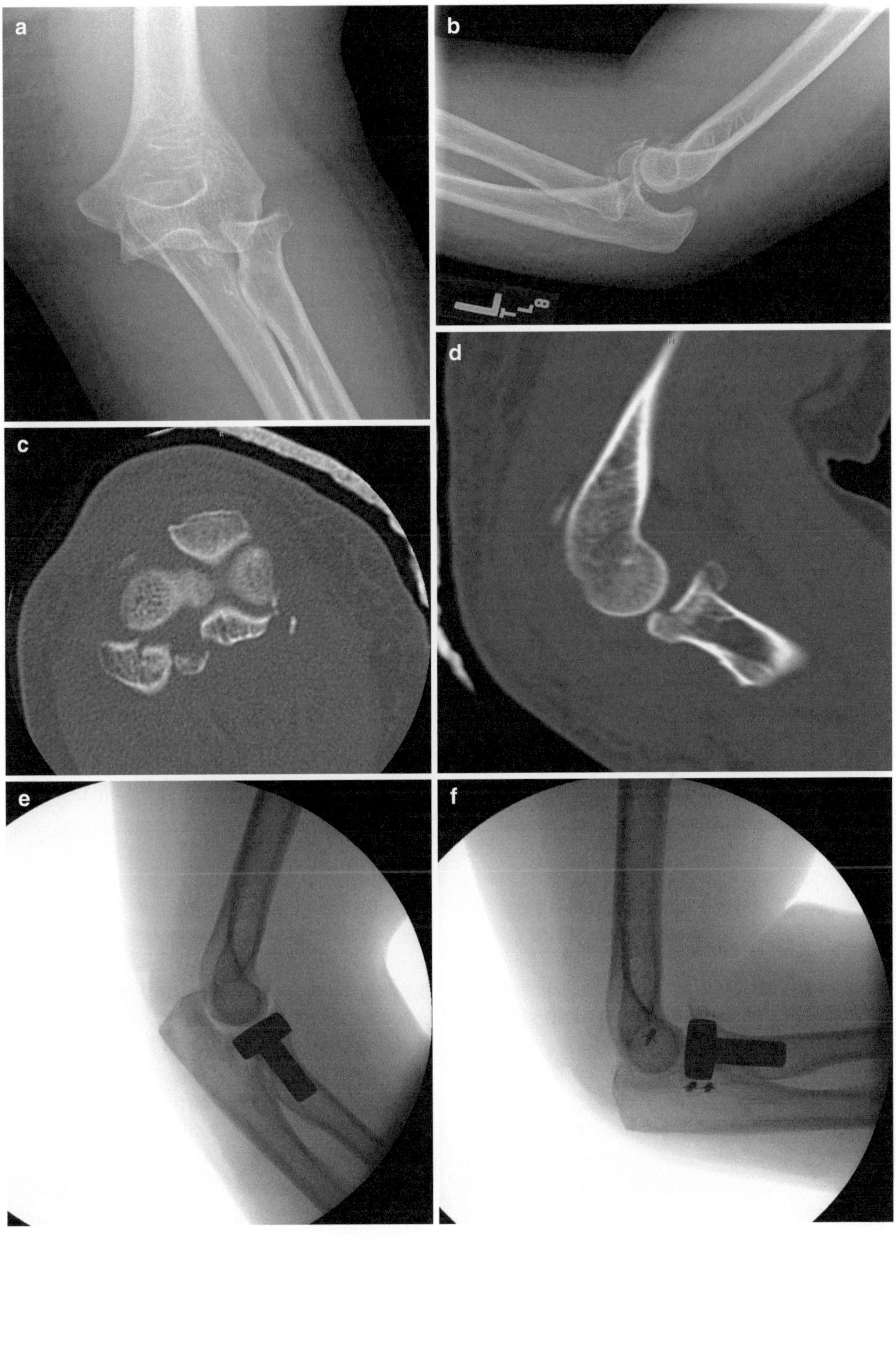
a
b
c
d
e
f

appropriate fracture or radiolucent table if needed and having a fluoroscopy machine available and optimally positioned relative to the table. The **patient setup** includes positioning on the table, padding of prominences, deciding on use of a tourniquet, and preparation/disinfection of the surgical site. It is important to remember the potential need to harvest bone, vein, or nerve grafts and have the appropriate sites prepared and draped.

The main **steps of the surgical procedure (tactic)** include the surgical approach, reduction of the fracture, and fixation of the fracture. Supplemental procedures, such as bone grafting, may be needed. The decisions are made working backwards, i.e., once the surgeon decides on the optimal fixation technique, and then he/she decides on the reduction technique, on the approach, and on patient positioning.

The **surgical approach** and the pertinent anatomy need to be reviewed preoperatively, especially if the surgeon does not have considerable expertise with the approach. The surgeon should be aware of the neurovascular structures at risk and has a specific plan to ensure that the risk is minimized, either by maintaining a safe distance from these structures or by identifying them so that they can be visualized and protected throughout the case. For example, once the surgeon has decided to fix a diaphyseal humeral fracture with an anterolateral plate using an anterolateral approach to the humerus, it is necessary to dissect and protect the radial nerve before reduction and fixation of the fracture.

Fracture reduction is an important part of the surgical tactic. The surgeon may consider direct open reduction techniques, for example, using a reduction forceps; indirect reduction techniques, for example, using a fracture table or a universal distractor device; or combinations of direct and indirect techniques. Provisional stabilization with Kirschner wires may be needed.

Selection of the **fixation implant** is a critical element of preoperative planning. It is not enough to determine whether fixation will be optimally accomplished with intramedullary nailing, plate and screw fixation, or external fixation. Selection of implant involves consideration of several details on the specific type and dimensions of an implant, as well as on the insertion and positioning of the implant.

For example, when considering intramedullary nailing of the femur, the surgeon has the options of antegrade versus retrograde insertion. Antegrade insertion options include cephalomedullary versus standard nail and piriformis versus trochanteric entry point. Once the type of nail is selected, the dimensions (length and diameter) need to be estimated based on imaging studies. Images of the uninjured extremity may be helpful in determining length and rotation in comminuted fractures.

When considering plate fixation, the surgeon needs to determine the need for anatomic plate versus a standard plate, the dimensions of the plate (thickness, width, and length), the type of the plate (non-locking versus locking versus combination of options), the insertion technique (minimally invasive insertion versus full surgical approach), the location of the plate on the bone, the number of screws needed on each side of the fracture, the order of screw insertion, and whether a specific screw should be locking or non-locking. The surgeon also may consider insertion of lag screw(s) outside or through the plate based on the fracture pattern.

When considering external fixation, the surgeon needs to decide on a half-pin unilateral frame versus a fine-wire frame, on the size and the exact insertion location of the half-pins or wires, and the details of frame construction.

Especially with plate fixation, planning has been traditionally done with the process of templating. Templating involves hand-tracing the final reduction and fracture fixation construct on paper based on hard copies of radiographs of the injured and contralateral intact bone utilizing a view box, tracing paper, pencils, and templates of the implants [3, 4, 6].

Templating helps the surgeon determine the required type and dimensions of the implant. This becomes very important when the characteristics of the bone and the fracture necessitate an implant that is not readily available and has to be called in, such as a very long plate to span an extensive area of comminution or an intramedullary nail of very small or large diameter to accommodate the patient's anatomy, (Fig. 8.2). Templating makes the surgeon mentally rehearse each step of the

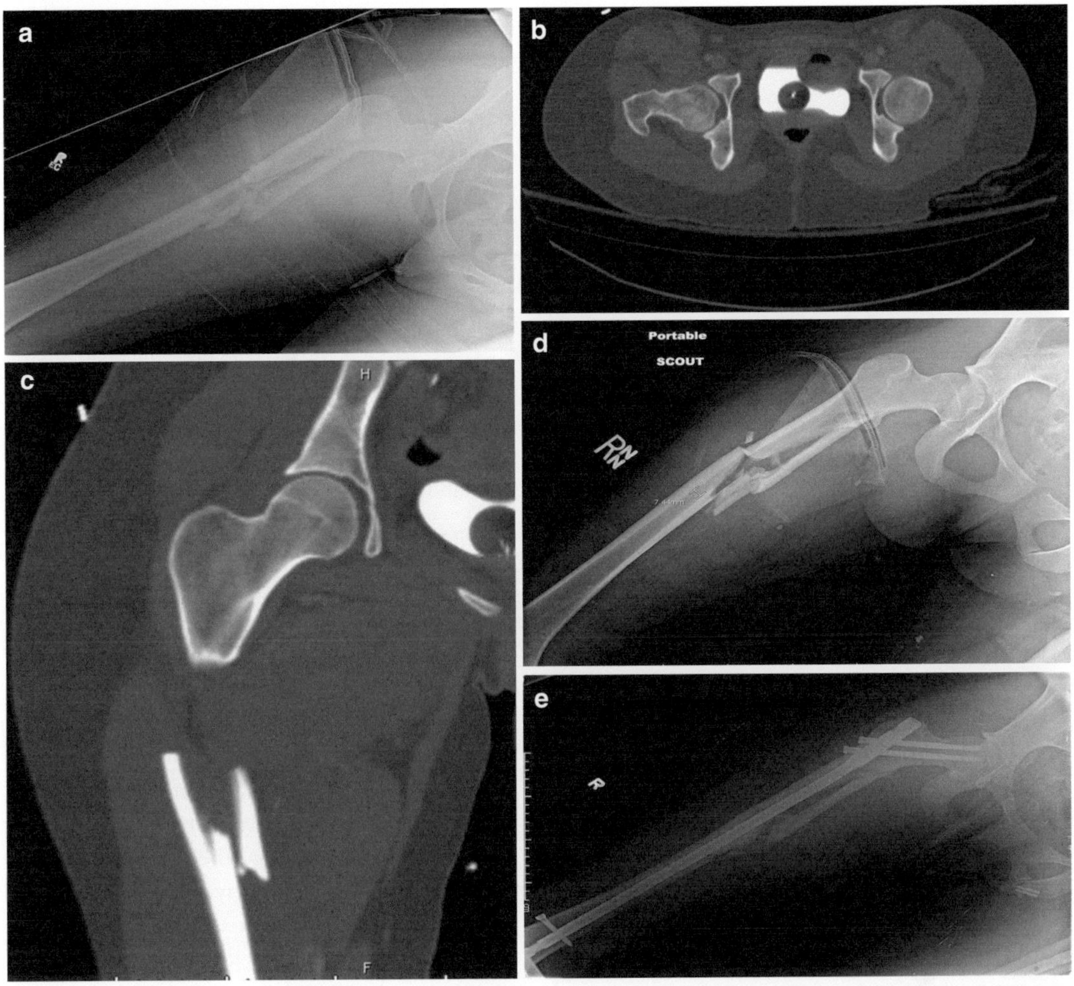

Fig. 8.2 An 18-year-old female patient was involved in a motor vehicle accident and sustained a right subtrochanteric femur fracture (**a**). Careful evaluation of the preoperative radiographs generates concerns about the proximal extension of the fracture and the integrity of the femoral neck. A CT scan did not demonstrate a femoral neck fracture or extension of the fracture to the piriformis fossa (**b**, **c**). A cephalomedullary nail was selected as implant of choice for fixation of this fracture. Preoperative planning and measurement of the canal diameter showed that the isthmus was less than 8 mm (**d**). The smallest diameter of the cephalomedullary nail readily available at the surgeon's institution was 10 mm, and the narrow canal alerted the surgeon to potential difficulties of extensive reaming of the canal to insert a 10 mm nail. An adolescent reconstruction nail of 8.5 mm diameter was called in and was ready to be used in this patient. Of note, this 8.5 mm reconstruction nail was only available as a trochanteric entry implant, in contrast to the larger diameter implants that were available as both trochanteric and piriformis entry implants. Postoperative anteroposterior and lateral radiographs are seen in panels **e** and **f**. Preoperative planning helped the surgeon avoid several pitfalls, such as (**a**) underestimating the complexity of the fracture and not using a cephalomedullary nail, (**b**) not recognizing the need for a smaller diameter implant and not having the optimal implant available during the case, and (**c**) establishing a piriformis entry point only to recognize afterwards that a trochanteric implant had to be used. Avoiding such pitfalls helps optimize patient care and improve outcomes. In this patient uneventful healing of the fracture took place as demonstrated in the anteroposterior radiograph at 2.5 months postoperatively (**g**)

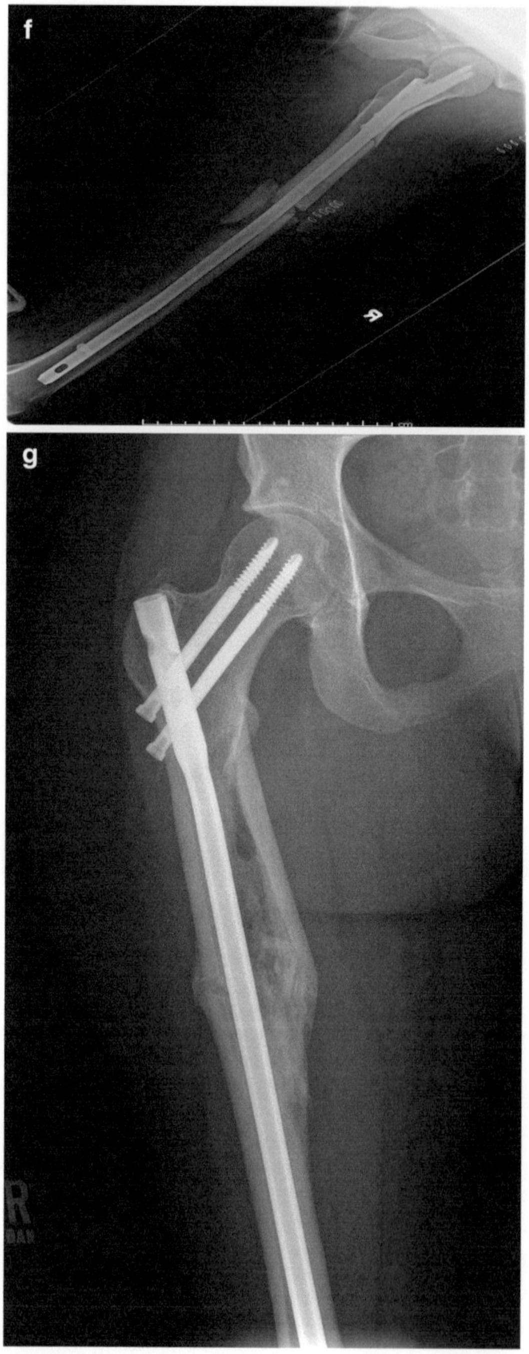

Fig. 8.2 (continued)

fixation and helps her/him prepare in advance. Templating also allows for a direct comparison of the postoperative radiographs with the preoperative plan. The surgeon can evaluate whether the preoperative plan was successfully followed and the desired end result was achieved, thereby achieving quality control.

The expanding use of digital radiographs and CT scans offers the possibility for novel digital preoperative planning techniques. Software programs using digital imaging studies allow 3-D reconstruction of fractures and malunions and preoperative planning of the surgical reduction and fixation, which may be enhanced by creation of real-size prototypes [6–11].

The surgical tactic also includes the need of supplemental procedures, such as harvesting of autogenous bone grafting or using allograft or bone substitutes, possible insertion of a drain, wound closure, and any form of splint or immobilization.

Postoperative Considerations

Postoperative considerations include the discharge of the patient (same-day surgery) versus admission or even need for an intensive care unit bed, need for thromboembolic prophylaxis, need for nutritional supplementation, plan for any weight bearing or activity restrictions, plan for physical and occupational therapy, and plan for follow-up. The need for any other interventions such as improved control of diabetes mellitus, cessation of smoking, and therapy for osteoporosis, needs to be considered as well.

3. *Implementation (logistics)*

As part of preoperative planning, the surgeon should make sure that all steps of the plan (surgical tactic) can be implemented smoothly without obstacles pertaining to resources, such as space, personnel, and implants/equipment/products.

Important elements of the logistics include ensuring the appropriate consultations for optimization of patient condition before surgery, the availability of an operative room with the required table and fluoroscopy support, and the availability of assistance. An experienced assistant may be very valuable in complex cases, and his/her availability should be confirmed beforehand.

Availability of all necessary or potentially useful implants, equipment, and products (e.g., blood products, allograft bone, bone graft substitutes, or other biologic products) is critical and needs to be confirmed in advance. During the development of the surgical tactic, the surgeon becomes aware of the specific type and size of implants that will be needed and the necessary instruments, but this is not enough, and potential problems may occur: (a) the specific type of implants may not be readily available at the surgeon's facility and may have to be ordered, delivered, and sterilized; (b) the specific type of implants may be available at the surgeon's facility, but a patient may need a specific size that is not in stock, for example, a very long plate or an intramedullary nail of very small or large diameter or length; and (c) the necessary implants and instruments may be available at the surgeon's facility, but another surgeon may be planning to simultaneously use them in a different room. These problems can compromise the outcome of the procedure but are all preventable, and attention to logistics will facilitate smooth execution of the surgical plan.

Clear communication and coordination with the operating room personnel well in advance are essential. In complex cases it is helpful to differentiate between the implants and equipment that will definitely be required (and should be opened and ready for use during the procedure) and the implants and equipment that should be stand-by in case they are needed. For example, if a preexisting plate needs to be removed prior to fixation of a new fracture, the surgeon should anticipate potential problems with removal of the implant, such as stripped or broken screws, and a broken screw removal set should be readily available to be opened in case such problems occur.

Summary

In fracture surgery, preoperative planning is a critical component of management as optimizes the patient outcome, the efficiency and operative performance of the surgeon, and the educational experience of everybody involved in the planning process. Preoperative planning starts with analysis of fracture, extremity, and patient characteristics in order to understand the current problem and determine the management goals. Potential solutions are evaluated, the optimal course of action is decided upon, and a step-by-step individualized management plan is developed and implemented. Traditional planning has involved hand-tracing the final reduction and fracture fixation construct on paper based on hard copies of radiographs. Modern digital imaging studies offer the possibility for digital preoperative planning techniques based on software.

References

1. https://www.ahdictionary.com/word/search.html?q=plan. Assessed 15 May 2017.
2. Graves ML. The value of preoperative planning. J Orthop Trauma. 2013;27(Suppl 1):S30–4.
3. Hak DJ, Rose J, Stahel PF. Preoperative planning in orthopedic trauma: benefits and contemporary uses. Orthopedics. 2010;33(8):581–4.
4. Ruedi TP, Buckley RE, Moran CG. AO principles of fracture management. Switzerland: AO Publishing; 2007.
5. Wade RH, Kevu J, Doyle J. Pre-operative planning in orthopaedics: a study of surgeons' opinions. Injury. 1998;29(10):785–6.
6. Atesok K, Galos D, Jazrawi LM, Egol KA. Preoperative planning in orthopaedic surgery. Current practice and evolving applications. Bull Hosp Jt Dis (2013). 2015;73(4):257–68.
7. Citak M, Gardner MJ, Kendoff D, Tarte S, Krettek C, Nolte LP, Hüfner T. Virtual 3D planning of acetabular fracture reduction. J Orthop Res. 2008;26(4):547–52.
8. Pilson HT, Reddix RN Jr, Mutty CE, Webb LX. The long lost art of preoperative planning–resurrected? Orthopedics. 2008;31(12):1–3.
9. Suero EM, Hüfner T, Stübig T, Krettek C, Citak M. Use of a virtual 3D software for planning of tibial plateau fracture reconstruction. Injury. 2010;41(6):589–91.
10. Wang H, Wang F, Newman S, Lin Y, Chen X, Xu L, Wang Q. Application of an innovative computerized virtual planning system in acetabular fracture surgery: a feasibility study. Injury. 2016;47(8):1698–701.
11. Fürnstahl P, Vlachopoulos L, Schweizer A, Fucentese SF, Koch PP. Complex osteotomies of tibial plateau malunions using computer-assisted planning and patient-specific surgical guides. J Orthop Trauma. 2015;29(8):e270–6.

Part III

An Anatomical Based Approach: Upper Extremity

9 Acromioclavicular Joint Dislocation

Paul Cowling

Anatomical Fracture Location: Radiograph of Fracture Pattern

Radiological views required to diagnose ACJ dislocations include standard anteroposterior shoulder views (Fig. 9.1), as well as axial views to determine any anteroposterior dislocation. A Zanca view can also be performed (a 15° cephalic view) to determine subtle superior subluxations. Stress views are also available where the patient is asked to hold a weight in the adducted injured arm, and comparison views are required with and without the weight, but this is often painful so rarely used. ACJ injuries are most commonly described using the Rockwood classification system. In general, types I and II will make a good recovery with conservative management including physiotherapy. Types III–VI, where the coracoclavicular (CC) ligaments are torn, may require surgical intervention, though the timing of any intervention remains controversial. Generally, a detailed discussion with the patient is required, including risks and benefits of surgery, their own expectations (including sports and any overhead manual work) and likely outcomes of both conservative and operative management.

P. Cowling, M.B.B.S., M.Sc., F.R.C.S. (Orth)
Leeds General Infirmary University Hospital, Leeds, UK
e-mail: paulcowling@nhs.net

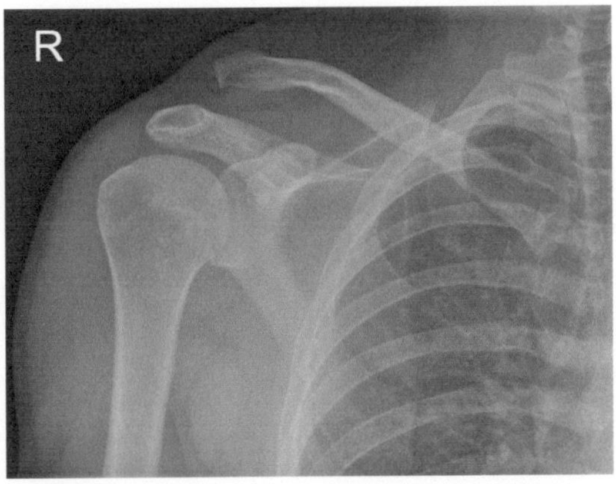

Fig. 9.1 AP radiograph of right shoulder demonstrating type V ACJ dislocation

Brief Preoperative Planning

Classically, a 'Weaver-Dunn' procedure and its modifications have been used, where the coracoacromial (CA) ligament is transferred to the distal clavicle to recreate the torn CC ligaments. More recently, surgeons favour internal fixation methods between the distal clavicle and coracoid. These often include a combination of suture or other material as a 'substitute' for the CC ligament and metalwork to provide the fixation into the clavicle and/or coracoid. Skilled arthroscopic surgeons have also become proficient at performing ACJ fixation arthroscopically.

P.V. Giannoudis (ed.), *Fracture Reduction and Fixation Techniques*,
https://doi.org/10.1007/978-3-319-68628-8_9

Patient Setup in Theatre

Though a standard beach-chair position can be used as for most upper limb procedures, this author prefers to elevate the head end of the table by only 30°, so the weight of the arm doesn't further exacerbate the deformity of the injury, to aid reduction. The head end of the table is also positioned away from the anaesthetic machine, either 90° or 180° from normal table positioning, to allow for easy access to the shoulder area. A radiolucent table is required (ideally a specific shoulder table to allow access to the shoulder from all angles) and the head supported in a head ring or other head-supporting device. Skin preparation covers the whole forequarter from sternum to the medial border of scapula, with a U-drape used to shut off the forequarter. The arm is draped free, using a stockinette to cover up to the level of the proximal humerus, to allow it to be manoeuvred to aid reduction. The surgeon would then stand at the side of the arm and assistant at the head end (Fig. 9.2). The image intensifier can then be brought in easily, usually from the head end with the screens across the patient.

Closed Reduction Manoeuvres

Generally, reduction of a type III ACJ dislocation requires pushing the humerus proximally towards the acromion, with a small amount of counter traction on the clavicle. Higher grades of ACJ dislocation are more difficult to reduce closed, as the trapezius muscle and/or deltotrapezial fascia may be interposed between the distal clavicle and acromion.

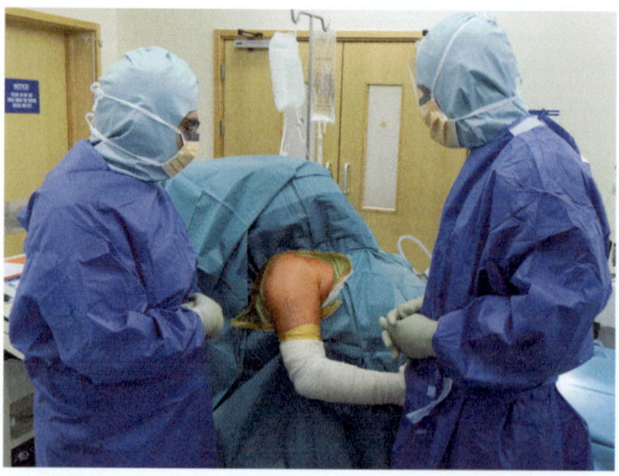

Fig. 9.2 Patient positioning at 30° head end elevation, draping of the upper extremity, with operating surgeon on the right, assistant at the head end on the left of the image

Reduction Instruments

Describe and show picture of exclusive instruments to be used for the specific procedure

- A basic shoulder set including small and large soft tissue retractors should be available (Fig. 9.3).
- If 'hooking' suture or other material under the coracoid to provide fixation, a passing device is required.
- The manufacturer's trays for the particular fixation device used are selected and checked to ensure all components required are present.

Surgical Approach

A number of approaches have been described, but a vertical sabre incision over the ACJ usually allows all the access required to the distal clavicle and coracoid and is cosmetically satisfactory for patients. Once the skin is incised, the distal clavicle and ACJ are exposed by mobilizing the overlying deltoid muscle. In higher grades of ACJ injury, trapezius may also require clearing from the distal clavicle. The coracoid is found inferior to the distal clavicle and should

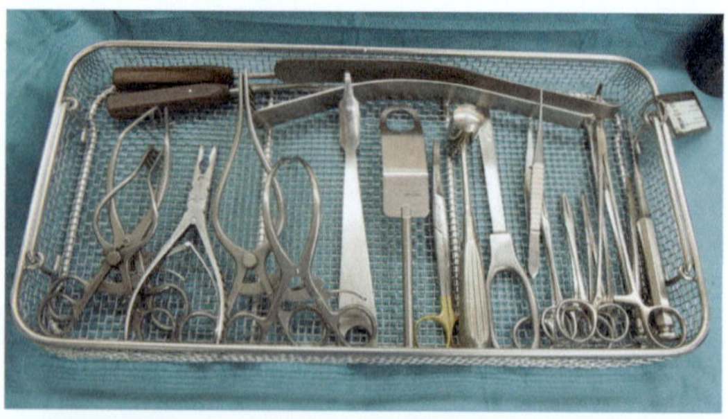

Fig. 9.3 Basic shoulder tray including retractors and curved suture passers if need to pass suture/material around the coracoid

be easily palpated throughout the operation. Remembering the musculocutaneous nerve enters the medial border of the conjoint tendon 2.5–8 cm distal to the coracoid provides exposure of the coracoid down to its base. The pectoralis minor (medially) and CA ligament (laterally) usually need not be divided. Some surgeons take the decision to excise up to 1 cm of the lateral end of the clavicle, especially in chronic cases, to ease reduction and prevent impingement, though there is no evidence to support preserving or resecting.

Open Reduction Manoeuvres

Reduction generally requires upward elevation of the humerus towards the acromion, with downward pressure on the distal clavicle. Once full surgical exposure is achieved, a reduction of the ACJ can be performed using pointed reduction forceps, with one arm placed inferior to the lateral coracoid and one arm superior to the distal clavicle. Care should be taken to ensure, as well as correcting the superior displacement, anteroposterior reduction is also achieved. Anteroposterior image intensifier views can now be taken to assess reduction, and a Zanca view can often be achieved.

Implant Insertion

The fixation device of choice can then be implanted. If this involved hooking suture or other material around the coracoid, this is usually performed from medial to lateral keeping the passing device on the undersurface bone of the coracoid at all times, to prevent nerve injury. If this involves placing drill holes through the coracoid, great care should be placed upon exposing the superior aspect of the coracoid to ensure the drill passes centrally on the horizontal limb of the coracoid. Again, anteroposterior image intensifier views can now be taken to assess reduction before the device selected is tightened and locked into place, and a Zanka view can often be achieved (Fig. 9.4).

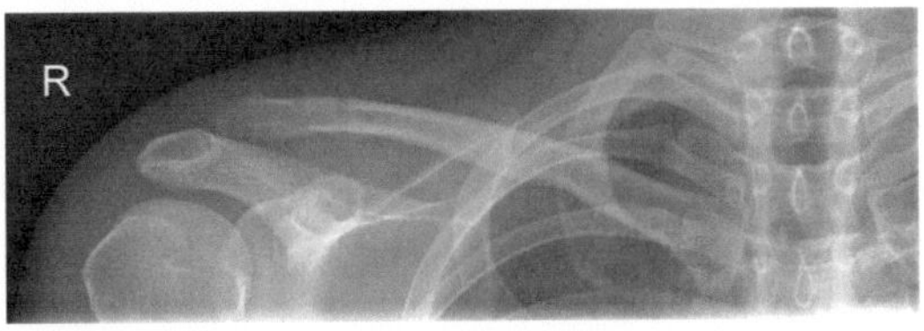

Fig. 9.4 AP radiograph of final fixation demonstrating ACJ fixation using two drill holes through clavicle and suture passed under coracoid

Summary of Tips, Tricks and Pitfalls

- As reduction is usually assessed under direct vision, as well as on image intensifier, it is imperative to ensure both superior displacement and anteroposterior reduction are achieved.
- To avoid fracture of the coracoid during the fixation, any sutures passed inferior to the coracoid should do so at the 'elbow' of this bony structure, deep to the conjoint tendon.
- Likewise, if the fixation device used requires a drill hole through the coracoid, this must be placed centrally on the horizontal part of the coracoid: any offset medially or laterally will eccentrically load this bone.
- The placement of the clavicle part of the fixation device, either via drill hole or placement on the superior clavicle, is also important in the success of the fixation: generally, this is at a point directly superior to the centre of the coracoid, as placement too medial or lateral may lead to eccentric loading and failure.

Further Reading

Modi CS, Beazley J, Lawrence TM, Veillette CJH. Controversies relating to the management of acromioclavicular joint dislocations. Bone Joint J. 2013;95-B:1595–602.

Rockwood CA, Williams GR, Young DC. Acromioclavicular injuries. In: Rockwood CA, Green DP, Bucholz RW, Heckman JD, editors. Fractures in adults, vol. I. 4th ed. Philadelphia, PA: Lippincott-Raven; 1996. p. 1341–413.

Weaver JK, Dunn HK. Treatment of acromioclavicular injuries, especially complete acromioclavicular separations. J Bone Joint Surg Am. 1972;54-A:1187.

10 Sternoclavicular Joint Dislocations

Harish Kapoor, Osman Riaz, and Adeel Aqil

Anatomical Fracture Location

Anteroposterior (AP) view including both sternoclavicular joints (Fig. 10.1). Difficult to visualise on AP therefore recommend serendipity views (Fig. 10.2), beam at 40 degree cephalic tilt. Anterior dislocation (much commoner)—affected clavicle above contralateral clavicle. Posterior dislocation—affected clavicle below contralateral clavicle. Computed tomography (CT), gold standard for investigation, axial views to determine position of medial end of clavicle in relation to mediastinal structures and associated injuries (Fig. 10.3). Posterior dislocation can present as an acute emergency with acute compression of mediastinal structures. Medial end clavicle last to fuse at 23–25 years and potentially growth plate injuries may occur.

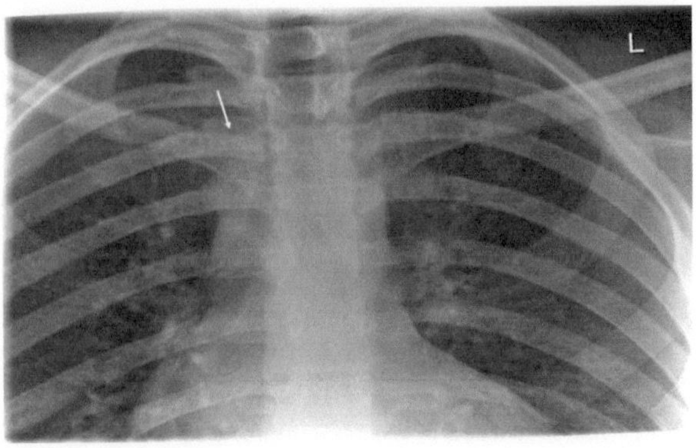

Fig. 10.1 AP radiograph showing inferior displacement of right medial end of clavicle (arrow); this suggests posterior dislocation

H. Kapoor, M.B.B.S., M.S.(Orth), D.N.B. (✉)
Consultant Trauma and Orthopaedics,
Leeds General Infirmary, Leeds, UK
e-mail: harish.kapoor@nhs.net

O. Riaz, M.B.B.S., M.R.C.S. • A. Aqil, M.B.B.S., M.R.C.S.
Department of Trauma and Orthopaedic Surgery,
Leeds General Infirmary, Leeds, UK

P.V. Giannoudis (ed.), *Fracture Reduction and Fixation Techniques*,
https://doi.org/10.1007/978-3-319-68628-8_10

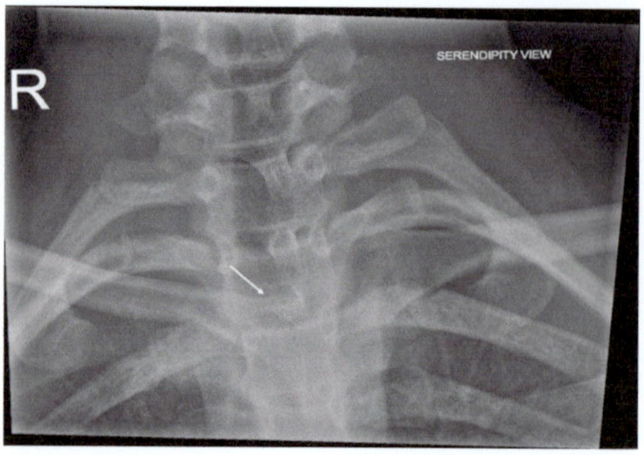

Fig. 10.2 Serendipity radiograph demonstrating right posterior dislocation (arrow)

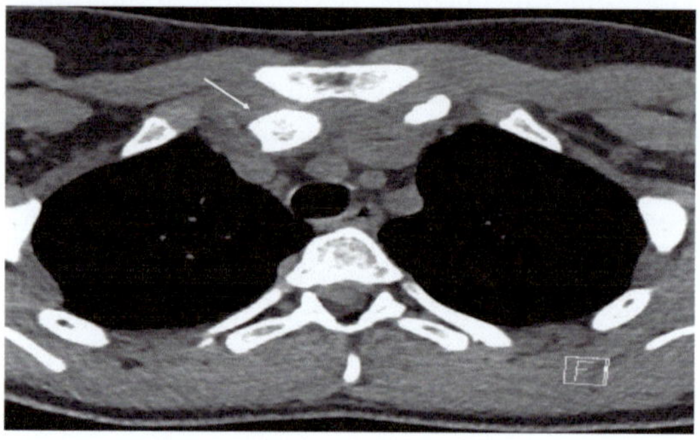

Fig. 10.3 Axial CT demonstrating posterior dislocation of right clavicle and its relationship to the structures in the mediastinum (arrow)

Pre-op Planning

Clinical assessment—usually high-energy injury (RTC, contact sports), deformity is present with ecchymosis, swelling, tenderness and crepitation. Anterior dislocation—palpable bump present, posterior dislocation can be associated with dyspnoea, dysphagia, tachypnoea and stridor which are worse on lying supine. Important to assess for pneumothorax or haemothorax. Assess and document vascular status of the upper arms and any difference in peripheral pulses between the injured and contralateral side. Assess neurological status to determine any injury to brachial plexus. Cardiothoracic/thoracic surgeon consult should be undertaken before any surgical intervention and should be on standby during procedure ideally. Anaesthesia—general anaesthetic at induction, administration of prophylactic antibiotics as per local hospital protocol. Would advise crossmatch of four units of packed red cells. Equipment—AO small fragment (3.5 mm) set, have FiberWire or Ethibond suture available. Would recommend sternotomy set to be available in the operating room.

Patient Setup in Theatre

Table setup—instrumentation is set up on the side of the operation. Image intensifier is from the contralateral side. Position table diagonally across the operating room so that the operating area lies in the clean air field. Place patient supine with arm at edge of the radiolucent table (OSI or equivalent) with side support (Fig. 10.4). Both surgeon and assistant will stand on the injured side.

Closed Reduction Manoeuvres (Anterior Dislocation)

Abduct and extend arm while applying axial traction, and simultaneously apply direct posterior pressure over medial clavicle. Manipulate medial clavicle with towel clip or fingers. Figure of eight bandage with sling post reduction for 6 weeks.

Surgical Approach

Skin preparation is carried out using usual antiseptic solution. Prepare the whole chest and both

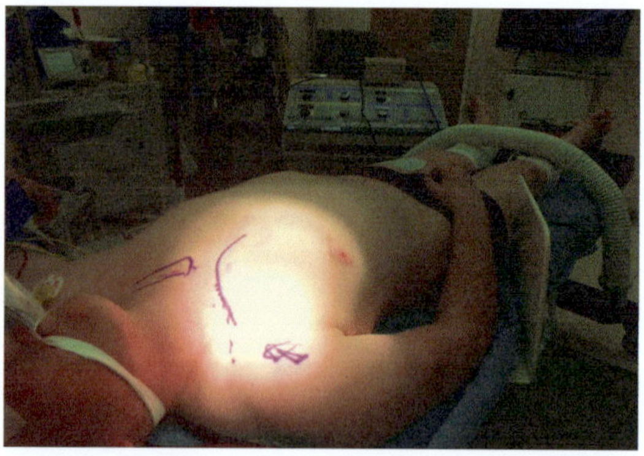

Fig. 10.4 Position of patient, supine with arm support on a radiolucent table

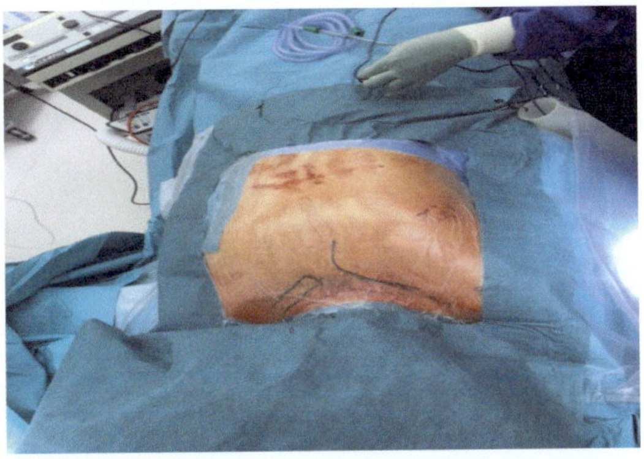

Fig. 10.5 Draping of patient allows access to perform sternotomy. Ensure curved incision of the clavicle is perform which is shown in this figure

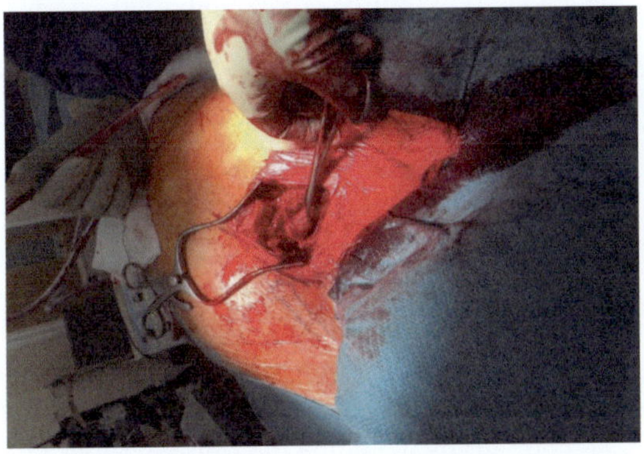

Fig. 10.6 Dissect down to the periosteum

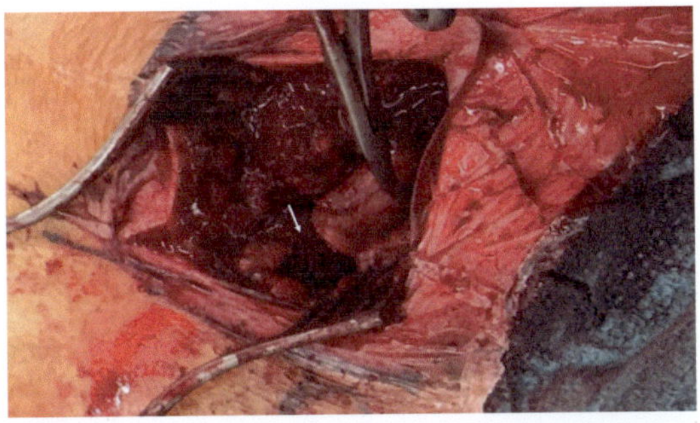

Fig. 10.7 Excise the articular disc to create space for reduction

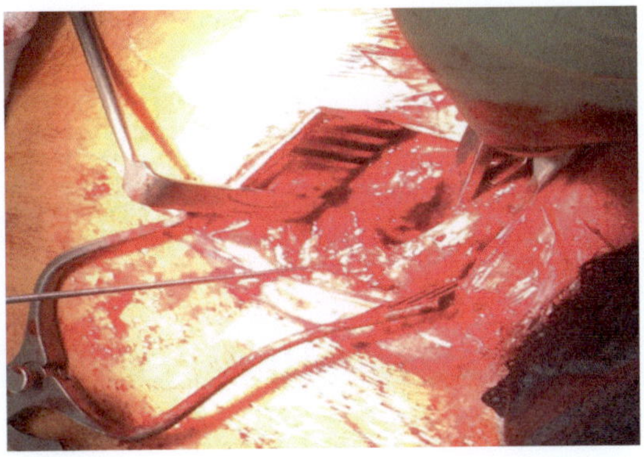

Fig. 10.8 Using a 2.5 mm drill, create a tunnel of the medial end of the clavicle around 2 cm lateral from SCJ

clavicle; clean up the anterior aspect of neck and to the lateral deltoid region. Use a sternotomy drape (like a DHS drape) to allow access to the mediastinal structures should it become necessary. Make an incision over the medial end of the clavicle, which curves inferiorly of the affected side (Fig. 10.5). Using the cutting diathermy, bring down the incision through the skin to the periosteum. Perform a subperiosteal dissection of the sternoclavicular joint (Fig. 10.6). Excise the fibrocartilage articular disc to expose the SCJ; this helps with reduction as it creates space (Fig. 10.7).

Open Reduction Manoeuvres

Ensure the medial end of the clavicle is not tethered to the structures of the mediastinum especially if old injury. If so, careful dissection is required with cardiothoracic team standby. Apply towel clip or serrated clamp to the end of the clavicle, and gently reduce the medial end onto the manubrium of the sternum. Gentle lifting of manubrium with a langenback can increase the view behind it to help deliver the clavicle. Use a 2.5 mm drill to create a tunnel of the medial end of the clavicle around 2 cm lateral from SCJ (Fig. 10.8). Create another tunnel in the articular surface of the sternum with a blunt malleable retractor posteriorly for protection. Create minimum two loops for stability. Pass FiberWire or Ethibond suture through the tunnels in a figure of eight configuration. While holding the joint reduced, tie the suture ensuring adequate reduction is maintained (Fig. 10.9). Assess dynamic stability by abducting, flexing and extending the arm at the shoulder joint. Obtain AP and serendipity views on the image intensifier to confirm

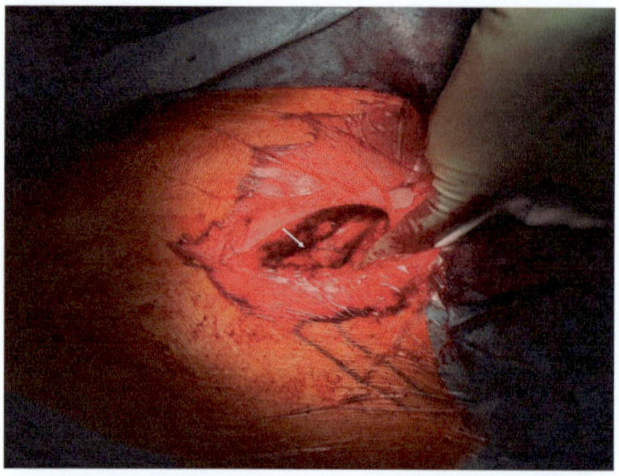

Fig. 10.9 FibeWire passed through drill tunnels and tied off maintaining reduction

reduction. Continue with wound closure using 1/0, 2/0 vicryl and 3/0 S/C to skin. Immobilise arm with a polysling. Protect arm for 6 weeks.

Summary of Tips and Tricks

- Always obtain preoperative CT scan with 3D reconstructions.
- Most anterior sternoclavicular subluxations can be treated closed/nonoperatively with a small percentage needing intervention and reconstruction for symptoms of instability.
- With posterior SCJ dislocations—have the cardiothoracic team on standby with presence of sternotomy kit in the operating theatre if proceeding to open reduction in case of a vascular emergency.
- Do not compromise on the incision as posterior dislocations can be difficult to visualise.
- Try closed reduction manoeuvres first which may be successful.
- Excise the articular disc of the SCJ to help create access to reduce posteriorly displaced clavicle.
- FibeWire is recommended as it provides good strength and hold. Other strong non-absorbable sutures like Ethibond/Ticron can be used.
- Repair of the posterior capsule/periosteal sleeve after delivering medial clavicle helps in preventing the medial end of clavicle falling into the dead space created.
- Always obtain intraoperatively serendipity views to confirm reduction and a CT postoperatively.
- Keep immobilised for 6 weeks and restriction of abduction and flexion beyond 90° and to avoid contact sports up to 4–6 months. Some swelling is likely to persist long term over the medial end of clavicle.
- Avoid metalwork due to the potential high risk of migration and implant failure and subsequently potentially disastrous consequences.
- I do not use grafts in my primary fixations, but tendon grafts including the sternomastoid fascia have been described in literature through intraosseous tunnels instead of non-absorbable sutures.
- Supplement additional suture/anchor fixation in the first rib for additional fixation as necessary.

Clavicle Fracture

11

Makoto Kobayashi and Takashi Matsushita

Fractures of the clavicle usually present in young males constituting approximately 2–4% of all fractures in adults [1]. The most common location of fractures is the midshaft area followed by the lateral and medial part. For many years, clavicle fractures have been managed nonoperatively, irrespective of the type of fracture. However, lately, new evidence has emerged indicating high incidence of nonunion with nonoperative treatment and a reduced functional capacity in up to 40% of patients [2]. Consequently more interest has been shown in operative interventions techniques. The Neer's and AO are the most commonly used fracture classifications.

Anatomical Fracture Location

A direct fall on the shoulder is the most common mechanism of injury. Clinical examination should assess the neurovascular status of the affected extremity. Anteroposterior and 15° cephalic tilt (ZANCA view) will allow determination of fracture pattern and superior/inferior displacement (Fig. 11.1). CT can assist in a detailed evaluation of the fracture pattern.

Preoperative Planning

Assess fracture pattern and degree of comminution. In this case it is appreciated that the intermediate fragments are small and would be difficult to reduce them anatomically without disturbing their blood supply. As the contact area between the main fragments was noted to be small, intramedullary wire fixation would not have been the ideal method to prevent shortening of the clavicle.

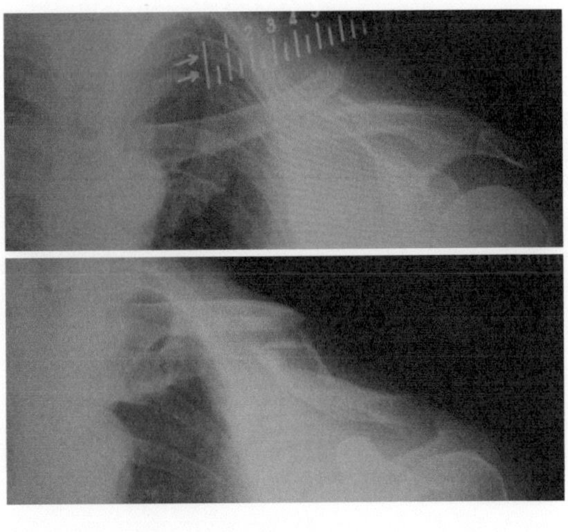

Fig. 11.1 Radiographs of a 48-year-old male with midshaft clavicle comminuted fracture. Top: cephalic view. Bottom: caudal view

M. Kobayashi
Department of Orthopaedic Surgery, Teikyo University School of Medicine, Tokyo, Japan

T. Matsushita (✉)
Department of Traumatology, Fukushima Medical University, Fukushima, Japan
e-mail: takashi@matsushita.net

P.V. Giannoudis (ed.), *Fracture Reduction and Fixation Techniques*,
https://doi.org/10.1007/978-3-319-68628-8_11

Consequently, it was decided to apply MIPO: minimally invasive plate osteosynthesis technique with an anatomically shaped locking plate [3].

Patient Setup in the Operating Theater

The patient is placed in the supine position on a radiolucent table. The arm does not need to be included in the operative field. A bolster can be placed under the spine to reduce the existing shortening of the clavicle. Image intensifier is positioned cephalad to the patient allowing acquisition of cephalic and caudal tilt views intraoperatively.

Surgical Approach

The entire shape of the clavicle is marked on the skin (Fig. 11.2). It is enough to fix only the two main fragments with a plate using two small incisions. Two 4 cm incisions are made, one on each, of the medial and lateral sides of the clavicle. Dedicated anatomical plates are available with either locking or non-locking screw options. Reduction instruments include K-wires, small pointed reduction forceps. The main fragments are manipulated and reduced directly with small pointed reduction forceps.

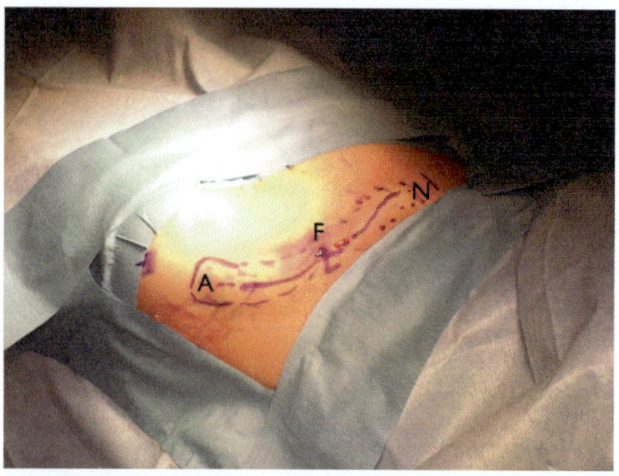

Fig. 11.2 Skin incision marking on the left clavicle. *A* acromion, *F* fracture site, *N* suprasternal notch

Open Reduction Maneuver

The main fragments are controlled directly with small pointed forceps. Thereafter, these fragments were temporarily fixed with an intramedullary Kirschner wire (1.8–2.0 mm), (Fig. 11.3). The "blunt" end of the K-wire is cut obliquely to make it a "double-tipped spear." One end of the K-wire is inserted into the medial fragment from the fracture end and is advanced through the bone fragment and out through the skin over the medial end of the medial fragment. Then the opposite end of the wire is pushed back into the lateral fragment from the fracture end. This "switchback insertion" is time saving. The alignment of the main fragments is checked with the image intensifier on two different views.

Implant Insertion (Figs. 11.4 and 11.5)

An anatomically shaped locking plate is convenient for MIPO [4]. The plate should be long enough so that three bicortical screws can be

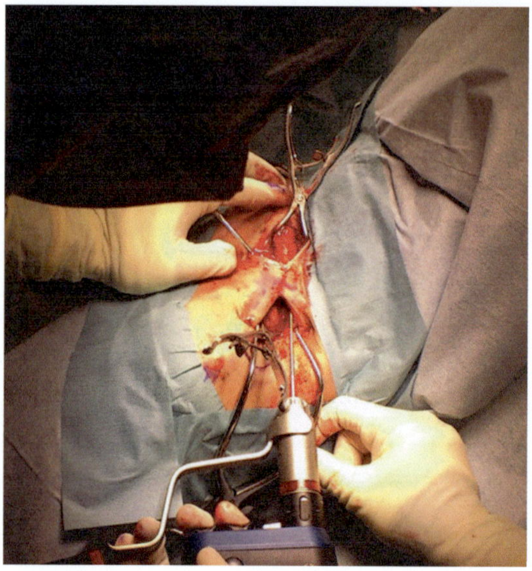

Fig. 11.3 K-wire insertion to the medial fragment. A "double-tipped spear" K-wire is inserted through the medial fragment from the fracture end. The main fragments are manipulated directly with small pointed forceps

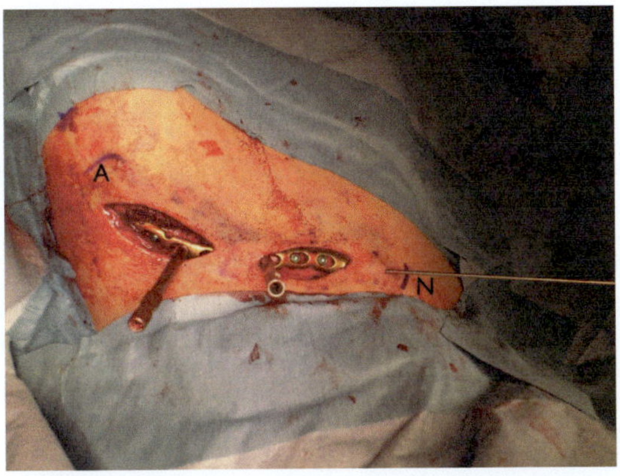

Fig. 11.4 Temporary K-wire fixation and plating. The "double-tipped spear" K-wire exits through the skin near the suprasternal notch. Then, the wire is pushed back such that opposite end goes into the lateral fragment in a "switchback" manner. An anatomically shaped locking plate is placed on the bone so that three consecutive screw holes are correctly over each fragment. *A* acromion, *N* suprasternal notch

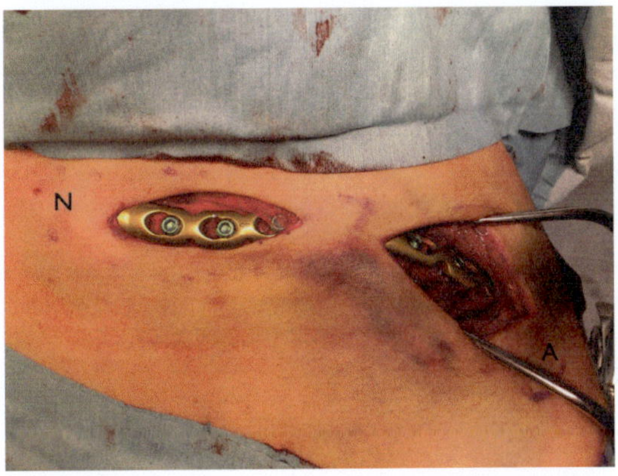

Fig. 11.5 Completion of plating. *A* acromion, *N* suprasternal notch

inserted into each main fragment. In this case, an eight-hole locking plate is chosen. The plate is inserted subcutaneously, and each main fragment is temporarily fixed using the plate with two 1.8 mm Kirschner wires (Fig. 11.4). The position of the plate on the bone is confirmed with the image intensifier. It is important to make sure that three consecutive screw holes are located on each fragment to optimize fracture stability. Then, three bicortical locking screws are inserted into

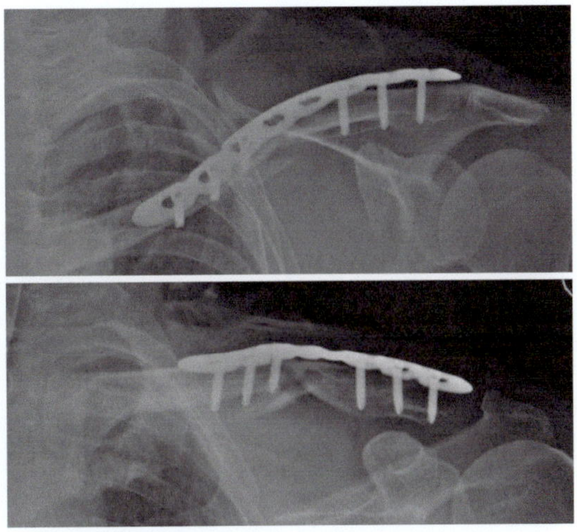

Fig. 11.6 Postoperative roentgenograms

each fragment (Fig. 11.5). Using 1, 2/0 vicryl and 3/0 s/c sutures, the wound is stitched. Postoperative radiographs are obtained prior to discharge (Fig. 11.6).

Postoperatively, a sling is worn for 1 week for comfort and to facilitate wound healing. Daily activities of living are not restricted, but manual labor is not allowed before callus formation is seen on the roentgenograms (Fig. 11.7).

Summary of Tips, Tricks, and Pitfalls

- "Switchback insertion" of K-wires is time saving as it maintains reduction.
- It is important to confirm by fluoroscopy that the plate is appropriately positioned on the bone prior to screw insertion.
- Three bicortical screws on each fragment are mandatory for optimum stability.
- Make sure that the length of the screws is not long enough to cause irritation/damage of the neurovascular structures underneath the clavicle [5].
- Take caution not to devitalize the bone fragments.
- Prevent iatrogenic damage to supraclavicular nerve endings [5].

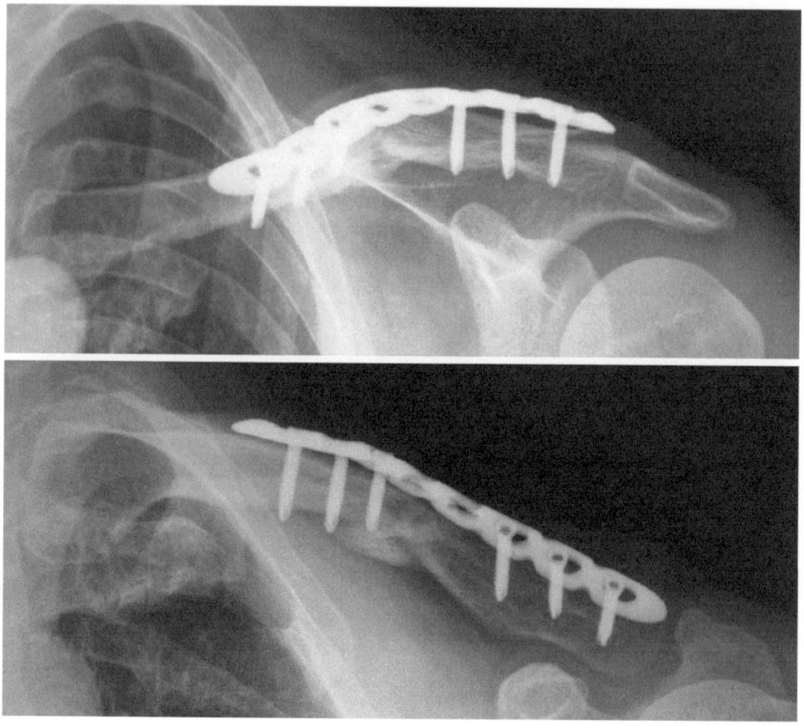

Fig. 11.7 8 weeks postoperative roentgenograms demonstrating fracture union

References

1. Postacchini F, Gumina S, De Santis P, Albo F. Epidemiology of clavicle fractures. J Shoulder Elb Surg. 2002;11(5):452–6.
2. Xu J, Xu L, Xu W, et al. Operative versus nonoperative treatment in the management of midshaft clavicular fractures: a meta-analysis of randomized controlled trials. J Shoulder Elb Surg. 2014;23:173–81.
3. van der Meijden OA, Houwert RM, Hulsmans M, Wijdicks FJ, Dijkgraaf MG, Meylaerts SA, et al. Operative treatment of dislocated midshaft clavicular fractures: plate or intramedullary nail fixation? A randomized controlled trial. J Bone Joint Surg Am. 2015;97:613–9.
4. VanBeek C, Boselli KJ, Cadet ER, Ahmad CS, Levine WN. Precontoured plating of clavicle fractures: decreased hardware-related complications? Clin Orthop Relat Res. 2011;469:3337–43.
5. Wijdicks FJ, Van der Meijden OA, Millett PJ, Verleisdonk EJ, Houwert RM. Systematic review of the complications of plate fixation of clavicle fractures. Arch Orthop Trauma Surg. 2012;132:617–25.

12 Scapula Fractures

David Limb

Anatomical Fracture Location: Radiograph of Fracture Pattern

Fractures of the body of the scapula are usually high-energy injuries resulting from a directly applied force. Fractures of the spine of the scapula and blade are therefore often associated with chest trauma and possibly abdominal and head injury. Fractures of the acromion result from a force applied to the point of the shoulder, and, if downwardly directed, the brachial plexus is vulnerable. High-energy forces directed to the front of the shoulder can tear the acromioclavicular joint apart and, in extreme cases, produce a scapulothoracic dissociation with vascular injury. If the force is transmitted to the scapula through the upper limb, then fractures of the glenoid fossa can occur, with or without glenohumeral dislocation. Of course, any combination of these injuries can occur depending on the energy delivered to the shoulder girdle and its vectors.

The surgical management of scapular fractures is most often indicated for displaced injuries including the glenoid fossa (Fig. 12.1), as this is assumed to have great potential for future impact on shoulder function. However, the approach differs significantly with fracture location—fractures of the blade and posteroinferior scapula often being approached from behind, whilst superior and anterior/anteroinferior fractures are usually approached from the front. The latter include anteroinferior fractures of the glenoid rim associated with shoulder dislocation. These may also occur with much lower energy injuries on the sports field, for example, and many are amenable to arthroscopic management but will not be considered further in this chapter, which will deal with open approaches for high-energy trauma. Given the significant differences between anterior and posterior approaches, both will be considered. Occasionally complex fracture patterns dictate a combined approach, whilst not uncommonly, fractures of the glenoid neck are associated with displaced clavicle fractures (the commonest variety of floating shoulder), and a decision has to be taken about whether to fix the clavicle and, if so, whether to reposition the patient or carry out both procedures in one position.

Preoperative Planning

The management of scapula fractures is not lifesaving in its own right and occurs in a planned fashion. The indications are not clear-cut but are often taken to include fractures of the glenoid that are associated with fixed subluxation or dislocation of the humeral head, often involving 5 mm or

D. Limb
Leeds Teaching Hospitals Trust, Chapel Allerton Hospital, Leeds LS7 4SA, UK
e-mail: david.limb@nhs.net

P.V. Giannoudis (ed.), *Fracture Reduction and Fixation Techniques*,
https://doi.org/10.1007/978-3-319-68628-8_12

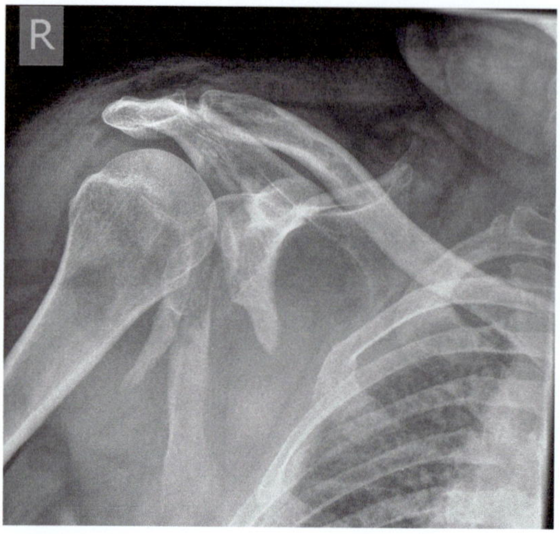

Fig. 12.1 An AP view of the scapula showing a fracture involving the glenoid neck and articular surface with medial displacement of the coracoid and glenoid fragments coupled with rotation

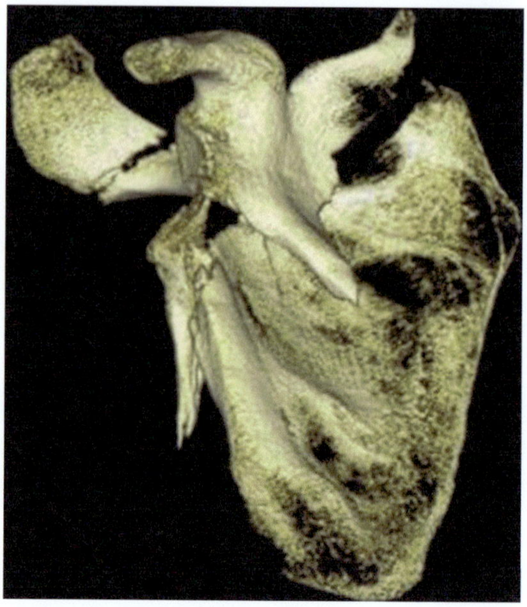

Fig. 12.2 3D reconstruction of CT data can be very useful in preoperative planning—in this case the data for the humeral head has been subtracted, allowing easier visualisation of the glenoid fracture

more of displacement at the articular surface. Very comminuted fractures may be impossible to fix but often demonstrate secondary congruence, with the many fragments aligning on the humeral head and healing there to form a socket against which articulation can occur. The trauma CT is useful in identifying the fracture, any associated joint subluxation or dislocation, any acromioclavicular or clavicle injury and indeed any other chest wall or thoracic trauma that might affect the timing of intervention.

If the trauma CT has sufficient data, 3D reconstruction is extremely useful for planning approaches and fixation (Fig. 12.2). If not, then a specific shoulder CT can be obtained once the patient is well enough. Plain radiographs are still useful for assessing the fracture, but these have to be centred on the injury—anteroposterior (AP), axial and scapula lateral views. Remember that the scapula faces forwards by approximately 30°, so an AP chest or direct AP including the shoulder images the scapula turned towards the film and is less useful.

Finally, timing is important—the patient has to be physiologically fit enough for surgery, and the fixation of scapula fractures is often delayed beyond the immediate period after trauma. However, the scapula is encased in a highly vascular muscle envelope, and fractures quickly form callus and heal—reduction of scapula blade fractures in particular can be difficult by 2 weeks after trauma and impossible by 3 weeks.

In general terms, fractures approached anteriorly are fractures involving a large segment of the glenoid fossa, usually superior or anteroinferior, and are fixed with lag screws after direct or arthroscopic observation of satisfactory reduction of the joint surface. Those approached from behind are displaced structural elements of the scapula, particularly the lateral column (often including part of the glenoid fossa, usually its interior half), spine and acromion, and are usually fixed with plates and screws.

Patient Setup in Theatre

For anterior approaches, the patient is set up in the beach chair position (Fig. 12.3). A gel pad or sandbag medial to the scapula and lateral to the spine helps push the scapula forwards. The arm is draped free and supported on a Mayo stand. The surgeon stands facing the shoulder, in the angle between the table and the Mayo stand. From this approach, direct reduction and lag screw fixation

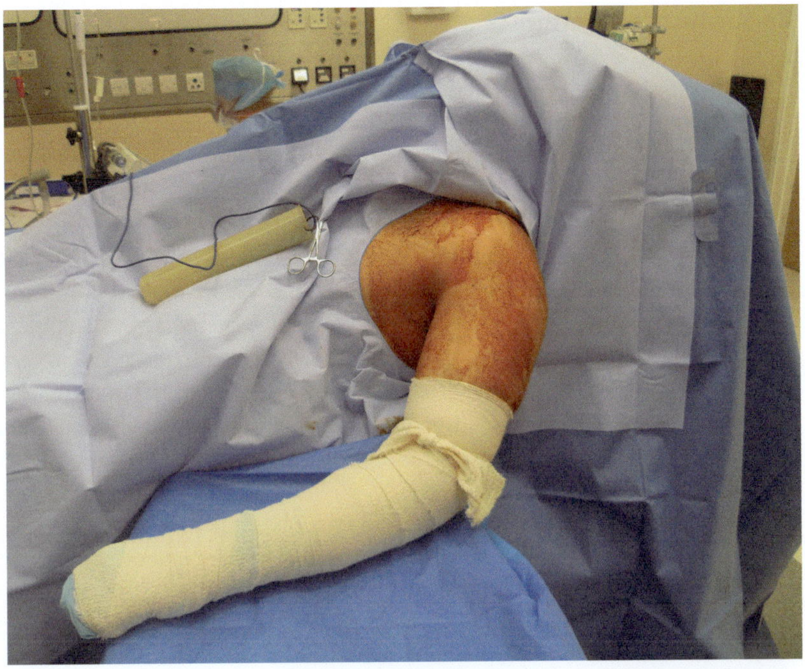

Fig. 12.3 The beach chair position is suitable for anterior approaches and allows easy intraoperative screening using the image intensifier

are often performed, and this can be facilitated by image intensifier (II) use. The II is brought in from behind the shoulder and raised to the top of its travel; then the 'C' arm is rotated over the shoulder—in this way the surgeon can operate without hindrance whilst using screening.

For posterior approaches, the patient is set up in a lateral position on a sandbag or between pelvic supports. Again, the affected arm is draped free and this time is rested on a Mayo table on the opposite site of the table to the surgeon (Fig. 12.4). The Mayo can be raised to abduct the arm and thus relax deltoid, facilitating exposure of the posterior glenoid.

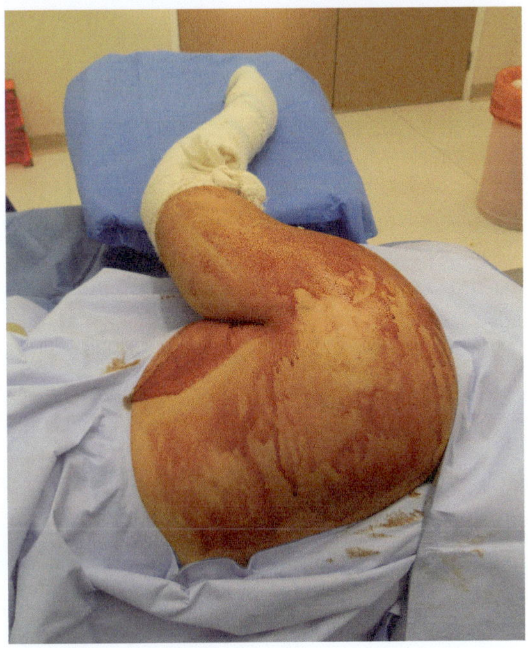

Fig. 12.4 The lateral position allows posterior approaches to the scapula. The arm is draped free so can be manipulated to allow indirect reduction of articular fragments with intact joint capsule attached

Closed Reduction Manoeuvres

Closed reduction manoeuvres have limited roles in the fixation of scapula fractures. However, the shoulder can be unstable and may need to be reduced to reduce fracture fragments. Manipulation of the arm also indirectly moves fragments of the glenoid that are attached to the humerus through the joint capsule, though this is more helpful once the shoulder is open. However, draping the arm free as described above allows traction, elevation, abduction, flexion, extension and rotation of the humerus, all of which can be used to help reduction at different steps in the operative procedure.

Reduction Instruments

By far the most useful aids to reduction are variations on the joystick—stout K-wires or long, small fragment screws that are inserted into fragments and used to manipulate them into place. For large fragments of the joint surface, especially from anterior approaches, the wires can be used from a cannulated screw set to allow definitive fixation over the wires. If a large superior glenoid fragment is contiguous with the coracoid process, which is easily visible through the deltopectoral approach if tackling a fracture from the front, then a bone clamp can be used to grasp the coracoid and manipulate the superior glenoid into place. Bone clamps from the small fragment set (pointed and crocodile) are also valuable in reducing fractures from a posterior approach (Fig. 12.5). However, the blade of the scapula is very thin, and the borders, which are strong enough for the application of clamps, are also the only areas suitable for the application of plates. Therefore, after pulling a fragment into a position of reduction, temporary K-wires might be possible around the glenoid fossa, but elsewhere wires and screws used as joysticks have to be removed before a plate can be applied. It is sometimes useful to have a drill and strong suture available to create a pair of holes through which suture can be passed simply to use to hold and manipulate fragments once they have been brought into reasonable alignment by a joystick or bone clamp technique.

Surgical Approach

From the front, the deltopectoral approach is the workhorse and does not interfere with any future surgery that might be needed for consequences of the shoulder injury. The incision can be a full deltopectoral exposure, or more limited. For example, a low deltopectoral approach allows a subscapularis split to give access to a single anteroinferior fragment that can be fixed with small fragment or cannulated screws. A higher limited deltopectoral approach allows the rotator interval to be opened and the glenoid surface to be inspected—through this approach the coracoid can also be grasped and used to manipulate the superior glenoid, to which it is often still attached. The coracoid can also be fixed itself through this approach if involved in the injury pattern.

From the back a Judet approach gives excellent visualisation of the whole of the scapula spine and the blade below it, elevating infraspinatus to expose medial and lateral columns. However, the thickness of the medial and lateral columns is such that even in stout individuals, screws of 14 mm or even less are all that can be inserted.

The Judet approach is, however, quite an injury in itself, and many fractures for which fixation is indicated affect principally the lateral column, glenoid neck and glenoid, and for these a more limited direct posterior approach can be used. The incision is placed from the joint line posteriorly and passes down the line of the lateral column of

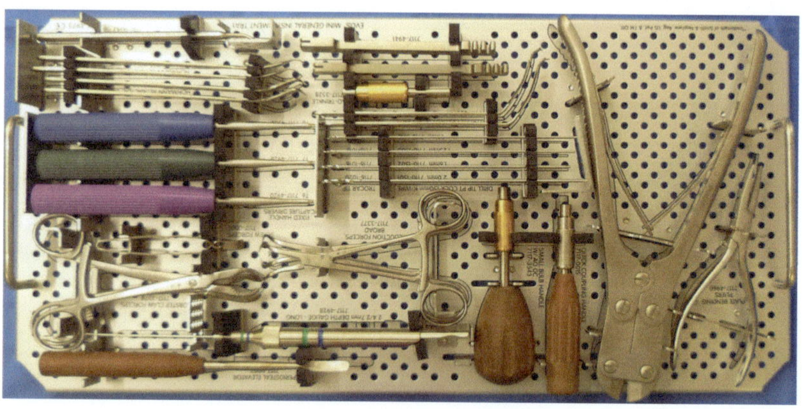

Fig. 12.5 Bone clamps, K-wires, pliers and a selection of retractors and screws can be used as reduction aids

the scapula (Fig. 12.6). The skin is very thick here and the fat layer quite fibrous and attached to the muscle fascia quite firmly. After separating the fat from muscle layers, the inferior edge of deltoid is identified and lifted towards the head, being relaxed by arm abduction, allowing the identification of infraspinatus and teres minor (Fig. 12.7). There is an internervous plane between the latter, which is exploited. It can be difficult to see but is usually easy to palpate as infraspinatus is sitting on the scapula blade, but teres is arising from the lateral column and running just off the lateral border as it passes up to the humeral head. Quite often the interval is easy to locate, as a displaced lateral column takes teres with it and leaves behind infraspinatus, tearing open the interval so that the fracture is immediately encountered. Once identified the interval is opened inferiorly, to the flat of the inferior angle of the scapula, and superiorly to the transition into rotator cuff tendons—a split developed here through the capsule opens the joint, but remember that the glenoid is facing forwards by about 30°, so the view of the joint surface is quite limited, though it may be palpated (it can also be inspected by inserting an arthroscope from the front, whilst carrying out the open procedure from the back). By elevating infraspinatus medially by about one centimetre, the whole lateral column is exposed, as well as the inferior half of the posterior glenoid, to the level of the spinoglenoid notch.

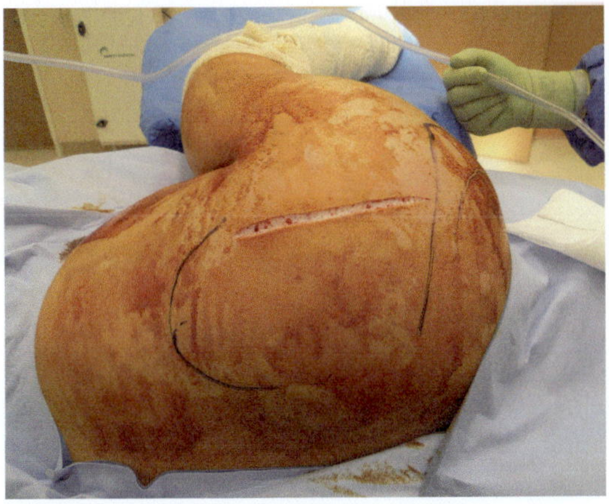

Fig. 12.6 A posterior approach starting over the posterior joint line and passing vertically down allows access to the lateral column through an internervous plane with minimal muscle stripping

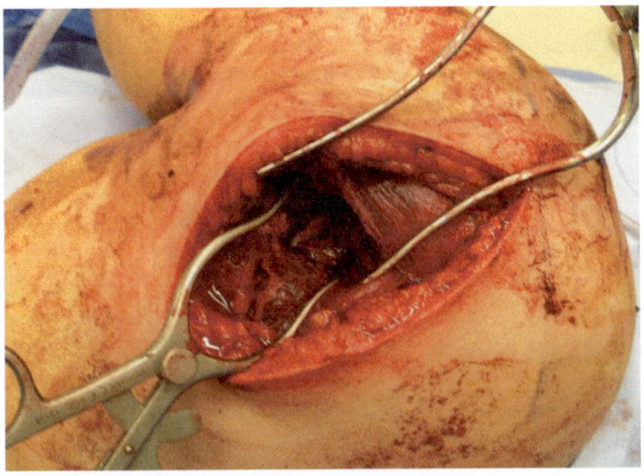

Fig. 12.7 The inferior edge of deltoid is identified, and below this infraspinatus and teres minor run side by side but are often separated by the injury. The interval can be developed and held open with a self-retaining retractor

Open Reduction Manoeuvres

An anteroinferior glenoid fragment, approached from the front, is best controlled initially by a 'K'-wire inserted about 5 mm from the joint margin, and the wire is then driven through, parallel to the glenoid surface, until it reaches the fracture surface. The wire is then used as a joystick to manipulate the fragment into position before driving it across to the posterior cortex of the glenoid. This can be done under direct vision if a deltopectoral approach has been used, but this is also exactly the same principle as is used for arthroscopic fixation of a large bony Bankart lesion. If there is room, a screw or second wire is passed through the fragment separately before replacing the wire with a screw. Alternatively, a cannulated screw can be inserted over the wire. Although 3.5 mm small fragment screws are perfectly adequate for holding such fragments, the guidewire for a 3.5 mm cannulated screw is very thin and flexible. When using an arthroscopic approach in particular, therefore, a larger screw diameter of at least 4.5 mm is chosen so that a thicker, stiffer K wire can be used, which is a better joystick for reducing the bone fragment before driving the wire across the fracture site.

Superior fragments attached to the coracoid can be manipulated by grasping the coracoid (Fig. 12.8), otherwise a long screw is inserted into the superior fragment from the anterior rim and

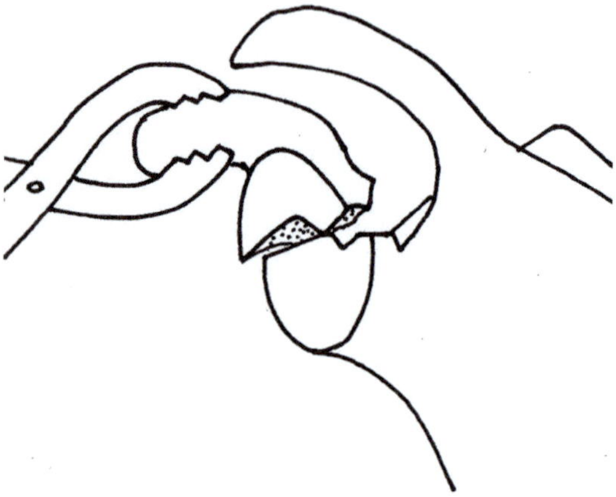

Fig. 12.8 If superior glenoid fragments remain attached to the base of the coracoid, the latter can be grasped and used to reduce the articular surface

used as a joystick to manipulate the fragment into place— a thin lever may also be used through the fracture site to help coax the superior fragment into place. Fixation then depends on the orientation of the fracture line. Oblique fractures may be amenable to lag screw fixation from the front, angling across the fracture line but being careful not to cause shear whilst compressing and lose reduction. Transverse fractures can be stabilised by passing a percutaneous wire under image intensifier control from superiorly (Fig. 12.9), behind the distal clavicle (a Nevassier portal in arthroscopic terms) to pass through supraspinatus muscle belly into the glenoid. Once happy with the position, a cannulated screw can be used over the wire to compress the fracture, after which the wire is removed.

Posterior fragments can be reduced under direct vision, but the lateral column and glenoid often disappear into muscle tissue anteriorly making safe grasping and manipulation a challenge. The posterior glenoid is usually visible, and there is sufficient room to insert a long screw (say a 50 m screw inserted only 10 mm into the bone, leaving a good length to use as a handle to manipulate the glenoid). This can then be used to lift and rotate the lateral column gently back into place, holding it with a crocodile clamp if sufficient is exposed or a second joystick screw if not (Fig. 12.10). Fortunately, the scapula is so vascular that healing still occurs even if one does not get good compression, though attempts should still be made to appropriately place screws in compression plates to achieve this. As noted above, if the lateral column tends to fall back into the wound once any holding device is removed, it can be useful to pass a '2' or '5' braided polyester suture through drill holes adjacent to the required plate position or around the lateral column itself so that the bone can be held up against the plate by traction on the sutures as fixation proceeds.

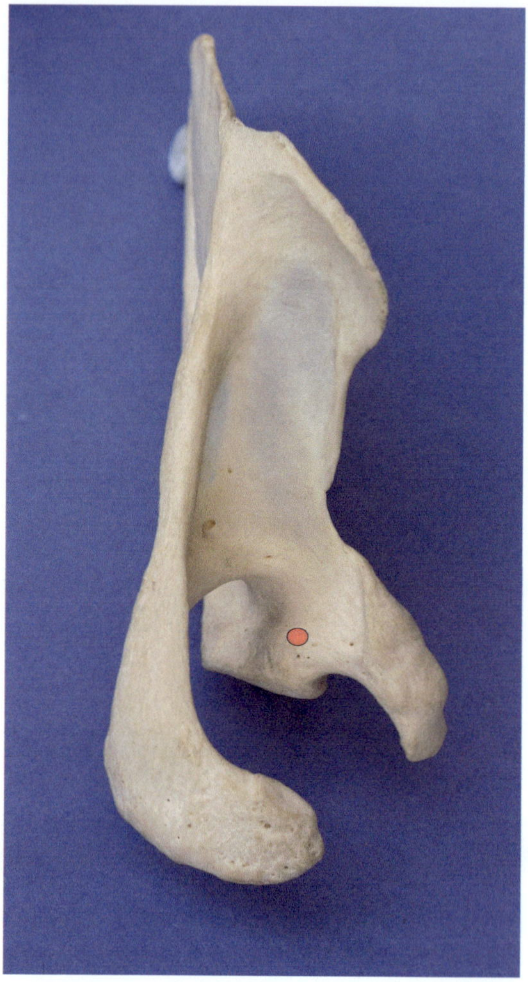

Fig. 12.9 The scapula seen from above—the coracoid can be gripped with a crocodile reduction clamp and be used to reduce attached superior glenoid fragments—a screw can be inserted from superior to inferior (entry point indicated by circle), whilst the reduction is maintained by grasping the coracoid

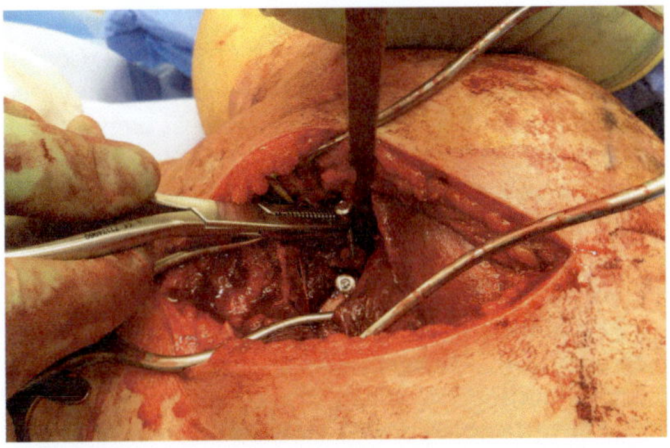

Fig. 12.10 The lateral column can be controlled and reduced by inserting long screws into the column either side of the fracture line and grasping these with pliers or reduction clamps to effect a reduction under direct vision

Implant Insertion

When inserting cannulated screws over wires anteriorly, always try to insert a second wire before drilling for the screw—the act of drilling abolishes any friction between the fragment and the wire and allows it to slide up the wire. Insertion of the screw can still push the fragment back down into the same place, but care has to be taken not to allow any rotation of the fragment in this case, or joint incongruency will result.

When inserting plates from a posterior approach (Fig. 12.11), remember that the glenoid articular surface is tilted forwards—a screw passing forwards in the sagittal plane of the patient will almost certainly be entering the glenohumeral joint. Take account of the scapular plane when inserting screws in glenoid fragments, and if necessary visualise either by posterior arthrotomy to allow direct vision or palpation, or insert an arthroscope from the front of the joint. Use the image intensifier to ensure satisfactory reduction without intra-articular penetration, and check by rotating the free arm and ensuring a smooth, full range of movement.

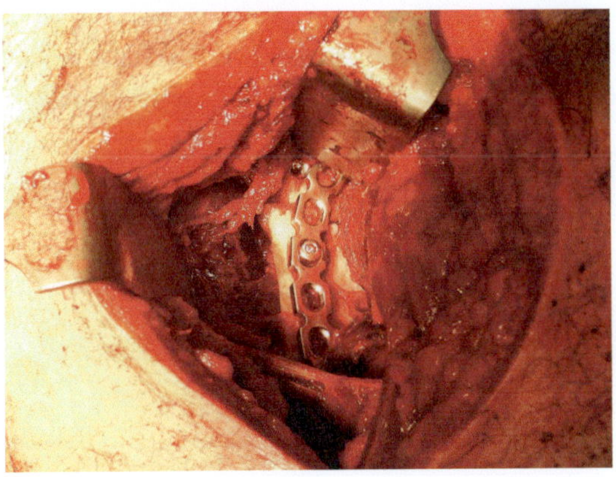

Fig. 12.11 The lateral column has been plated, being contoured away from the articular surface. A separate lag screw is compressing two large glenoid fragments

Summary: Tips, Tricks and Pitfalls

- Scapula fractures are high-energy injuries and are usually fixed as a planned procedure, though rapid healing makes reduction very difficult much beyond 2 weeks after injury. CT and 3D reconstruction are useful preoperative planning tools. Superior and anteroinferior displaced glenoid fossa fragments are approached most usually from an anterior approach, whilst other scapula fractures and glenoid fractures involving the interior and posterior glenoid are usually approached from posterior.
- Views of the joint surface are relatively good from anterior approaches but more difficult from posterior as the glenoid faces approximately 30° forwards from the coronal plane. An arthroscope can be used as an adjunct for joint visualisation, whilst some anterior fractures can be fixed entirely by an arthroscopic approach.
- Approaches that use internervous planes and involve minimal muscle stripping allow rapid healing and rehabilitation after surgery. However, access is more difficult, and reduction can be tricky—inserting long screws a short distance into the posteroinferior glenoid and lateral column is a useful trick as these screws can then be grasped with instruments and used to reduce fracture fragments.
- Aim to create a congruent glenoid that is supported on the scapular blade and in particular the lateral column of the scapula (Fig. 12.12), which fortunately is the strongest segment of bone for the attachment of plates. Aim to allow immediate mobilisation—the long-term complication that is almost inevitable to a degree is stiffness, and immobilisation will make this worse.

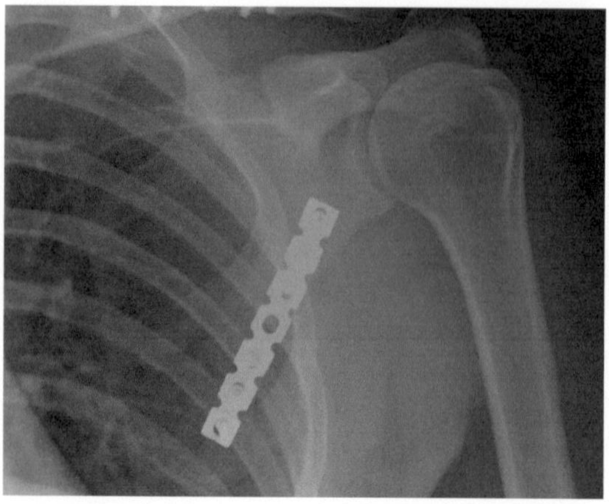

Fig. 12.12 Aim for a congruent glenoid supported by a stable lateral column—comminution of the blade of the scapula itself rarely needs any intervention or stabilisation

Further Reading

Bartoníček J, Tuček M, Frič V, Obruba P. Fractures of the scapular neck: diagnosis, classifications and treatment. Int Orthop. 2014;38(10):2163–73.

Lewis S, Argintar E, Jahn R, Zusmanovich M, Itamura J, Rick Hatch GF. Intra-articular scapular fractures: outcomes after internal fixation. J Orthop. 2013;10(4):188–92.

Mighell MA, Hatzidakis AM, Otto RJ, Watson JT, Cottrell BJ, Cusick MC, Pappou IP. Complex trauma to the shoulder girdle, including the proximal humerus, the clavicle, and the scapula: current concepts in diagnosis and treatment. Instr Course Lect. 2015;64:121–37.

Pizanis A, Tosounidis G, Braun C, Pohlemann T, Wirbel RJ. The posterior two-portal approach for reconstruction of scapula fractures: results of 39 patients. Injury. 2013;44(11):1630–5.

Schroder LK, Gauger EM, Gilbertson JA, Cole PA. Functional outcomes after operative management of extra-articular glenoid neck and scapular body fractures. J Bone Joint Surg Am. 2016;98(19):1623–30.

Zlowodzki M, Bhandari M, Zelle BA, Kregor PJ, Cole PA. Treatment of scapular fractures: Systematic review of 520 fractures in 22 case series. J Orthop Trauma. 2006;20-3:230–3.

13 Humeral Head Avulsion of Greater Tuberosity

Mark Philipson

Indications for Surgery and Preoperative Planning

Surgical management of displaced isolated fractures involving the greater tuberosity is not controversial. I will offer surgical fixation to all fit patients with an isolated greater tuberosity fracture displaced more than 5 mm.

I approach these as I would an open cuff repair not as an osteosynthesis procedure. My experience is that simple screw fixation often fails even when the bone quality appears to be good. My objective is to repair the rotator cuff with the tuberosity fragment restored to the fracture bed.

Patient Setup in Theatre

The patient is sat up in the beach chair position. The arm is draped free and rests on a Mayo stand, typically in an abducted position to reduce the tension in deltoid. The surgeon stands facing the shoulder. While others may do, I do not routinely utilise an image intensifier.

Closed Reduction Manoeuvres

There is no role for closed reduction except to relocate the humerus in cases of glenohumeral dislocation (Fig. 13.1).

Surgical Approach

I utilise a coronal incision, extending from the ACJ to 3–4 cm distal to the acromion (Fig. 13.2). I take the coracoacromial ligament off the acromion. I perform an acromioplasty using a saw or osteotome if the acromion is hooked. I find the tendinous raphe at the anterolateral corner of the

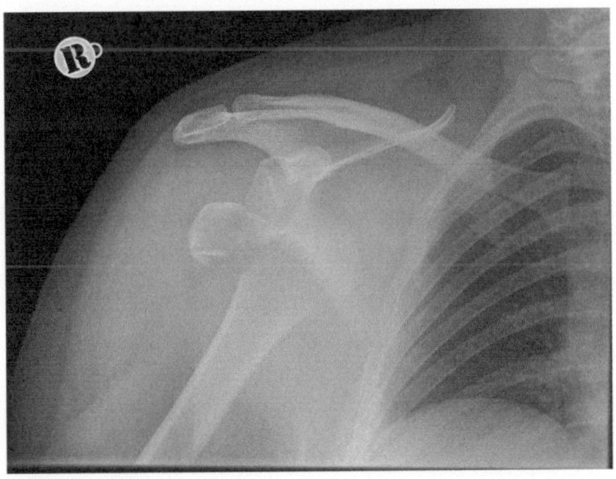

Fig. 13.1 An X-ray image of an isolated greater tuberosity fracture associated with anterior dislocation of the glenohumeral joint

M. Philipson
Leeds General Infirmary, Leeds, UK
e-mail: mark.philipson@nhs.net

P.V. Giannoudis (ed.), *Fracture Reduction and Fixation Techniques*,
https://doi.org/10.1007/978-3-319-68628-8_13

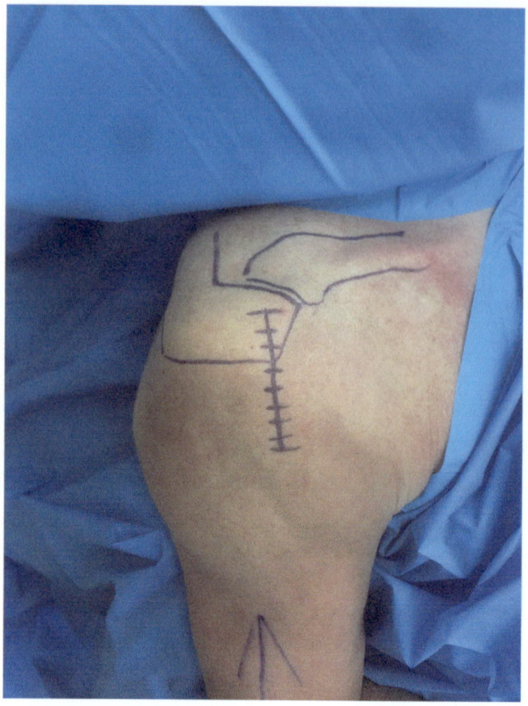

Fig. 13.2 The skin incision for a superolateral deltoid-splitting approach

acromion and split deltoid at this point for a distance of approximately 4 cm. The humerus can be rotated to facilitate access.

Open Reduction Manoeuvres

An assistant elevates the acromion utilising a large Langenbeck retractor. The surgeon applies traction to the humerus to open the subacromial space and retrieves the retracted posterosuperior cuff tendon and tuberosity fragment(s) with forceps. A stay suture is placed in supraspinatus.

In cases of locked anterior dislocation associated with a greater tuberosity fracture, I still utilise the same superolateral approach described above. This gives excellent access to the empty glenoid so that any debris can be removed from the joint and facilitating direct digital manipulation of the humeral head. If relocation remains difficult, then a bone hook can be used on the strong bone of the proximal humeral shaft to manipulate the humerus in to joint.

Implant Insertion

I utilise two anchors designed for labral repair in the hard cortical bone at the posterior edge of the bicipital groove. An effective repair can be achieved using transosseous sutures through drill holes in the metaphysis; however I find that access for the drill holes and suture passing is challenging through my preferred superolateral approach. Each anchor is double loaded with abrasion-resistant suture material. Utilising the four available sutures, I place four simple horizontal mattress sutures spread out evenly from front to back in the injured cuff. Before tensioning and tying these sutures, I place a stitch to secure the most anterolateral portion of the free edge of supraspinatus to rotator interval tissue at the most posterolateral portion of subscapularis. In other words, I secure the cuff over the top of the bicipital groove. This is to help achieve anatomic tension in the cuff when the four mattress sutures are tied using a sliding locking knot (Figs. 13.3 and 13.4). It is easy to inadvertently over-tension the cuff in a fresh injury.

Post-op Instructions

In cases involving a fresh injury with minimal tension in the cuff and the anchors are in good bone, then this is a very secure repair, and I am

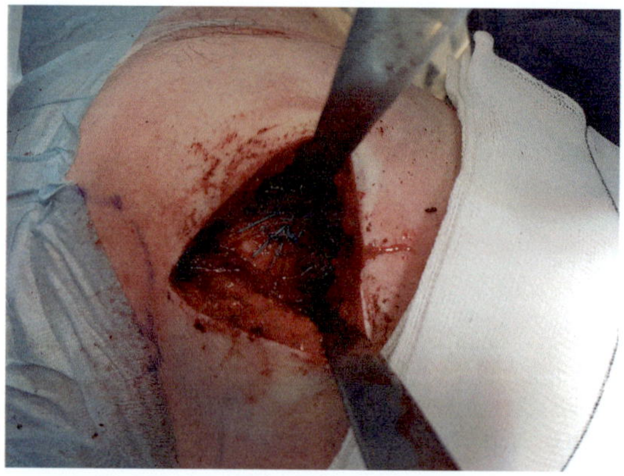

Fig. 13.3 A large isolated greater tuberosity fracture has been repaired using two double-loaded anchors

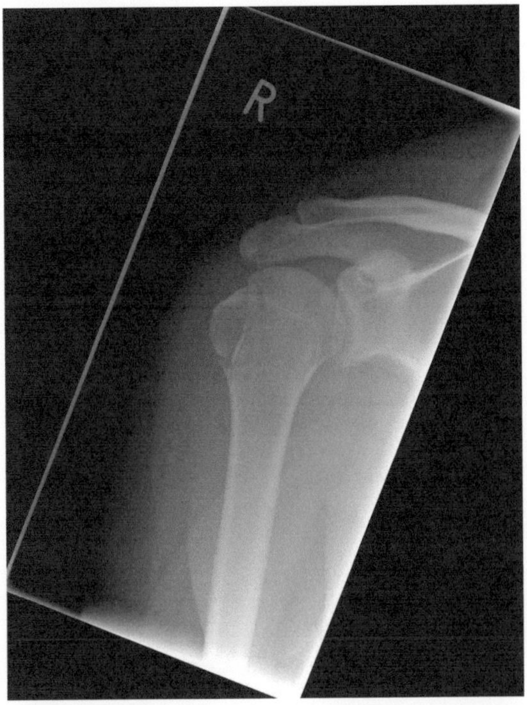

Fig. 13.4 A post-op X-ray image of the same case (the anchors are radiolucent)

happy for the patient to commence active-assisted exercises immediately. The patient wears a simple sling for 4–6 weeks.

Tips, Tricks and Pitfalls

- Always try and repair these earlier rather than later. At 2 weeks the reduction is easy. At 6 weeks it is challenging because of retraction of the cuff. Beyond 6 weeks it can be impossible even with extensive releases.
- Avoid using screw fixation alone. Think of it as a cuff repair.
- The use of double-loaded anchors rather than transosseous sutures facilitates a smaller superolateral exposure.
- Avoid over-tensioning the cuff.

14 Fractures of Proximal Humerus Open Reduction and Internal Fixation

Harish Kapoor, Adeel Aqil, and Osman Riaz

Initial Assessment

It is crucial that all proximal humerus fractures are assessed with an anteroposterior (AP) Fig. 14.1 and axial view (Figs. 14.2 and 14.3) X-rays. Axial views in most cases can be obtained; however in some instances where pain restricts shoulder movement, a modified angled axial view should be undertaken to ensure a dislocation is not missed. A scapular lateral view may also be useful. In complex injuries, computed tomography (CT) may assist in diagnosis and surgical planning. CT scans can help to determine whether the humeral head is intact and to assess the position and comminution of the tuberosities (Fig. 14.4).

The decision as to whether to treat three- or four-part fractures by internal fixation or with an arthroplasty solution can be very difficult. Patients can potentially retain better function if they retain their own humeral heads and in the presence of intact rotator cuff muscles.

Open reduction in the presence of severely comminuted fractures is more challenging as the head, both tuberosities and the shaft are separated from one another. However, an arthroplasty solution in the form of a hemiarthroplasty or total or reverse shoulder arthroplasty may be indicated when the fracture is deemed unreconstructable especially in an older population group. Internal fixation is preferable in younger group as far as possible in three- or even four-part fractures.

Clinically always assess for neurovascular status especially in reference to axillary nerve and brachial plexus.

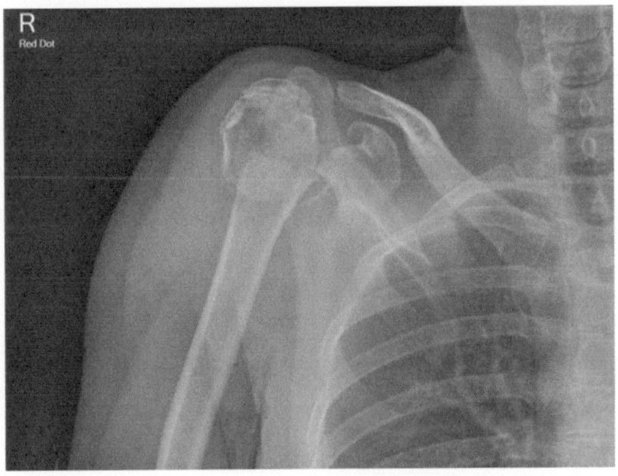

Fig. 14.1 AP radiograph of a right proximal humeral fracture

H. Kapoor, M.B.B.S., M.S.(Orth), D.N.B. (✉)
Consultant Trauma and Orthopaedics,
Leeds General Infirmary, Leeds, UK
e-mail: harish.kapoor@nhs.net

A. Aqil, M.B.B.S., M.R.C.S. • O. Riaz, M.B.B.S., M.R.C.S.
Department of Trauma and Orthopaedic Surgery,
Leeds General Infirmary, Leeds, UK

P.V. Giannoudis (ed.), *Fracture Reduction and Fixation Techniques*,
https://doi.org/10.1007/978-3-319-68628-8_14

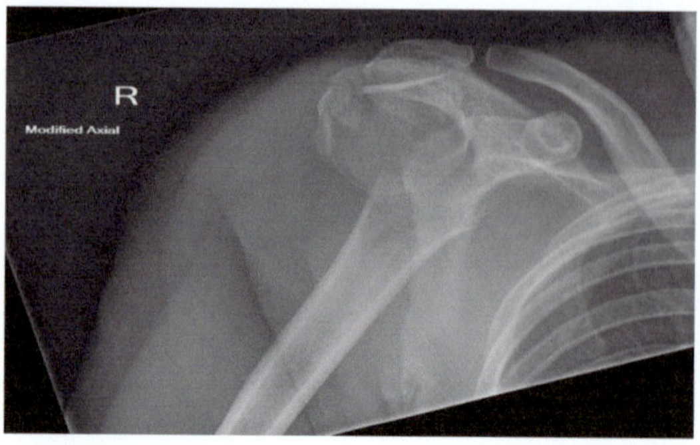

Fig. 14.2 Modified axial view of a right proximal humeral fracture

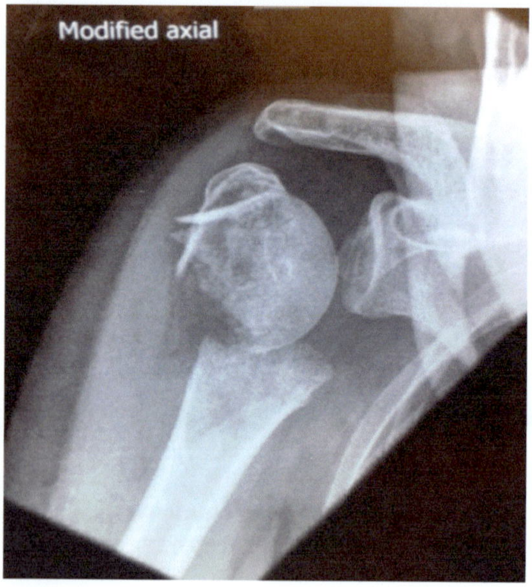

Fig. 14.3 Modified axial view of a right proximal humeral fracture

Preoperative Planning and Anaesthesia Considerations

A general anaesthesia with or without an intrascalene block is commonly used. Blocks are very useful in providing effective post-operative analgesia; however they introduce additional risks including pneumothorax or phrenic nerve injury paralysis. An experienced anaesthetist in upper limb surgery is extremely helpful.

Due to proximity of the surgical site to the airway, anaesthetic tubes should be secured and positioned, so they are not unnecessarily close to avoid displacement or getting in the way of the surgeon.

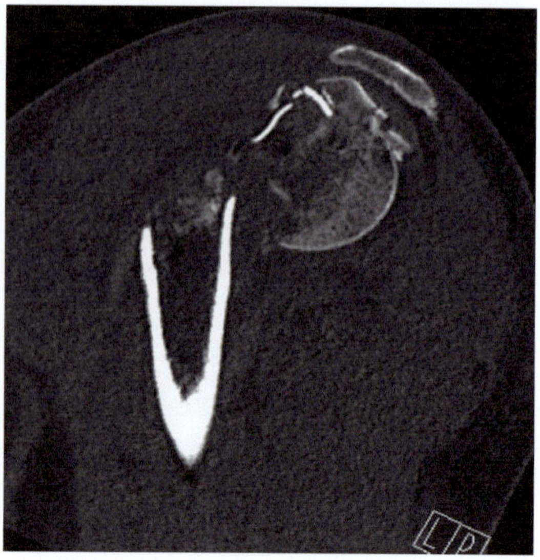

Fig. 14.4 Preoperative CT scan

Therefore, a definitive airway that is well secured is our preference, as the head and face are usually well covered from the sight of the anaesthetist. I do not like laryngeal masks especially in a semi-reclining beach chair position due to the tendency to dislodge.

Prophylactic antibiotics should be administered, as per institutional guidelines.

A general set for the surgical approach, including suitable retractors (a West and Norfolk and Norwich self-retaining retractor), are adequate, but specially designed shoulder retractors can improve the exposure.

Plates of different lengths should be available with the set including the jig for correct aiming of the locking screws. Small fragment set, K-wires and Ethibond sutures should also be available.

Patient Setup in Theatre

Given the methodical staged process of patient setup and surgical exposure for clarity, these steps are given in list and bullet point format.

- Shoulder table attachments are available which convert normal operating table to permit patient positioning into a beach chair position (Fig 14.5).

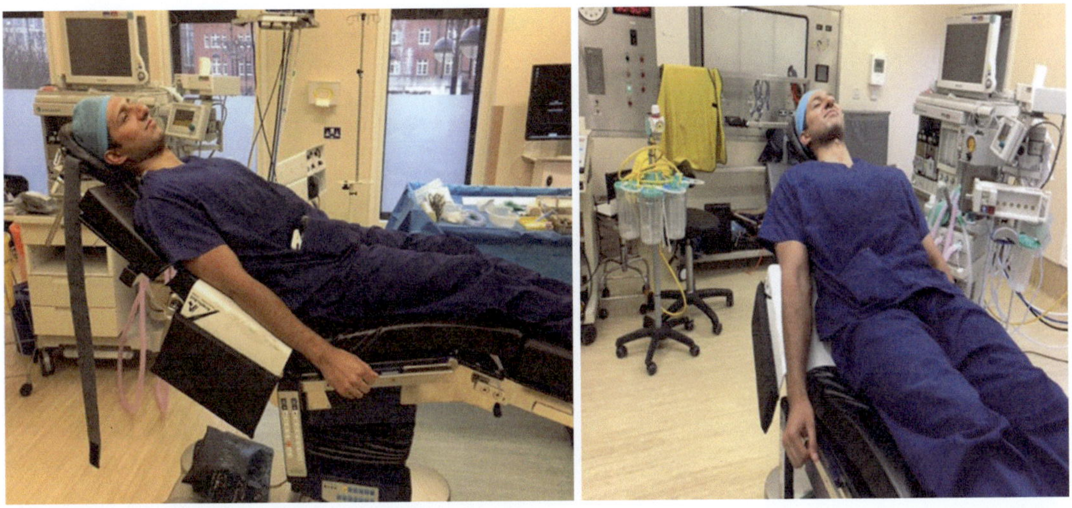

Fig. 14.5 Simulated patient positioning (model)—see reversed arm support

- The patient should be sat up at the hips into a beach chair position. The torso is normally 40 degrees from the horizontal, but if access of the shoulder is needed from the back or front, then an upright position is more appropriate. Spine and the head need to be supported, but at the same time, access to the whole shoulder needs to be maintained.
- Patient feet are tilted up to avoid patient sliding down. Knees are flexed with a pillow behind them.
- Table needs to be radiolucent as it can interfere with the C-arm when using the image intensifier.
- Proximal humerus surgery requires the surgeon to be in the axilla of the patient on the affected side. The assistant or the C-arm can be positioned above the patient's shoulder.
- It is preferable the head of the table to be away from the anaesthetic machine which should be at the foot end. Extension tubing will be required for this.
- The scrub nurse can work from behind of the surgeon as along the instruments are within the laminar flow.
- Skin preparation is carried out using usual antiseptic solutions.
- Prepare up to the midline of the chest to the medial border of the scapula. Clean up to the root of the neck and down level of the nipple. The arm is prepared down to the wrist.
- A U-drape is used to shut off, and a separate impervious stocking is rolled up the arm to above the level of the elbow. This leaves the draped arm free for manipulation.
- Both ends of the C-arm are covered with sterile drapes (Fig. 14.6).

Closed Reduction Techniques and Manoeuvres

Reduction can be achieved by external manoeuvres with traction, adduction and internal rotation of the arm. Displacement of the distal fragment is usually medially and anteriorly, and pushing laterally and posteriorly helps in lining up the most common displacement. To complete the reduction, a bone lever can be introduced via a small incision to correct varus/valgus angulation by pushing on the superolateral portion of the head. If needed, a hook instrument can be introduced into the subacromial space and used to complete the reduction of the greater tuberosity by pulling the tuberosity forwards and downwards. Three- or four-part fracture dislocations may be impacted or non-impacted. In impacted fractures, cautious reduction via external manoeuvres in the operating room under anaesthetic and image intensifier can be attempted. There is a risk of disimpaction, an event consistently followed by AVN in four-part fractures. The lifting of the impacted head should be gentle in open procedures.

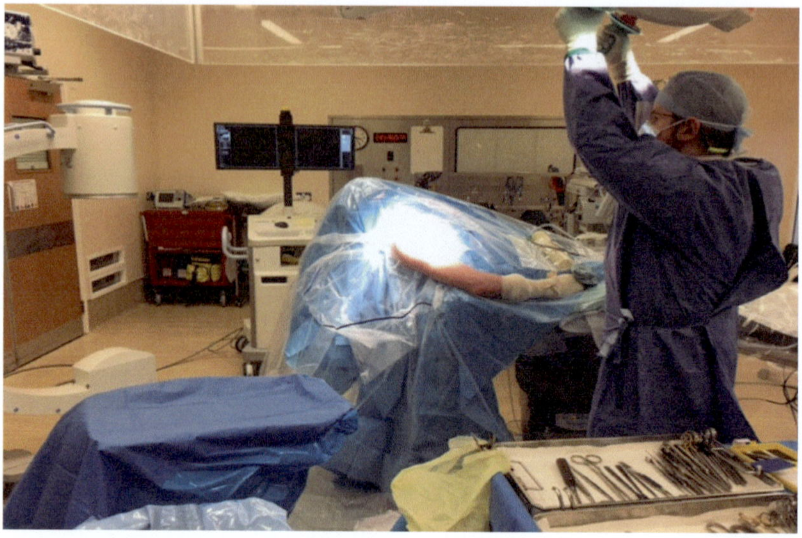

Fig. 14.6 Theatre setup

Overall though, these closed reduction manoeuvres are useful if one was to use minimally invasive fixation using intramedullary nails, for example. They are less important when aiming to internally fix the fracture as reduction is more easily achieved following open surgical exposure. If using an intramedullary nail and with a fracture where the head is in varus malposition, part of the reduction can be achieved by slightly medialising the entry point of the nail. Note, however, that this will not correct gross varus malposition. One should only use this to correct mild varus malreductions and take care not to encroach too much on to the articular surface. My preference is to use locking proximal humeral plates; rarely, I use an IM nail in a low metaphyseal neck fracture or a pathological fracture. I am aware that humeral nailing is used for complex two, three and even four part fractures with similar results in some centres to good affect.

Reduction Instruments

Tools useful in fracture reduction: your finger, pointed reduction clamps, bone hook, blunt bone retractors and large Bristow-like elevator. Intraoperative X-rays can then give further visual feedback as to what your finger has been trying to achieve. Care must be taken when using your finger. However, fracture fragments are sharp and can pierce your glove, endangering you and the patient. Therefore, we only recommend using your finger as a last resort. K-wires are extremely useful as levers and for transfixing fragments once reduced. However, stout wires should be used to prevent bending and to avoid deviating from the intended trajectory when being inserted. We favour minimum 2 mm wires as a general rule. Other general instruments such as Trethowan bone levers should be available to free up fragments to allow easier manipulation. Strong sutures should also be available to grab the superior cuff and subscapularis tendons. Once attached they can be used to pull the tuberosities down and tied to the plate or each other. Occasionally a 5 mm bone anchor can be used to pull both lesser and greater tuberosities and associated tendons down to the required positions, thus acting as a reduction and fixation tool. I prefer to use transosseous sutures to recreate the shape of the head with the tuberosities reattached before application of plate in three- or four-part fractures.

Surgical Approach

The deltopectoral approach is the workhorse approach to the shoulder in fracture fixation. It allows adequate exposure to the joint and allows easier access to head fragments which may have been left behind when anterior fracture dislocations of the shoulder have occurred. In deltopectoral approach, incision extends from the clavicle across the lateral edge of the coracoid process and down to the arm in the groove between anterior edge of the deltoid muscle and the biceps muscle. Length of incision is depending on the extent of exposure required (Fig. 14.7). The deltoid and pectoralis major muscle are separated, retracting the cephalic vein either laterally or medially depending on available anatomy (Fig. 14.8 (a,b,c)). Fascia is exposed deep in the deltopectoral interval. It is opened vertically, adjacent to the lateral border of the conjoint tendon. Using your finger, sweep under the conjoint tendon to ensure axillary nerve is not in close proximity. Then insert self-retaining retractors. The proximal humerus is now visible, which the rotator cuff tendon surrounds (Fig. 14.9). I use the direct lateral approach with deltoid split in fresh/relatively new up to 7–10 days old displaced two-part fractures in suitable patients where the plate is used as a reduction tool with putting a non-locking first screw in the shaft after positioning the plate at the right height depending on implant design.

Open Reduction Manoeuvres

It is important that the reduction process does not further compromise the blood supply to the humeral head. Detachment of cuff tendons and capsule is not advised; image intensifier should be used to check reduction (Fig. 14.10 (a,b)). Any fracture involving the tuberosities heavy no. 5 Ethibond suture should be placed, to bring the supraspinatus and infraspinatus onto the greater tuberosity and subscapularis onto the lesser tuberosity. Traction can be applied to bring these fragments down to the humeral head. Varus angulation—the head is separated from the shaft and pulled into varus by the superior rotator cuff muscles that are still attached. If only the lesser tuberosity is attached to the head, then the head is pulled in medial rotation by the subscapularis tendon. Impacted fractures—overlap exists between the medial part of the head and shaft. The lateral periosteum is normally intact. The stability provided by the intact lateral periosteum allows medial hinge reduction via external manoeuvres involving abduction and traction of the shoulder. A Bristow or a similar instrument can be introduced between the tuberosities and elevating the supero-lateral edge of the head upwards. The medial periosteum acts as a hinge that prevents medial translation of the head.

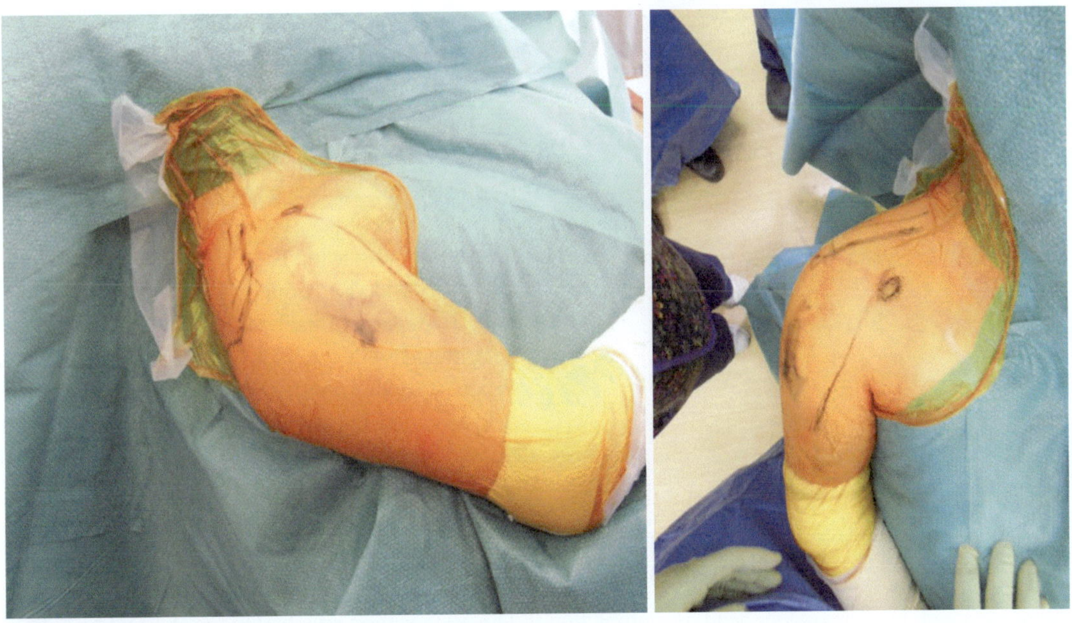

Fig. 14.7 Deltopectoral marked incision for the surgical exposure

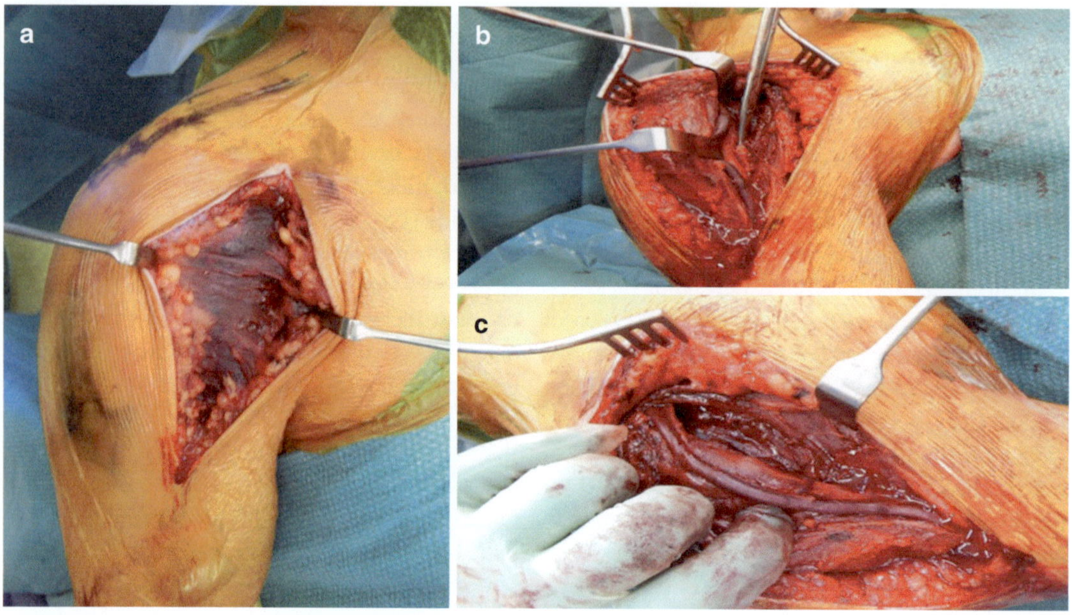

Fig. 14.8 (**a**–**c**) The deltoid and pectoralis major muscle are separated, retracting the cephalic vein either laterally or medially depending on available anatomy

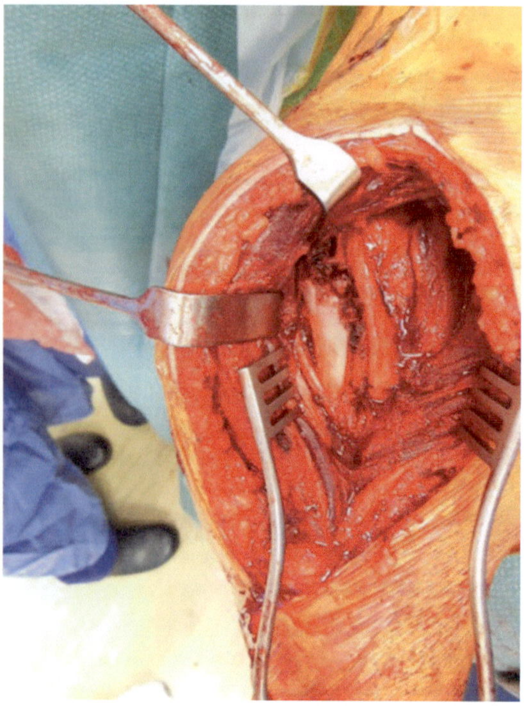

Fig. 14.9 Exposure of proximal humerus

Non-impacted fractures—the head is completely separated from the shaft and the lateral periosteum is torn. Reduction is considerably more challenging in this. The first step consists in aligning the head on the shaft. With the arm in traction, an instrument such as a blunt elevator is introduced at the medial edge of the anatomic neck to reduce the medial hinge. Medial rotation of the head can be corrected by looping a suture around the bone tendon junction of the subscapularis then pulling it in the medial to lateral direction. Valgus angulation—lateral impaction of the head on the shaft. The fractured tuberosities remain aligned with the head and shaft, and the lateral periosteum connecting the four fragments is intact. The medial hinge should be assessed; it may or may not be intact. Fracture-dislocation—percutaneous pinning using K-wires of the head can help aid with reduction prior to opening the shoulder joint. Reduction of the head and tuberosities can be determined with the arm held in neutral rotation. When acceptable reduction is attained, it can be held using tension band sutures which can be passed through the locking plate.

Implant Position

The plate is then attached to the shaft using slotted hole for adjustment of height (Fig. 14.11 (a,b)). The locking plate should sit on/below the cuff

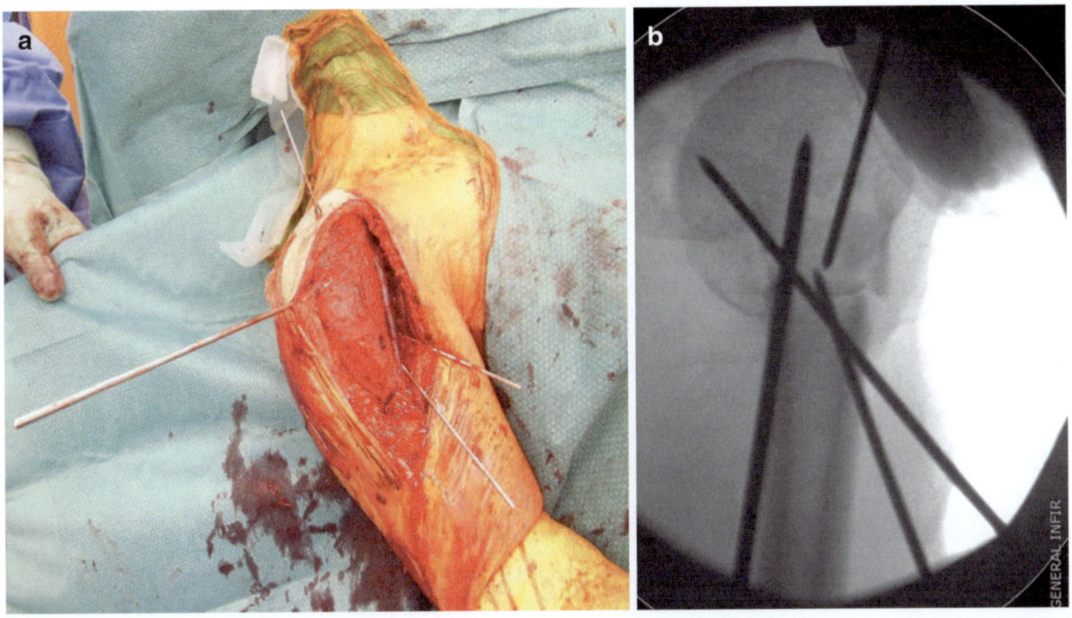

Fig. 14.10 (**a**) Intraoperative picture and (**b**) image intensifier view demonstrating reduction of fracture using K-wires

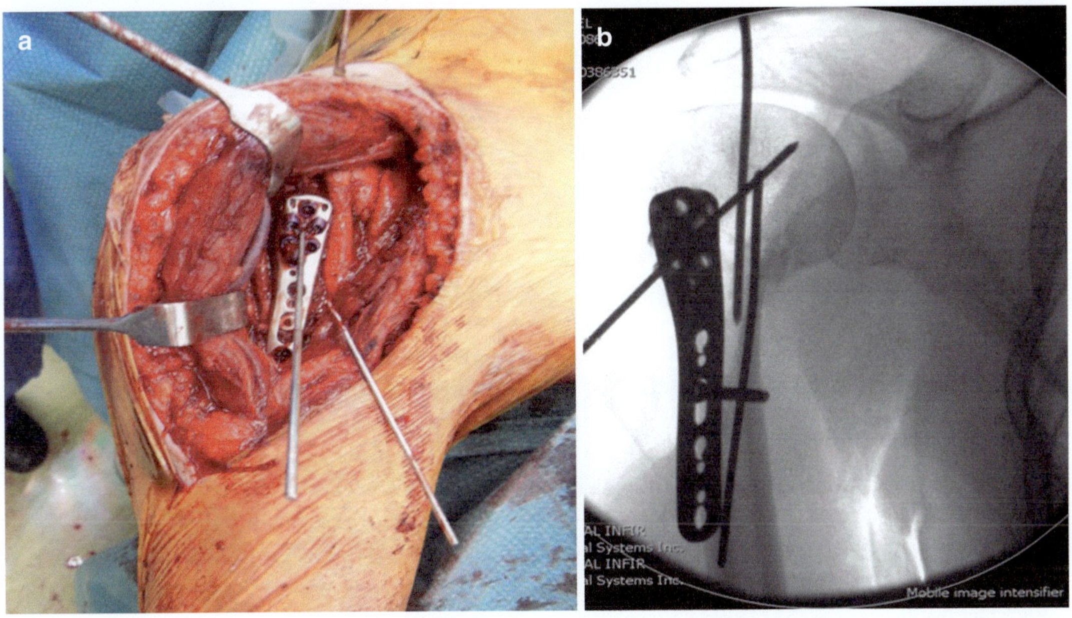

Fig. 14.11 (**a**) Intraoperative image and (**b**) fluoroscopic view demonstrating application of the plate on the humeral shaft

insertion on the greater tuberosity; any higher will cause impingement. Plate can be fixed onto the shaft using K-wires through the small holes on the plate. The anterior edge of the plate should be about half a cm behind the posterior lip of bicipital groove to avoid impinging the biceps tendon. The fracture can then be stabilised by the placement of locking screws/pegs through the head and tuberosities. Try to catch the greater tuberosity under the plate if possible depending on the fracture pattern and implant design. Check AP and axial views on the image intensifier to see if reduction is main-

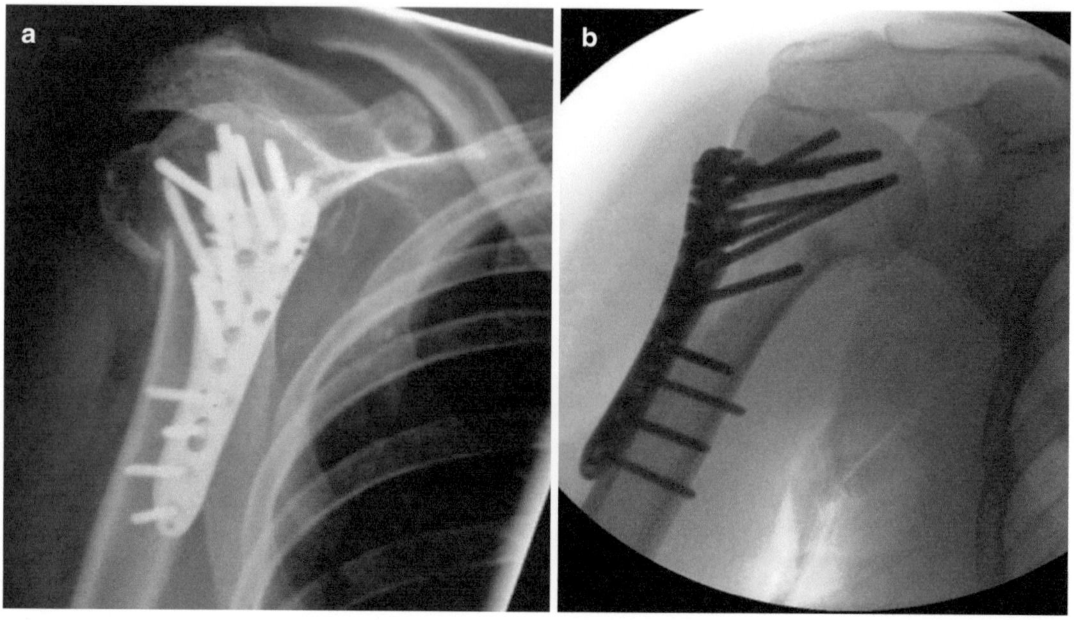

Fig. 14.12 (a) Lateral and (b) anteroposterior image intensifier views of the proximal humerus showing definite fixation of the fracture

tained on dynamic testing. Ensure the implant is well centred on AP and lateral views (Fig. 14.12 (a,b)). Minimal eight cortices are necessary distally with proximal head pegs/screws as per implant design (prefer six minimum pegs if possible). I prefer locked pegs, but additional threaded screws can be used in young strong bone or large head fragments for additional compression.

Summary of Tips, Tricks and Pitfalls

- Ensure proper positioning of the patient ensuring no interference in the surgical field from anaesthetic equipment.
- Positioning of the C-arm with a good radiographer will make the operation easier, before draping test the position of the C-arm.
- Avoid detaching capsular and rotator cuff muscles as it further compromises blood supply and preserve blood supply to head fragment with minimal dissection for reduction as necessary.
- Use non-absorbable sutures like Ethibond sutures to bring down the tuberosities and reattach to the screw holes in plates.
- Ensure good reduction with adequate release and mobilisation and control of tuberosities in complex three- or four-part fractures recreating humeral head before plate application.
- Restore Gothic arch akin to the Shenton's line in the pelvis.
- Medial calcar contract/restoration key. Calcar screw and pegs important to prevent secondary collapse.
- Locking plates always as majority in osteoporotic bone in elderly patients.
- High risk of screw penetration intraoperatively. Screen in all positions including live imaging to avoid screw penetration after nearly every screw insertion proximally.
- Balance between good subchondral fix and too far insertion of pegs/head screws. Safe distance between 5 and 8 mm.

Humeral Shaft Fractures (Transverse, Oblique, Butterfly, Bifocal)

15

Anthony Howard, Theodoros Tosounidis, and Peter V. Giannoudis

Anatomical Fracture Location

The humeral shaft commences inferior to the surgical neck, having a cylindrical cross section, which flatters in the coronal plane towards the condyles distally.

Mid-shaft humerus fractures (Fig. 15.1 (a,b)) make up 3–5% of all fractures, with a bimodal age distribution, occurring through high-energy trauma in the young and lower-energy mechanism in the elderly patients [1, 2].

The majority of these types of fractures can be managed nonoperatively [3]. It has been established that good function is retained where there is less than 3 cm shortening, <20 in the sagittal plane and <30° varus/valgus angulation [4].

The prevalence of radial nerve palsy after fractures of the humeral shaft is in the region of 12%, particularly in transverse and spiral fractures; thus closer observation of the radial nerve is essential [1]. It is imperative that in any surgical fixation, the nerve is identified and protected.

Fractures are classified according to the AO classification system. Type A1 fractures are mid-shaft spiral fractures, type A2 fractures are oblique fractures, and type A3 are transverse fractures. Butterfly fractures are classified B1–3 and bifocal fractures C1–3 dependent on their configuration.

Brief Preoperative Planning

Anatomic reduction and stable fixation are the goals of surgical management, although many of these fractures can be managed nonoperatively (Figs. 15.2 (a,b) and 15.3 (a,b,c)). Indications for surgery include failure of nonoperative management, open fractures, neurovascular injury, high-energy injury, ipsilateral radial/ulna fixation, impending pathological fractures, bilateral humeral fractures, fractures of the humeral shaft that are associated with displaced intra-articular fracture extension, obesity and polytrauma.

In comminuted fractures, a CT scan is advisable to assist in preoperative planning. In intramedullary fixation, canal size, nail length and diameter can all be estimated from radiographs of the uninjured humerus.

If there is severe comminution at the fracture site, lack of soft tissue coverage or gross swelling, an external fixation may be required as a temporizing measure; 4–5 mm pin should be employed (Figs. 15.4 and 15.5).

A. Howard • T. Tosounidis • P.V. Giannoudis (✉)
Academic Department of Trauma and Orthopaedic Surgery, University of Leeds, Leeds, UK
e-mail: pgiannoudi@aol.com

P.V. Giannoudis (ed.), *Fracture Reduction and Fixation Techniques*,
https://doi.org/10.1007/978-3-319-68628-8_15

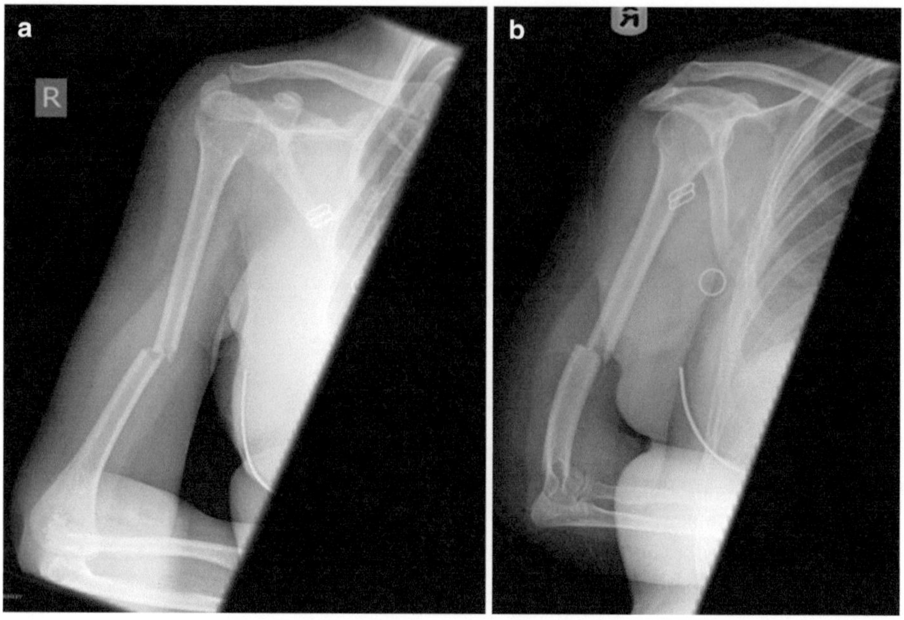

Fig. 15.1 (**a**) AP radiograph. (**b**) Lateral radiograph of right mid-shaft humeral fracture

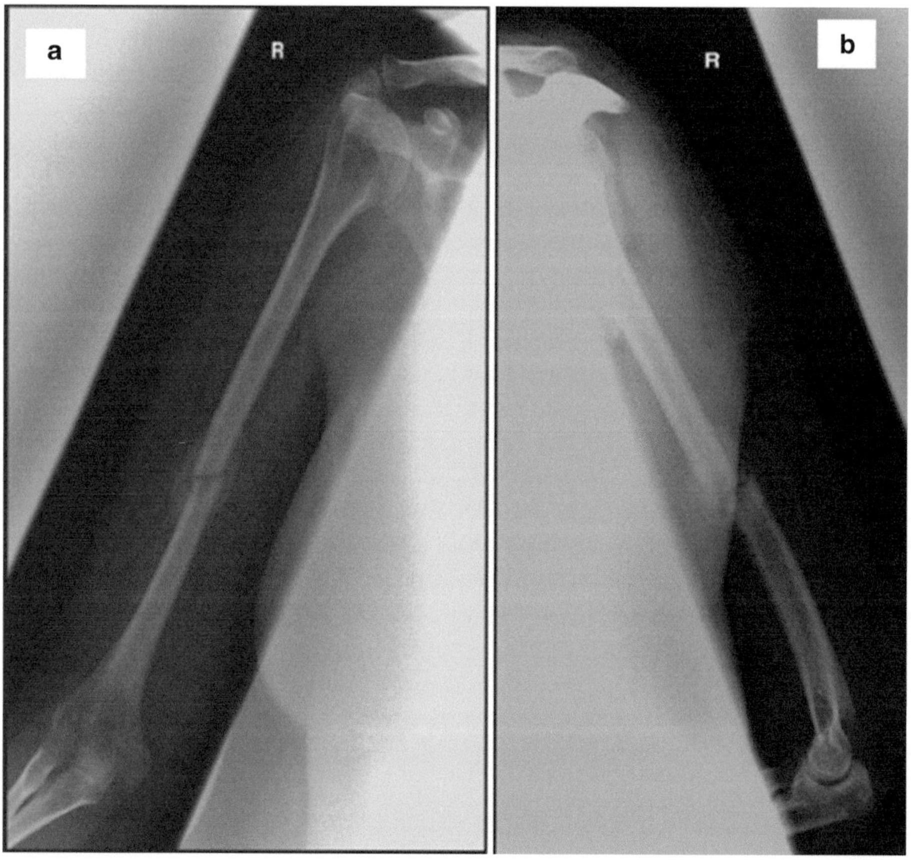

Fig. 15.2 (**a**) AP radiograph. (**b**) Lateral radiograph of a right mid-shaft humeral fracture treated with nonoperatively with a functional brace demonstrating healing 6 weeks after injury

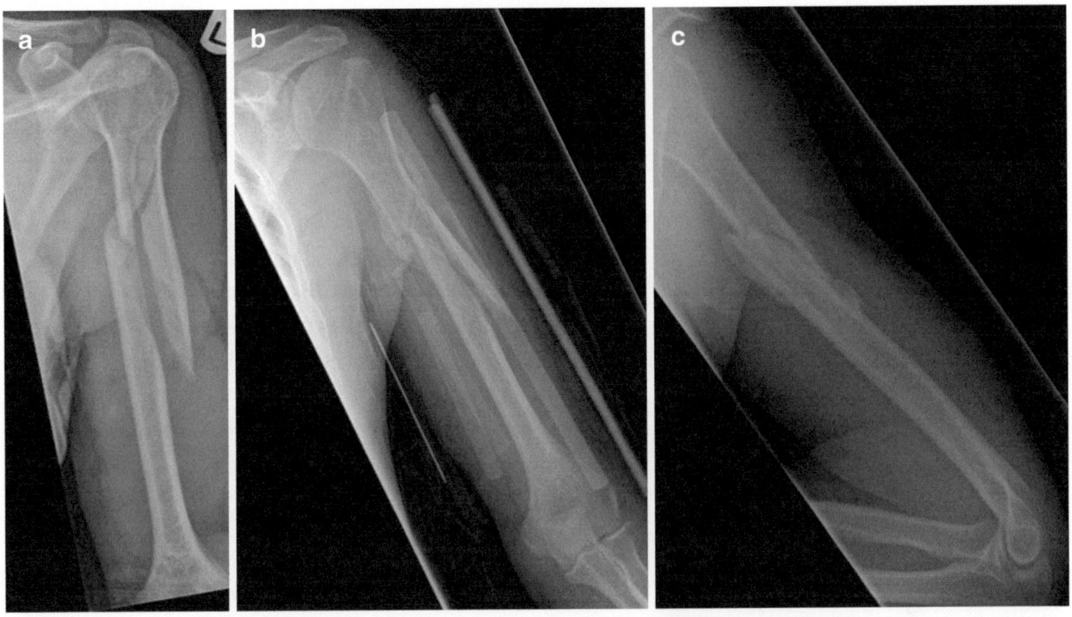

Fig. 15.3 (**a**) AP view of spiral left humeral fracture with comminution; (**b**) AP radiograph showing fracture position treated nonoperatively with a brace; (**c**) lateral view 6 weeks after injury showing fracture healing

Patient Setup in Theatre

Predominately the procedures will be undertaken under general anaesthesia, although regional blocks afford early mobilization and pain relief. Given the high incidence of radial nerve palsy and the potential for compartment syndrome, regional blocks, which mask both of these symptoms, have to be approached with caution.

The selection of fixation method and surgical approach will dictate the patient position in theatre. The beach chair or supine position can be used for antegrade nailing/anterior approach (Fig. 15.6). Whereas for retrograde nailing/posterior approach, the patient is placed in a prone position with the arm placed onto an arm board or lateral decubitus position (Fig. 15.7).

A c-arm image intensifier will need adequate access to the relevant positions, and a radiotranslucent arm board/table will be required.

Closed Reduction Manoeuvres

These are indicated when nonoperative management has been decided as the method of treatment. Closed techniques available include traction, hanging arm cast, Velpeau dressing (polysling) (Fig. 15.8) and functional brace amongst others. Usually, the initial application of a hanging cast is replaced after 3 weeks with a functional brace. Nonoperative treatment is more effective when the patient remains upright (standing or sitting) allowing the exerted gravitational force to assist in fracture reduction.

For many of the nonoperative treatments (e.g. functional bracing, hanging arm casts, polysling) in order to work most effectively, the patient should remain upright, either standing or sitting, and should avoid leaning on the elbow for support. This allows gravitational force to assist in fracture reduction. Range of motion exercises of the shoulder, elbow, wrist or fingers should com-

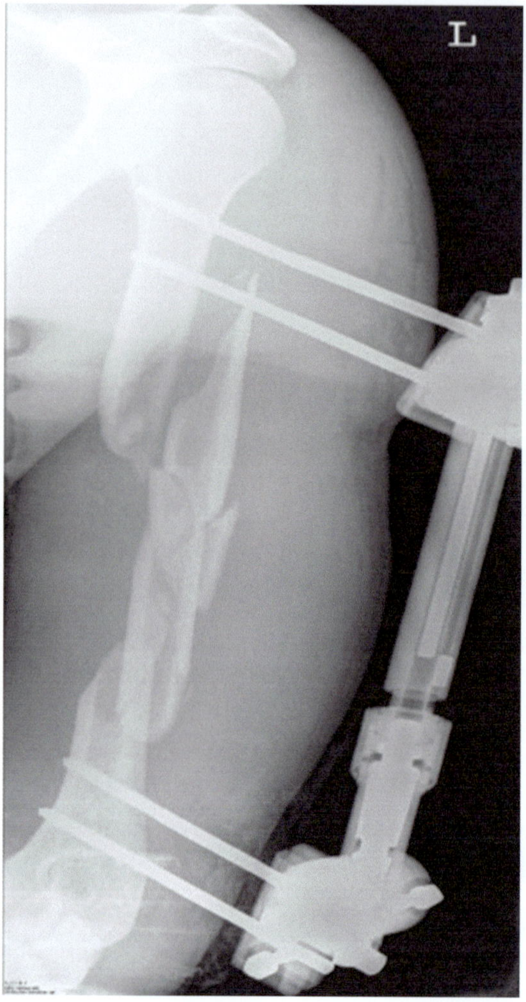

Fig. 15.4 Segmental left mid-shaft humeral fracture initially managed with an external fixator

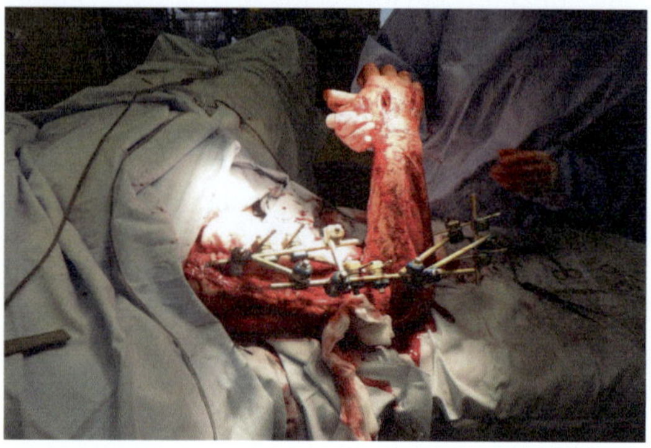

Fig. 15.5 Open right humeral shaft fracture following industrial accident stabilized with external fixator. Forearm and hand fasciotomies were performed due to compartment syndrome

mence as soon as these can be tolerated. Serial radiographic imaging is essential to ensure that satisfactory reduction can be maintained. Where this is proven difficult, then operative intervention is indicated.

Intramedullary fixation of humeral shaft fractures may be advantageous in osteoporosis and impending pathological fractures. The antegrade intramedullary nail is recommended for this type of fracture, although this has the disadvantage of damaging the rotator cuff [5]. The patient is placed in the beach chair or supine position with the head off the table, elevated at 40°. The surface anatomy is identified and marked. The incision for the nail insertion is the anterolateral corner of the acromion centred over the top of the greater tuberosity, which is extended distally no greater than 5 cm to avoid damaging the axillary nerve. Under an image intensifier, the entry point (medial to the top of the greater tuberosity/lateral to the articular margin/5 mm posterior to the bicipital groove) is identified using a K-wire. The entry point and intramedullary canal are developed in a manner appropriate to the design of nail being deployed (Fig. 15.9 (a,b)) [6, 7].

Retrograde intramedullary nail insertion requires a distal triceps-splitting approach. An entry point, 1 cm wide and 2 cm long, is made 2.5 cm proximal to the olecranon fossa. The nail can be locked proximally, either lateromedially (placing the axillary nerve at risk) or anteroposteriorly (placing the biceps tendon at risk).

For both antegrade and retrograde intramedullary nailing procedures, no residual fracture gap must be left after fixation as this will increase the risk of fracture non-union. Finally, if difficulty is noted during passage of the nail either antegrade or retrograde, thought should be given to creating an incision to safeguard that the radial nerve is not entrapped in the fracture site.

Reduction Instruments

For the humerus, reduction tools that can be used are as follows: small Hohmann retractors, small periosteal elevators, Howarth elevator,

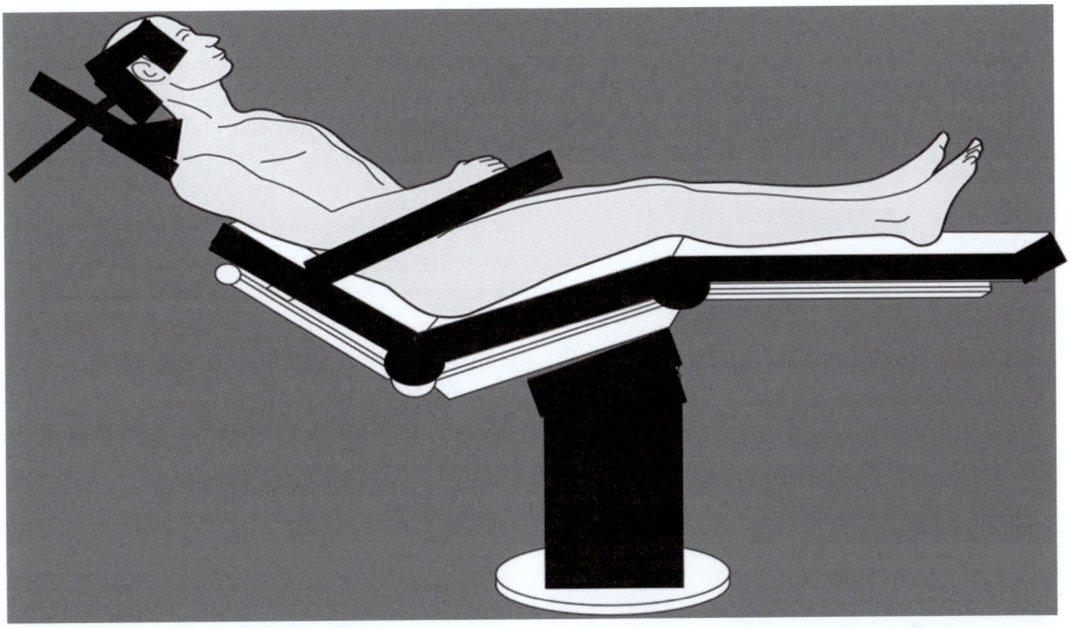

Fig. 15.6 The beach chair patient position

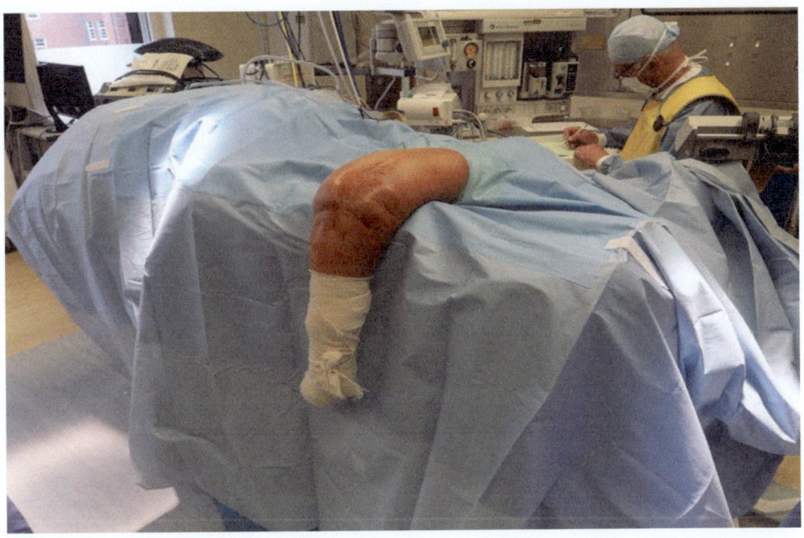

Fig. 15.7 The lateral decubitus patient position

pointed reduction clamps, blunt/serrated bone holding forceps/clamps (small "crocodile" clamps), articulated tension device and K-wires to joystick.

If severely comminuted or minimally invasive plate osteosynthesis is being adopted, then the use of an external fixation is required to reduce the risk of malalignment or mal-union [8].

Surgical Approach

The anterior lateral approach is used for proximal and mid-shaft fractures, whereas for more distal shaft fractures, the posterior approach is preferred, exploiting the flat posterior surface of the distal humerus for plate placement [9].

The anterior lateral approach is a distal extension of the deltopectoral approach, coursing along the lateral aspect of the biceps and splits the brachialis muscle. It is critical to identify the radial nerve, which is located in the lateral aspect of brachialis, and the lateral antebrachial cutaneous nerve located in the distal aspect of the incision (Fig. 15.10) [10].

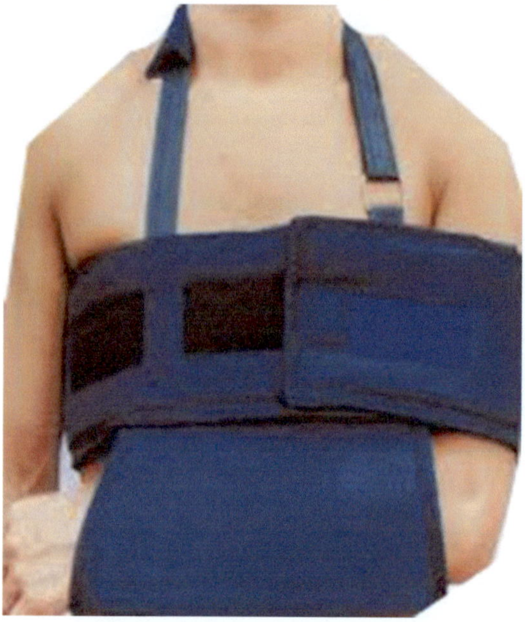

Fig. 15.8 Polysling immobilization device for nonoperatively treated humeral shaft fractures

The posterior approach with triceps splitting and radial nerve mobilization enables visualization of 76% of the humerus [11]. A large incision is made over the midline of the posterior arm extending to the olecranon fossa. Initially a plane is developed between the long and lateral heads of triceps brachii, until the deeper medial head comes into view. The medial head is then incised allowing dissection onto the humeral shaft (Fig. 15.11 (a,b,c)). The radial nerve crosses the posterior aspect of the humerus, where it is, on average, 20.7 (±1.2) cm proximal to the medial epicondyle and 14.2 (±0.6) cm proximal to the lateral condyle.

Open Reduction Manoeuvres

The fracture location relative to the deltoid and pectoralis major insertions will influence how the fracture is reduced, if the fracture is in between:

1. Rotator cuff and pectoralis major, the humeral head will abduct and internally rotate.

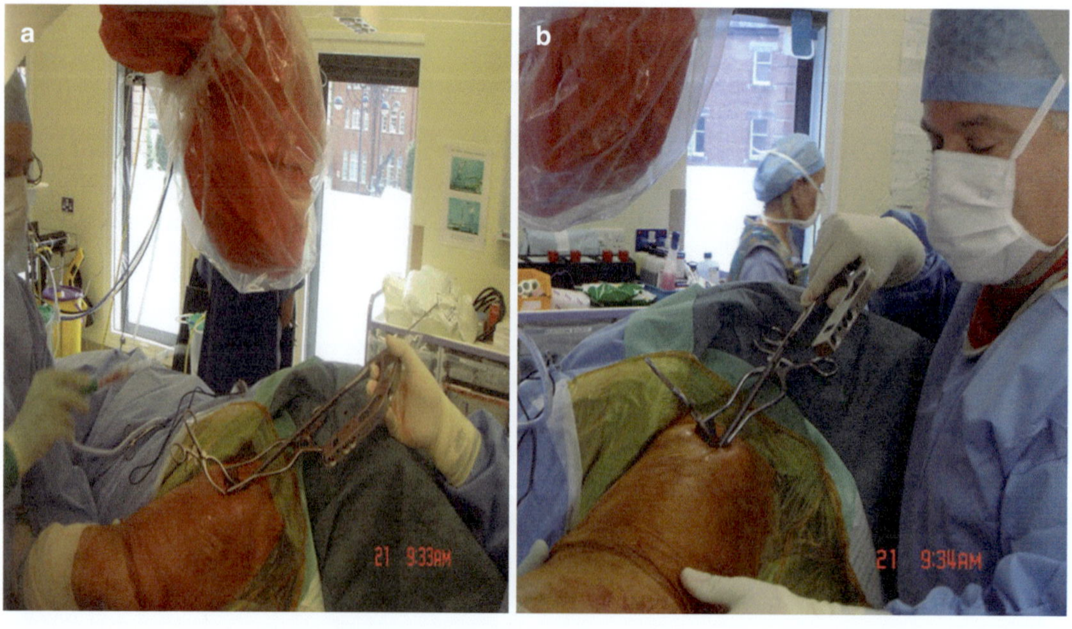

Fig. 15.9 (**a**) Humeral nail is inserted into the intramedullary canal of the humerus; (**b**) whilst closed fracture reduction is maintained, the nail is advanced to the distal fragment

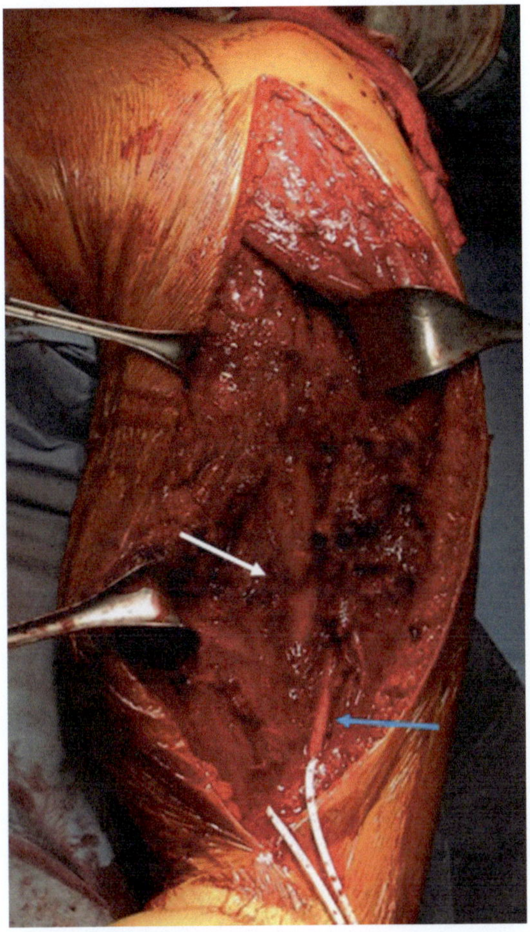

Fig. 15.10 Anterolateral approach used to expose left humeral fracture (white arrow). Blue arrow illustrates radial nerve

2. Pectoralis major and deltoid insertion, the distal fragment will shift laterally and the proximal segment will adduct.
3. Distal to the deltoid insertion the proximal segment will adduct [12].

Understanding and counteracting the respective deforming forces caused by the muscles acting on the fractured humerus will enable an easier and better reduction.

The reduction needs to be maintained until the plate fixation is secured (Fig. 15.12); for spiral or butterfly fractures, this can be achieved with a lag compression screw. The alternative is to use a small plate or cerclage wires around the definitive plate to maintain the reduction.

If there is a high degree of comminution, an external fixation may be deployed. Proximally, the pins should be inserted along the anterior margin of the deltoid insertion from anterolateral direction, Fig. 15.13 [13]. The distal pins are applied to the posterior surface of the humerus inferior to the radial groove.

Open Reduction and Fixation

The fracture fragments are released from the surrounding soft tissue to enable inspection of fracture site and to achieve a good reduction. Both ends of the fractures are held in crocodile clamps to allow rotation of the two ends into the appropriate orientation to achieve reduction. The rotation to achieve this reduction is often the reverse of the deforming forces that caused the fracture or muscle forces acting on the now fractured humerus, Fig. 15.14 (a,b,c,d).

It is critical that a good reduction is achieved and maintained; in spiral or oblique fractures, this reduction and compression can be achieved by using a lag screw. If the humeral fracture is transverse or an oblique angle of less than 30°, then the reduction and compression can be achieved by using a DCP plate in compression mode. As a minimum six cortices of fixation proximal and distal to the fracture site should be achieved, Fig. 15.15 (a,b). Care needs to be taken to ensure the plate does not impinge on the shoulder joint [14]. Further, it is also important to pay attention to the working length created by the construct. If early mobilization is desired or there may be poor patient compliance anticipated, then the placement of a secondary plate at 90°, in the transverse plane, is advisable.

In highly comminuted fracture, distraction needs to be applied to achieve restoration of length and a long plate employed in a bridging mode configuration. With the appropriate expertise, a minimally invasive percutaneous osteosynthesis technique can be used in these circumstances, having the advantage of reducing biological disruption and soft tissue dissection. In a recent network meta-analysis found comparative to plates, intramedullary nails are more advantageous [14].

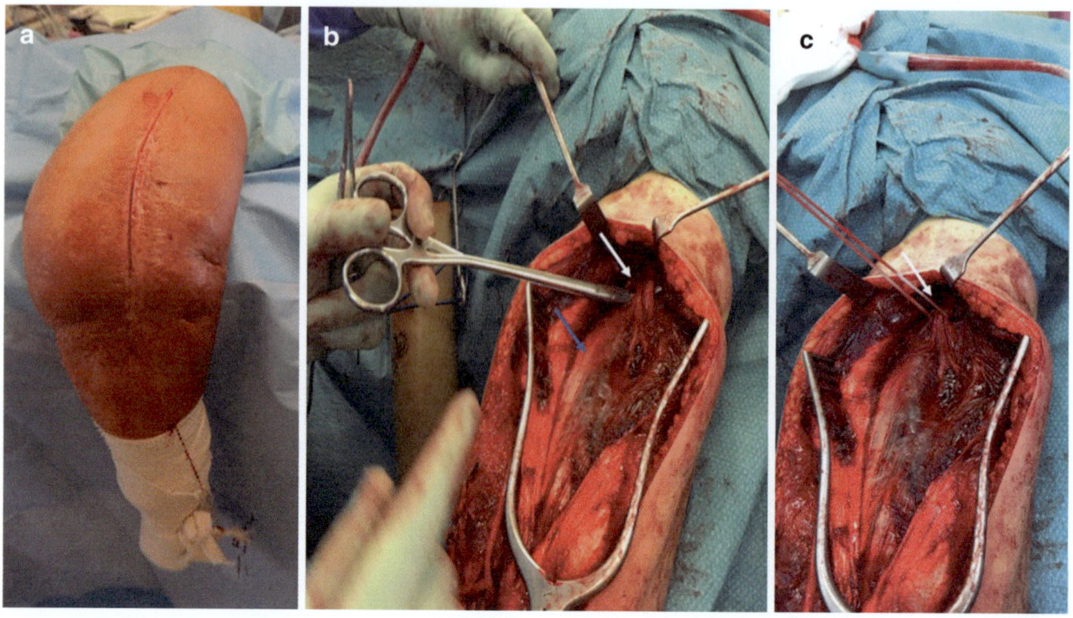

Fig. 15.11 (**a**) A large incision is made over the midline of the posterior arm extending to the olecranon fossa. (**b**) A plane is developed between the long and lateral heads of triceps brachii, until the deeper medial head comes into view. Note mobilization of radial nerve with artery clip forceps (white arrow points to radial nerve; blue arrow points to medial head of triceps). (**c**) Image illustrates isolation of radial nerve

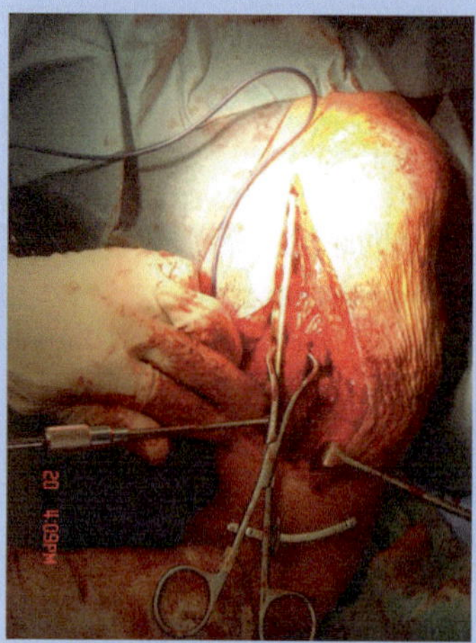

Fig. 15.12 Using the anterolateral approach, the humeral fracture has been reduced with reduction forceps with the plate to use for fixation place in position to continue with fixation whilst maintaining reduction

During the procedure, if feasible, the nerve needs to be identified and protected, with careful movement of the arm during fixation to avoid iatrogenic injury.

Summary of Tips and Tricks-Pitfalls

- If the fracture is managed in a brace, this will need to be tightened periodically over the initial 2 weeks to account for the reduction in swelling.
- Pendulum exercises should be encouraged regardless of the type of management to promote shoulder joint flexibility.
- The humerus needs to be treated as a full load-bearing structure, in terms of the fixation decision-making.
- During the posterior approach, identify and isolate the radial nerve to avoid iatrogenic nerve damage. Ensure that the nerve can sit freely over the plate (Fig. 15.16).

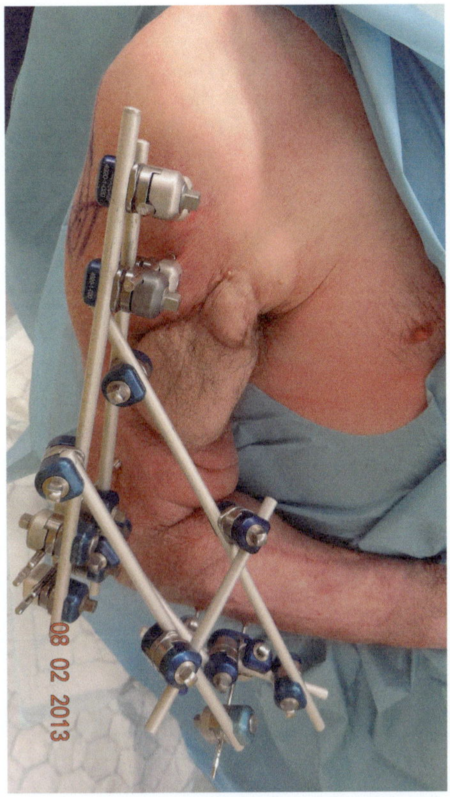

Fig. 15.13 An open humeral fracture that was treated with a rectus abdominal free flap and an external fixator

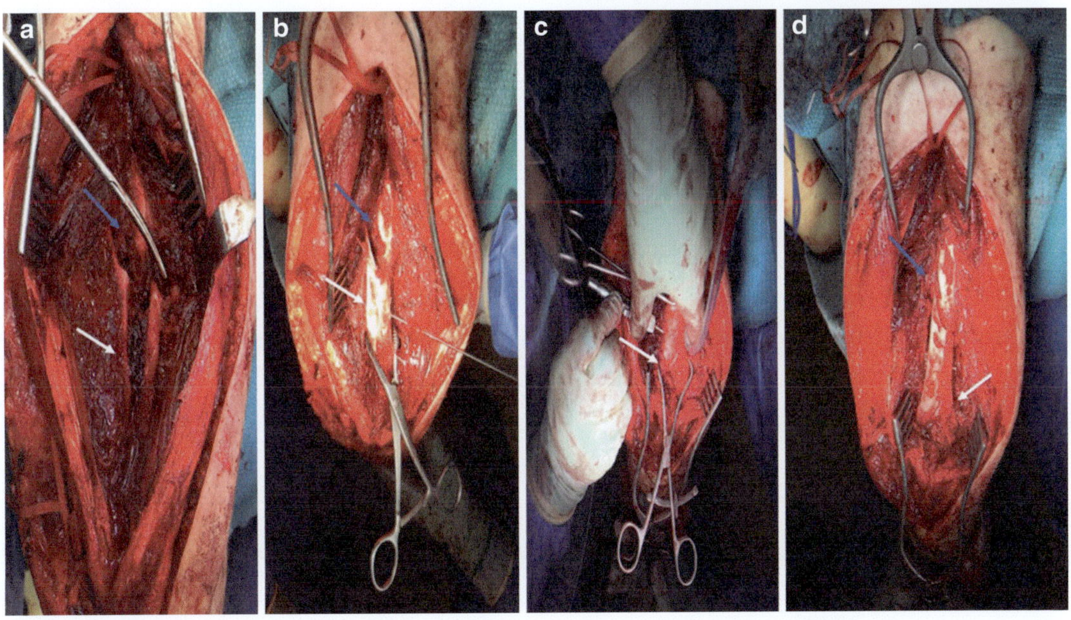

Fig. 15.14 (**a**) Using a posterior approach, the distal 1/3 shaft of the humeral fracture has been exposed. White arrow demonstrates the two-part split of the distal fragment. Blue arrow illustrates fracture line. (**b**) Split of distal fragment has been reduced with a reduction forceps and a K-wire (white arrow). Blue arrow is the fracture line. (**c**) A lag screw is inserted into the split distal fragment to convert it to one piece. (**d**) Following insertion of lag screw, distal fragment moves as one unit (white arrow). It can now be connected to the proximal fragment. Blue arrow represents the fracture line

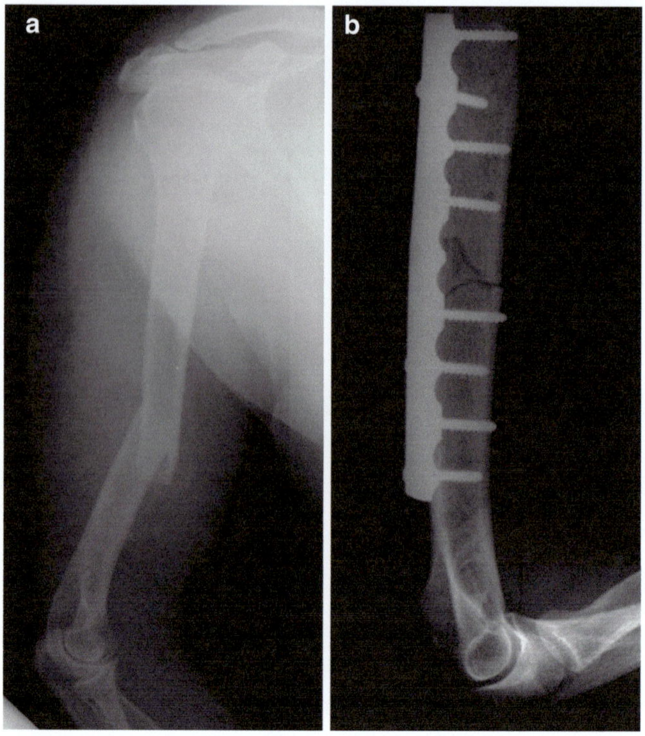

Fig. 15.15 (**a**) AP and (**b**) lateral radiographs of a mid-shaft humeral fracture stabilized with a plate using a posterior approach. Note that there are four screws supporting each fragment

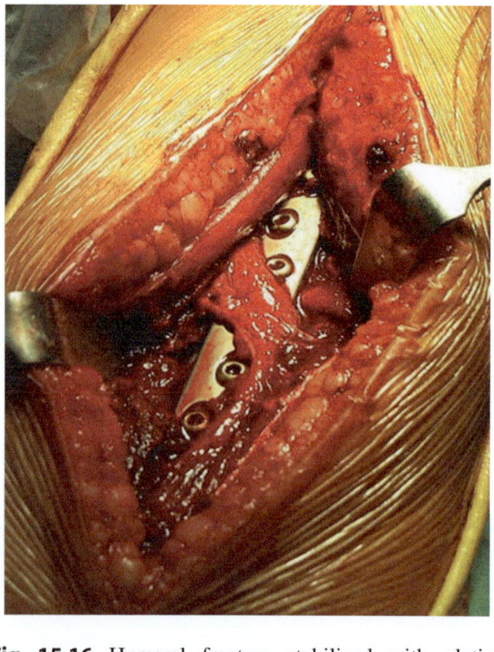

Fig. 15.16 Humeral fracture stabilized with plating using posterior approach. Note the radial never sitting freely above the plate

- Ensure that the image intensifier is rotated during surgical fixation rather than the arm, reducing the risk of iatrogenic injury.
- Compression plating is the preferred method of fixation compared to intramedullary nailing.

References

1. Shao YC, Harwood P, Grotz MR, Limb D, Giannoudis PV. Radial nerve palsy associated with fractures of the shaft of the humerus. J Bone Joint Surg Br. 2005;87-B(12):1647–52.
2. Humeral Shaft Fractures. https://www.orthobullets.com/trauma/1016/humeral-shaft-fractures.
3. Walker MPB, Badman B, Brooks J, Van Gelderen J, Mighell M. Humeral shaft fractures: a review. J Shoulder Elb Surg. 2011;20(5):833–44.
4. Klenerman L. Fractures of the shaft of the humerus. J Bone Joint Surg Br. 1966;48(1):105–11.
5. Bencic I, Cengic T, Prenc J, Bulatovic N, Matejcic A. Humeral nail: comparison of the antegrade and retrograde application. Acta Clin Croat. 2016;55(1):110–6.

6. Euler SA, Petri M, Venderley MB, Dornan GJ, Schmoelz W, Turnbull TL, Plecko M, Kralinger FS, Millett PJ. Biomechanical evaluation of straight antegrade nailing in proximal humeral fractures: the rationale of the "proximal anchoring point". Int Orthop. 2017;41(9):1715–21.
7. Langer P, Born C. Intramedullary fixation of humeral shaft fractures. In: Wiesel S, editor. Operative techniques in orthopaedic surgery. London: Lippincott Williams & Wilkins; 2011.
8. Lee H-J, C-W O, J-K O, Apivatthakakul T, Kim J-W, Yoon J-P, Lee D-J, Jung J-W. Minimally invasive plate osteosynthesis for humeral shaft fracture: a reproducible technique with the assistance of an external fixator. Arch Orthop Trauma Surg. 2013;133(5):649–57.
9. Garberina M, Getz C. Plate fixation of humeral shaft fractures. In: Wiesel S, editors. Operative techniques in orthopaedic surgery. London:Lippincott Williams & Wilkins.
10. Carroll EA, Schweppe M, Langfitt M, Miller AN, Halvorson JJ. Management of humeral shaft fractures. J Am Acad Orthop Surg. 2012;20(7):423–33.
11. Gerwin M, Hotchkiss RN, Weiland AJ. Alternative operative exposures of the posterior aspect of the humeral diaphysis with reference to the radial nerve. J Bone Joint Surg Am. 1996;78(11):1690–5.
12. Higgs D. Humeral shaft fractures - principles of management. In: Bentley G, editor. European surgical orthopaedics and traumatology. Berlin: Springer; 2014.
13. Crenshaw A. Fractures of shoulder, arm and forearm. In: Canale ST, Beaty JH, Campbell WC, editors. Campbell's operative orthopaedics, vol. 3. London: Mowby; 2003.
14. Zhao JG, Wang J, Meng XH, Zeng XT, Kan SL. Surgical interventions to treat humerus shaft fractures: a network meta-analysis of randomized controlled trials. PLoS One. 2017;12(3):e0173634.

16 Distal Humerus Fracture

Stefaan Nijs

Anatomical Fracture Location

Distal humerus fractures are fractures of the distal metaphysis of the humerus with or without involvement of the articular surface.

The distal metaphysis of the humerus can be considered as a triangle, consisting of a radial and an ulnar column, between which the joint block is positioned (Fig. 16.1). The joint block consists of the hemispheric capitellum humeri on the radial side and the spool-shaped trochlea on the ulnar side.

In the frontal plane, the axis of the trochlea makes an angle of 94°–98°, relative to the humeral diaphyseal axis (Fig. 16.2). Therefore, the forearm is not in line with the arm. The angle between both is what we call the 'carrying angle'. The axis of rotation, a line drawn between the centre of the capitellum and the centre of the trochlear sulcus, exits medially just anterior and inferior to the medial epicondyle. It has the same angulation as the axis of the trochlea.

In the sagittal plane, the medial (ulnar) column angulates 10°–20° to the longitudinal axis of

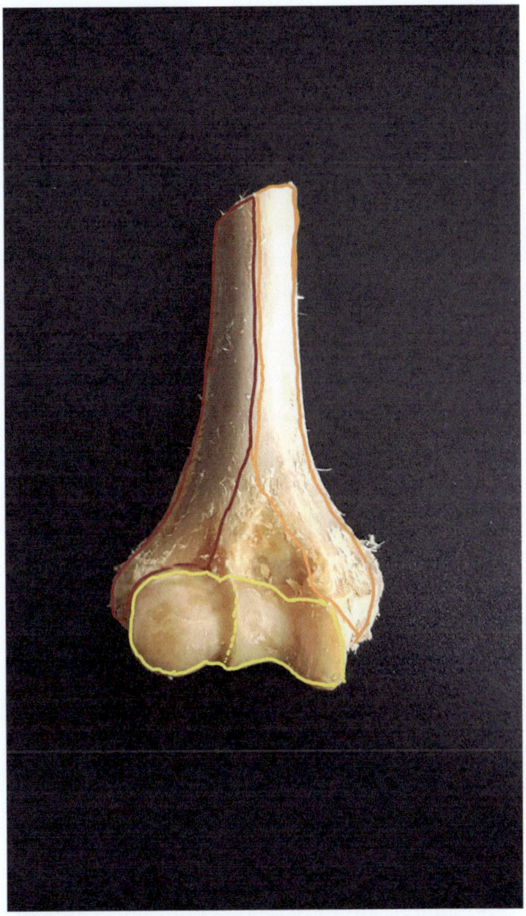

Fig. 16.1 AP view of the distal humerus, showing the radial column (dark red), the ulnar column (orange) and the interposed articular block (yellow)

S. Nijs
Department Trauma Surgery, UZ Leuven, Leuven, Belgium

Department Development and Regeneration, KU Leuven, Leuven, Belgium
e-mail: stefaan.nijs@uzleuven.be

P.V. Giannoudis (ed.), *Fracture Reduction and Fixation Techniques*,
https://doi.org/10.1007/978-3-319-68628-8_16

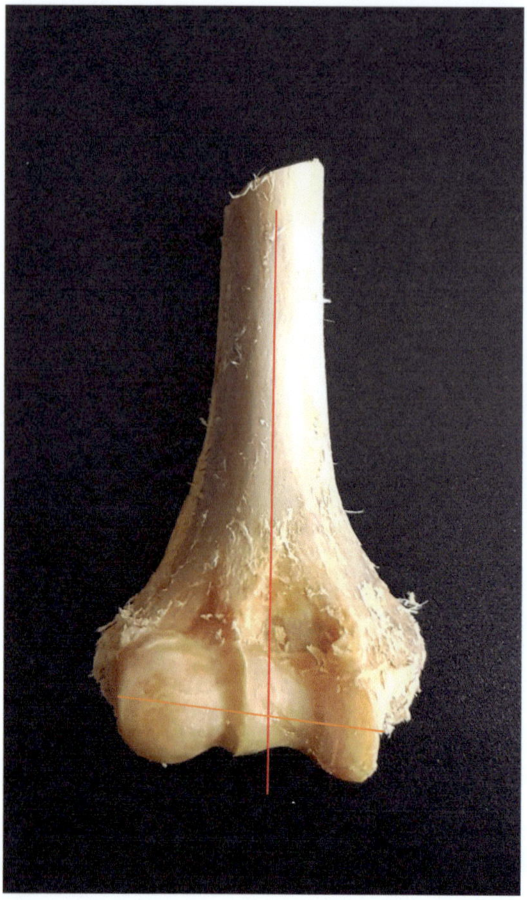

Fig. 16.2 AP view of the distal humerus. There is a 94°–98° angle between the longitudinal axis of the humerus (red) and the trochlear axis (orange)

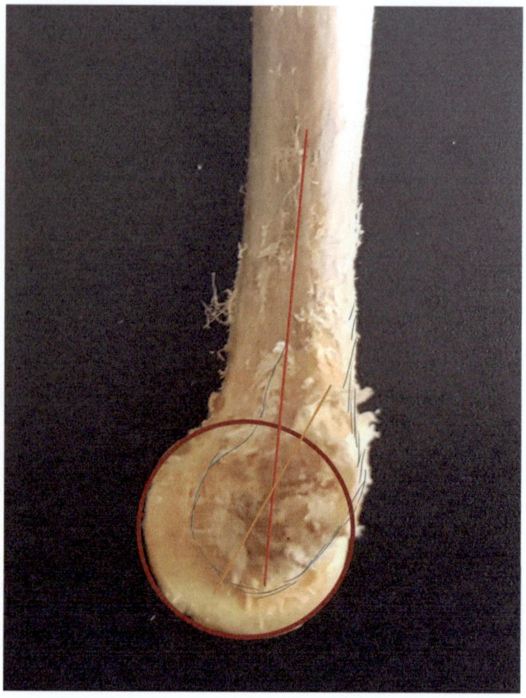

Fig. 16.3 Medial view of the distal humerus. The medial column (orange) makes a 10° angulation to the longitudinal humerus axis (red), positioning the trochlea slightly in front of the humeral shaft

the humerus (Fig. 16.3). The lateral column (radial) angulates 30°–40° to the longitudinal axis of the humerus (Fig. 16.4).

In physiological circumstances, about 60% of the forearm load is transmitted to the humerus through the radio-capitellar joint. This load transmission however is influenced by the relative position of both forearm bones in elbow flexion and/or elbow extension.

Fractures are classified according to the AO classification system. A-type fractures are extra-articular fractures. B-type fractures are partial-articular, mono-column fractures. C-type fractures are articular, bi-column fractures.

Brief Preoperative Planning

Anatomic reduction and stable fixation are the goals of surgical management of distal humerus fractures. For the articular component, absolute stability is the aim for stability; for the metaphyseal components, relative stability is the goal.

This mandates for open reduction and internal fixation. Indirect and minimal reduction and fixation techniques yield suboptimal result and should be avoided. Standard open reduction and internal fixation techniques with meticulous soft tissue handling should be employed.

In order to evaluate the fracture and to adequately plan, CT scan with 3D reconstruction is preferred (Fig. 16.5). Preoperative planning should take into account the comminution of the articular surface and of both columns. Furthermore, CT is extremely useful to determine the presence of capitellar shear fractures (Fig. 16.6).

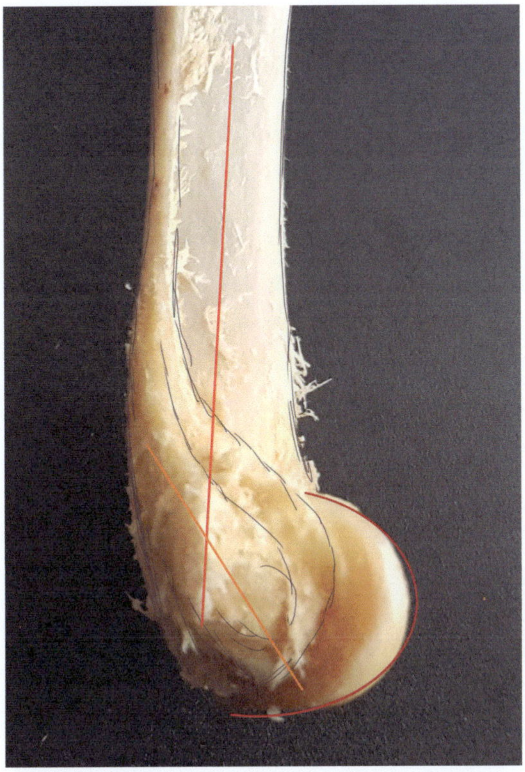

Fig. 16.4 Lateral view of the distal humerus. The lateral column makes a 30° angulation to the humeral axis. Therefore, the capitellum is positioned in front of the humeral diaphysis

Anatomically preshaped plates are available for the fixation of the humerus with 3.5 mm screws in the metadiaphyseal part and 2.7 mm screws in the articular area. One should be able to choose between cortical and angular stable screw options (preferably variable angle angular stability). For metaphyseal and/or articular fractures, a double plating system, i.e. a medial plate combined to a posterolateral or lateral plate, is preferred. In AO B-type fractures, a mono-plate fixation in combination to a lag screw can be used.

Traditionally (AO philosophy) distal humerus fractures have been instrumented by a medial and a posterolateral plate (90° construct). This has been challenged by O'Driscoll, proposing a fixation by medial and lateral plates (180° construct) [1]. No clinical study could prove a benefit of one construct over the other [2]. Biomechanically 180° constructs are more stiff under axial loading [3], but both constructs show loads to failure well above clinical loads [4]. Based upon these observations, we developed a treatment strategy as in Algorithm 16.1.

For extra-articular fractures at the metadiaphyseal transition or with diaphyseal extension, a single posterolateral 3.5 mm angular stable plate can be used.

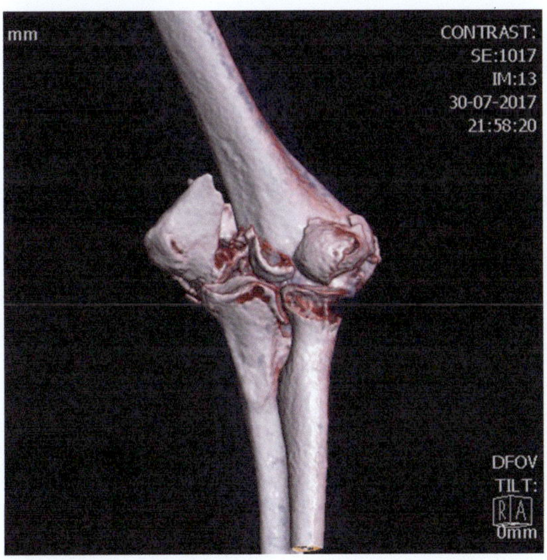

Fig. 16.5 3D CT shows the extension of articular comminution and fragment displacement

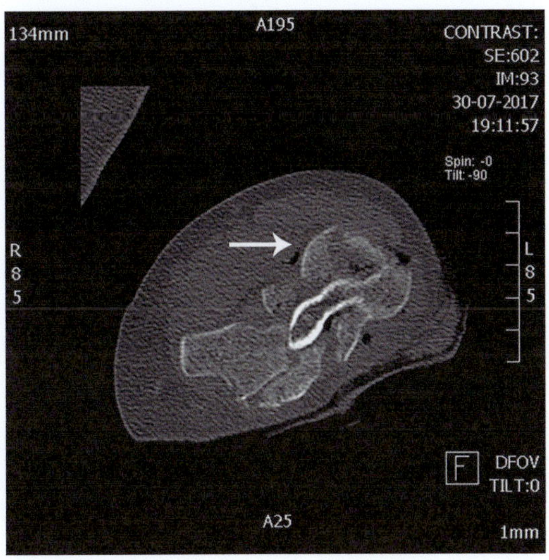

Fig. 16.6 Axial CT scan image showing the coronal shear fragment (arrow)

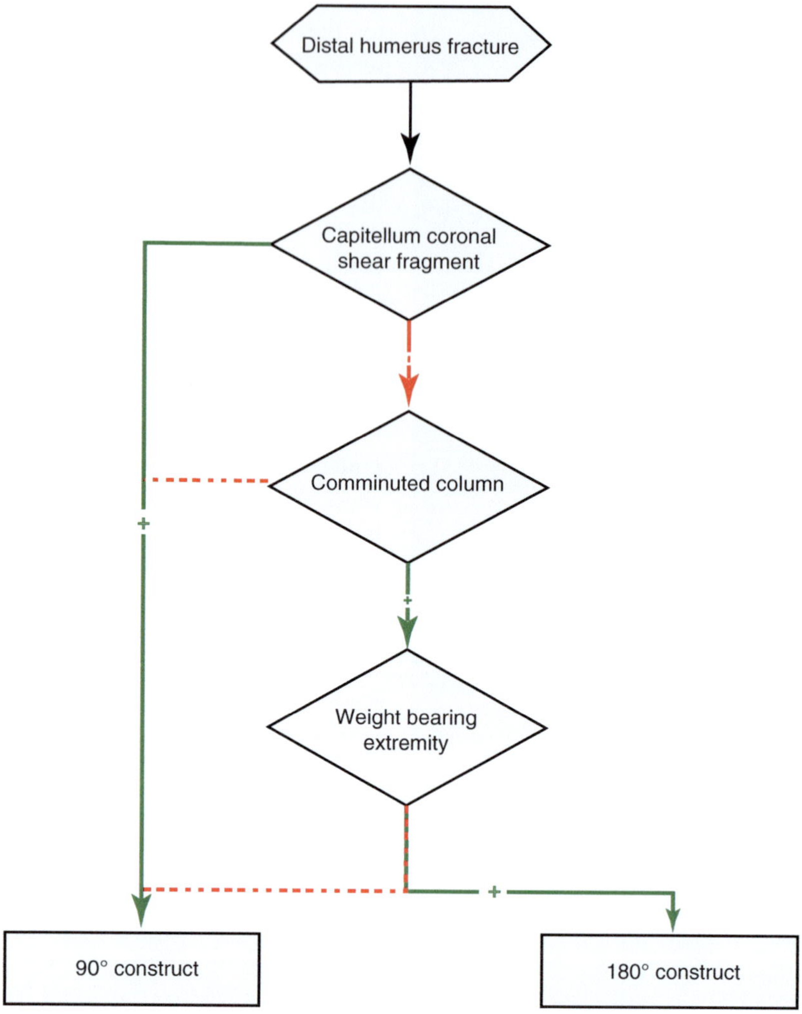

Algorithm 16.1 Plate-positioning algorithm

To fix small articular fragments, headless compression screws and/or resorbable pins can be used.

For temporary fixation, 1.6 mm and 2 mm K-wires can be used.

Fixation of an eventual olecranon osteotomy would require 2 mm K-wires and metal wire (1.25 mm) or anatomical preshaped plates.

Patient Set-up in Theatre

General anaesthesia is preferred as the procedure can be of longer duration. A regional block can be used to reduce postoperative pain and allow for early mobilization. Attention should be given not to mask a compartment syndrome and/or neural (ulnar nerve) injury.

The patient is positioned prone or in lateral decubitus on a standard table, and the affected arm is placed on a radiolucent side table. One should check prior to draping that free flexion of the elbow, well over 90°, is possible so that visualization of the anterior compartment of the elbow (capitellum and anterior half of the trochlea) is guaranteed. The table is placed in such a way that unobstructed intraoperative imaging can be performed. This usually requires rotation of the table 90° so that the affected extremity is

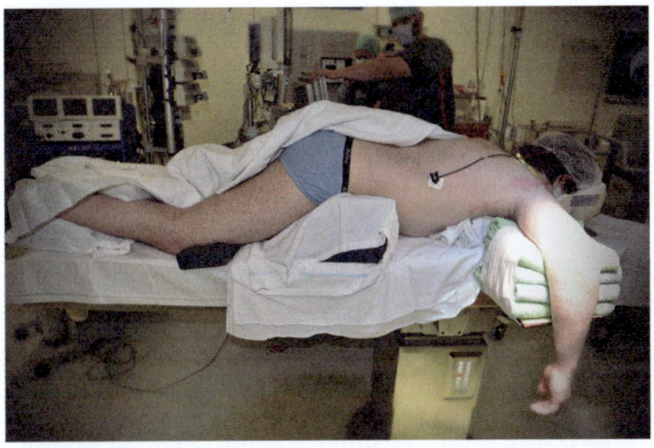

Fig. 16.7 The patient is positioned prone on a standard table, and the affected arm is placed on a radiolucent side table

placed at the centre of the operating theatre (Fig. 16.7). A tourniquet is placed, and the affected extremity is prepped and draped following the administration of intravenous antibiotics. Some people prefer not to use a tourniquet because they fear the procedural time exceeds that of allowed tourniquet use. However, this causes more blood loss, and because of the blurred visualization, caused by excessive bleeding, surgical time increases. The image intensifier is brought from the top of the patient.

Closed Reduction Manoeuvres

Closed reduction manoeuvres are not used for distal humerus fractures. In cases with extreme soft tissue situations (swelling, bruising), a temporary external fixator can be used until subsidence of the swelling. In those circumstances, a fixation in extension allows for easier and more stable fixation, than a 90° fixation.

Reduction Instruments

For the humerus, reduction tools that can be used are the following: small Hohmann retractors, small periosteal elevators, Howarth elevator, pointed reduction clamps, blunt/serrated bone holding forceps/clamps (small 'crocodile' clamps), articulated tension device, K-wires to joystick and temporarily fixing fragments.

Surgical Approach

A straight posterior incision over the distal humerus, aiming at the posterior crest of the ulna, is made. This incision curves around the tip of the olecranon, avoiding excessive pressure at the wound after closure (Fig. 16.8). The skin and subcuticular tissue are taken down as one to the level of the fascia overlying the triceps, creating two big skin flaps (Fig. 16.9).

We start creating a lateral window. The triceps muscle is mobilized off the humerus at its lateral edge (Fig. 16.10). If needed, this approach can be extended proximal up to the level of the deltoid insertion (Fig. 16.11). Along the lateral border of the triceps, we can identify the posterior antebrachial cutaneous nerve. Following this nerve proximally will guide us to the radial nerve. In cases of fractures with proximal extension towards the diaphysis, identifying and protecting the radial nerve while reflecting it medially are a must requirement (Fig. 16.12).

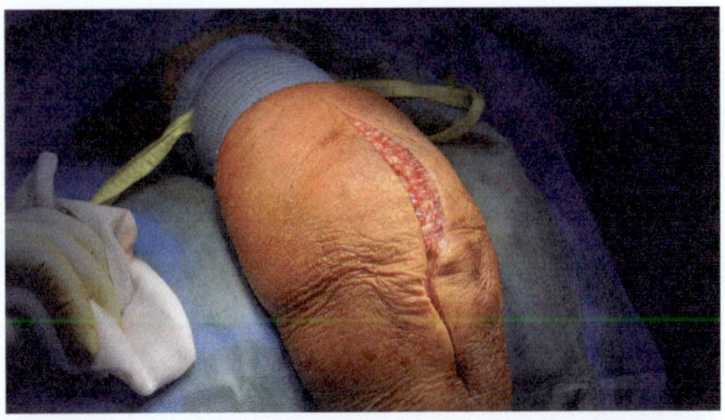

Fig. 16.8 Straight posterior incision, making a curve around the olecranon tip

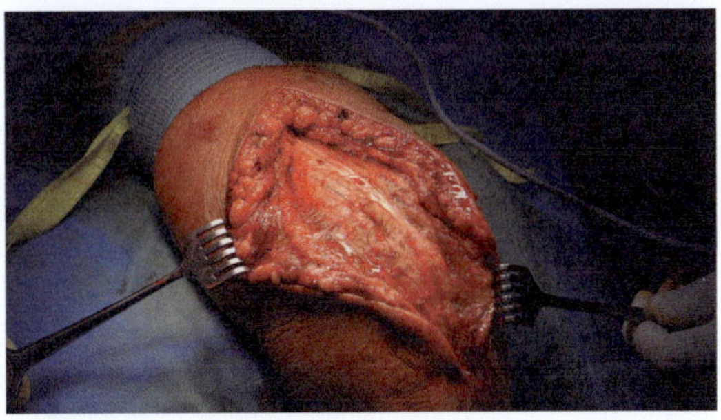

Fig. 16.9 The incision is taken down to the triceps fascia, creating big skin-subcutaneous flaps medially and laterally

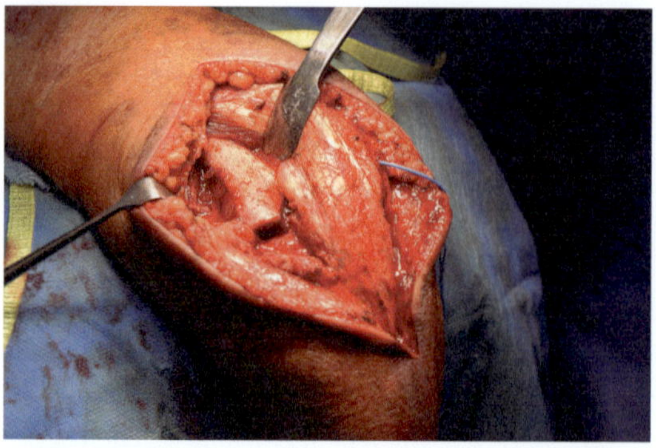

Fig. 16.10 After creating a lateral window, releasing the triceps of the lateral septum, extending distally in Kocher's interval (between anconeus and extensor carpi ulnaris), the lateral column can be visualized

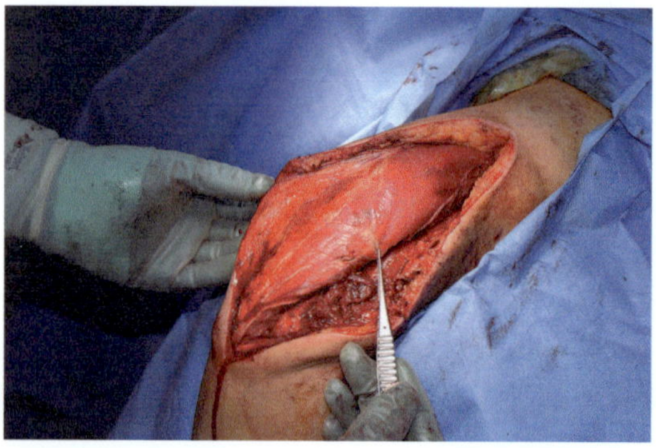

Fig. 16.11 Proximal extension of the release to the level of the deltoid insertion. The posterior antebrachial cutaneous nerve can be recognized and guide us to the radial nerve

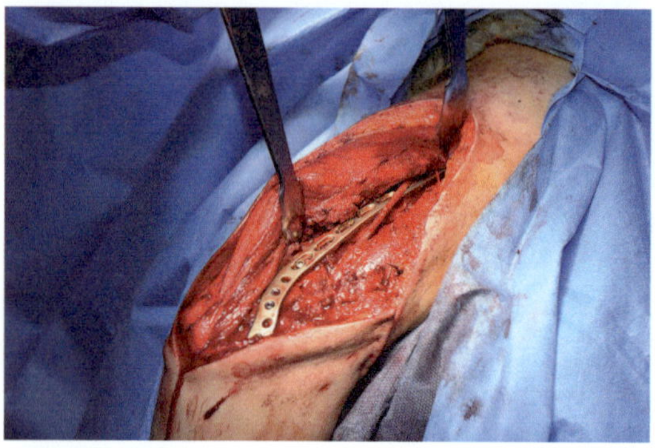

Fig. 16.12 Reflecting the entire triceps laterally visualizes the humeral diaphysis and the radial nerve. Implants need to be positioned underneath the nerve. A thin layer of soft tissue should be positioned between the nerve and the implant to avoid adherence

To visualize the distal part of the radial column and the posterior surface, the approach can be extended in the interval between the anconeus and extensor carpi ulnaris muscle (Kocher's interval) (Fig. 16.13).

For more distal and intra-articular fractures, a second window is created. The ulnar nerve is dissected on the medial side (Fig. 16.14). It is important to leave the nerve together with its vascularization and a layer of soft tissue around it, to cover later implants, avoiding direct contact between the implant and the nerve (Fig. 16.15).

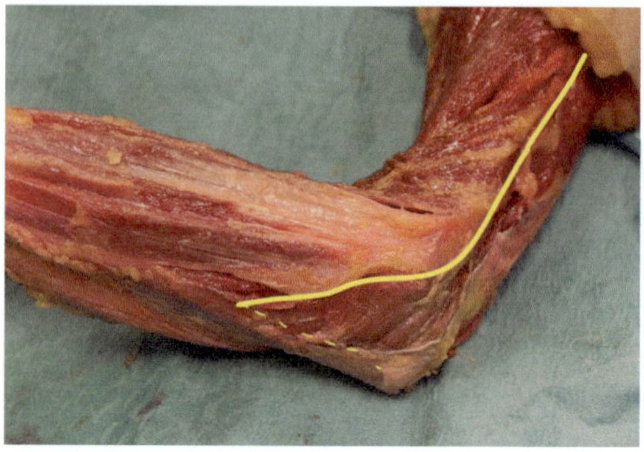

Fig. 16.13 The radial incision can be extended in Kocher's interval (yellow line). When an osteotomy becomes necessary, the anconeus can be mobilized of its ulnar insertion, reflecting the anconeus together with the triceps, respecting its innervation that comes of a radial nerve branch, going through the triceps

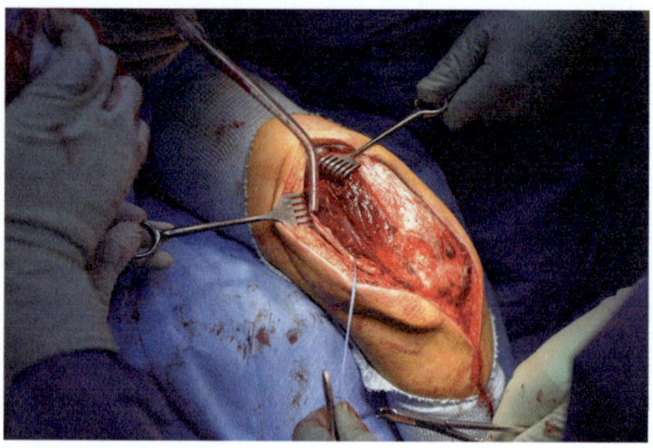

Fig. 16.14 Medially the ulnar nerve should be mobilized from above the arcade of Struthers to the level of the deep flexor-pronator aponeurosis, opening the cubital retinaculum and Osborne's ligament and identifying the first motor branch to the flexor carpi ulnaris

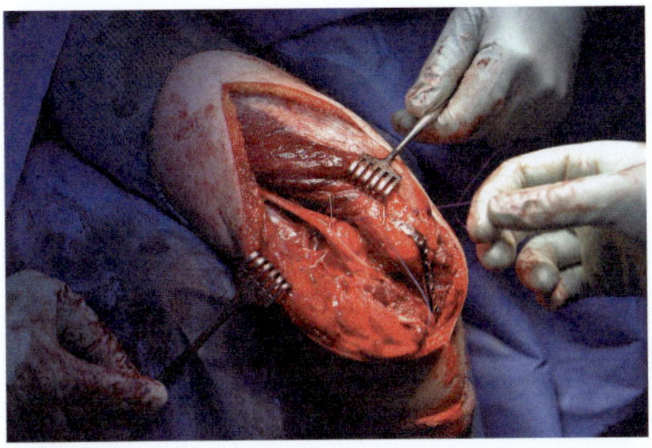

Fig. 16.15 A thin layer of soft tissue, containing among others the nerve blood supply, should be left together with the nerve. This makes it possible to reposition this layer between the nerve and the implant, avoiding adhesion. It is important to preserve the nerve vascularization, as post-op ischemia is an important cause of neuritis

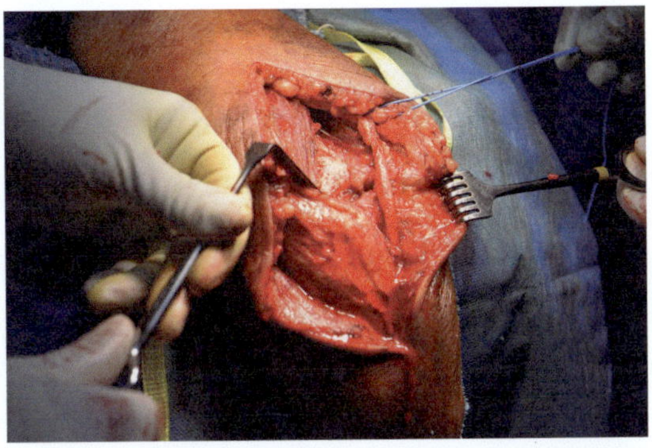

Fig. 16.16 After mobilization of the medial triceps, a second medial window can be created that allows visualization of the medial column

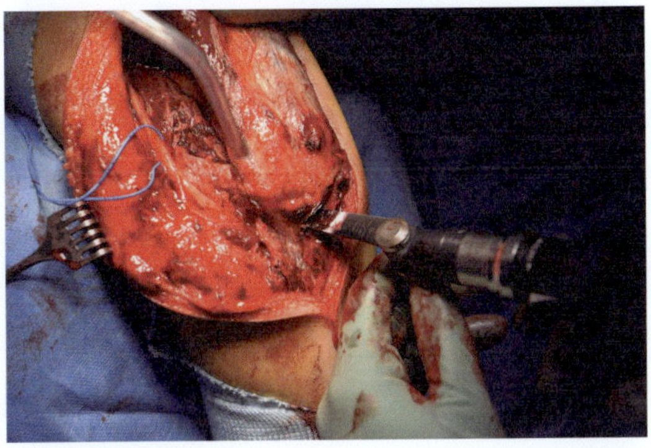

Fig. 16.17 In complex articular fractures, a Chevron osteotomy is performed. The apex lays at the bare area of the olecranon fossa, between the coronoid and the olecranon process

The nerve should be mobilized from above the arcade of Struthers to the level of the deep flexor-pronator aponeurosis, opening the cubital retinaculum and Osborne's ligament and identifying the first motor branch to the flexor carpi ulnaris. In cases where anterior transposition of the nerve is performed, a piece of the medial intermuscular septum should be resected, avoiding kinking of the nerve over the septum after transposition. After mobilization of the nerve, a window to the humerus can be created, medial to the nerve, mobilizing the triceps of the humerus (Fig. 16.16).

Both windows will be sufficient to treat extra-articular and simple intra-articular fractures. In cases of extensive intra-articular comminution however, more visualization of the articular surface is necessary. Many approaches have been described; however, the approach giving the most extensile visualization of the joint surface is the olecranon osteotomy. A chevron osteotomy, apex distal, is performed (Fig. 16.17). We release the anconeus first of its ulnar insertion, leaving it in continuity to the triceps, and reflect it, together with the triceps proximally. This TRAP approach avoids denervation, and subsequent atrophy, of the anconeus. The anconeus is an active stabilizing muscle to the elbow (posterior stability radial head). The osteotomy is performed with its apex at the level of the bare area, between the olecranon and the coronoid processes [5].

Open Reduction Manoeuvres

The fracture is identified, and it is debrided from soft tissue debris and hematoma (Fig. 16.18).

In most cases, the fracture of one of both columns is simple. If this is the case, this column is reduced first. It is held in its reduced position using K-wires and reduction clamps (Fig. 16.19). In case of articular fracture, the articular surface is reconstructed next. Perfect anatomical reduction is aimed for. In case of simple articular fracture, a large reduction clamp is used across the fracture to put it under compression. In comminuted cases, this should be avoided, as overcompression could result in loss of articular width and therefore in joint incongruency. Again, the

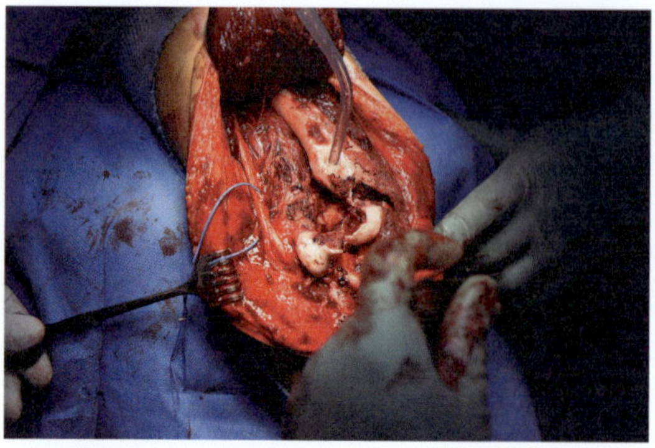

Fig. 16.18 After osteotomy we visualize the fracture. Fracture haematoma is rinsed and removed

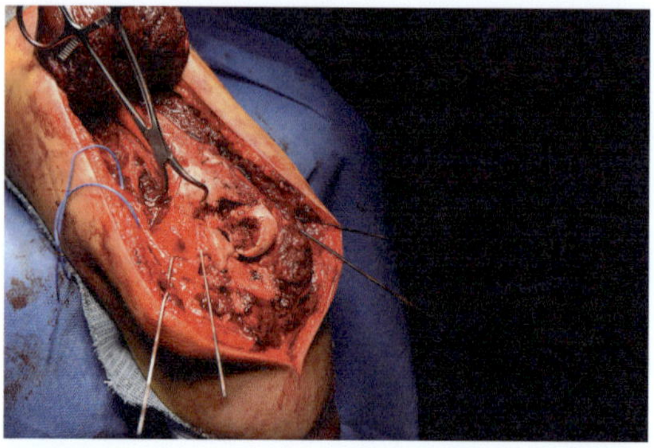

Fig. 16.19 The column(s) are repositioned and temporarily hold by K-wires and reduction clamps

reduction is held with multiple small K-wires (Fig. 16.20). Finally the second column is reconstructed. If this fracture is simple, it should reduce perfectly. In case of comminution, the joint block should be aligned, reconstructing both the frontal and sagittal angulation of the joint surface relative to the longitudinal axis of the humerus.

In cases with severe comminution of both columns, one should reconstruct the articular block first and then align it to the frontal and sagittal longitudinal axis of the humerus. In cases of severe comminution, some shortening of the columns can be accepted to reconstruct bone contact, if the axes are respected and the olecranon fossa remains of adequate volume to accept the olecranon tip.

In cases of metadiaphyseal fractures, without articular involvement, a single posterolateral

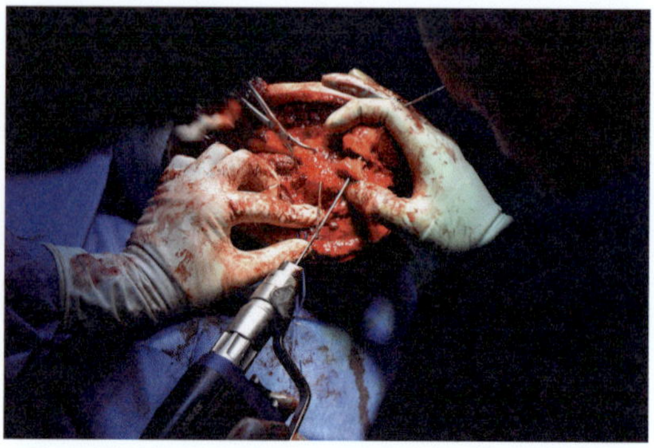

Fig. 16.20 The articular surface is reconstructed

plate can be used. In these cases, only the lateral window of the approach should be used. Fracture fixation can be either using absolute stability in simple fractures or bridging in complex fractures (Fig. 16.12).

Open Reduction and Fixation

After temporary fixation with K-wires and clamps, fluoroscopic control is performed to confirm reconstruction of the alignment, both in AP and lateral direction (Figs. 16.21 and 16.22).

We use Algorithm 16.1 to determine plate positioning. First, we look for the presence of a coronal shear fracture of the capitellum. If present, postero-anterior screws, going through a plate, should be used to fix this fracture to the column. Therefore, the radial-sided plate should be positioned posteriorly. If there is no coronal shear, we look for the presence of column comminution. If absent there is no proven advantage of either construct. The choice is then depending on the surgeon's preference. A 180° construct, however, involves a more extensive soft tissue release at the lateral side of the elbow, with a theoretical risk of devascularisation and iatrogenic ligament injury (lateral collateral ligament complex, with the lateral ulnar collateral ligament being most at risk). For these reasons, my personal preference goes to a 90° construct. If there is a/are comminuted columns, angular stable bridging is preferred. Under physiologic loads, both 90° and 180° constructs accept loads

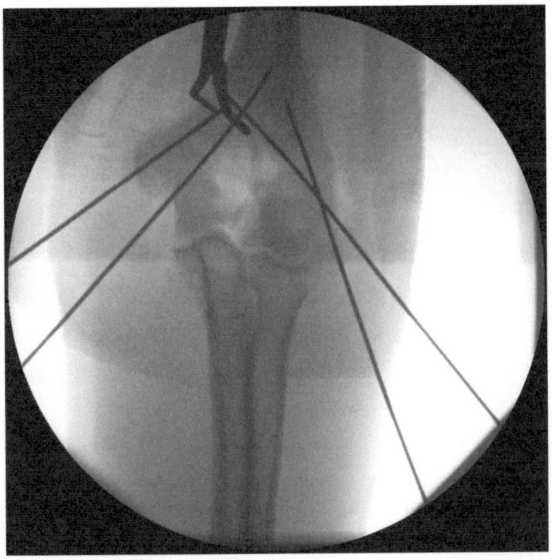

Fig. 16.21 The axes of the distal humerus after reconstruction and temporary fixation are evaluated under fluoroscopic control

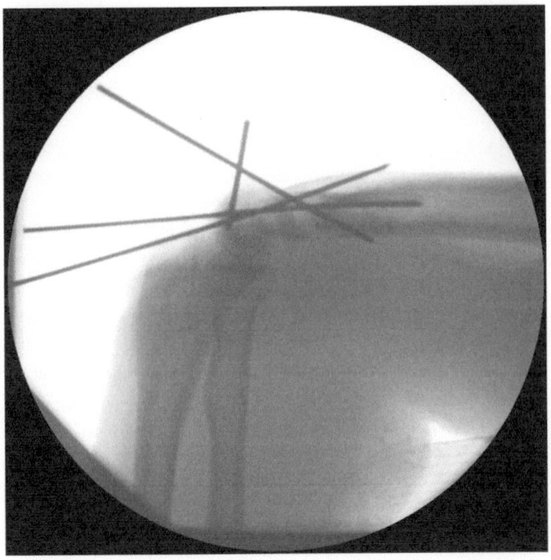

Fig. 16.22 The axes of the distal humerus after reconstruction and temporary fixation are evaluated under fluoroscopic control

well above these. In axial loading (weight bearing of the upper extremity), biomechanical studies have shown the superiority of a 180° construct. Thus, for patients in need of crutches or a walker (because of pre-existing conditions or concomitant injuries to the lower extremities), a 180° construct is preferred.

In cases of articular fracture, again a distinction between simple and complex fracture patterns guides fixation principles. In simple fractures, anatomical reduction and absolute stable fixation (compression by interfragmentary lag screws) are the golden standards. In comminuted fractures, using lag screws however bears a risk of overcompression and subsequent narrowing of the articular surface, resulting in incongruence of the humeroulnar and/or humeroradial joint. In comminuted fractures, a three-dimensional scaffold of interdigitating 2.7 mm screws is used to support the fragments in their reduced position. Each screw should engage as many fragments as possible and certainly a fragment on the opposite side to increase stability (Fig. 16.23).

The ulnar nerve is not transposed anteriorly routinely. We leave it in its natural position, but put a thin layer of soft tissue between the plate and the nerve (Fig. 16.15).

If an olecranon osteotomy has been performed, this needs to be stabilized after fixation of the distal humerus fracture. The most often used technique of osteosynthesis for olecranon osteotomies is the K-wire and cerclage fixation. This has a high complication rate, especially in osteoporotic bone. We prefer an angular stable plate to fix the osteotomy. This is positioned next

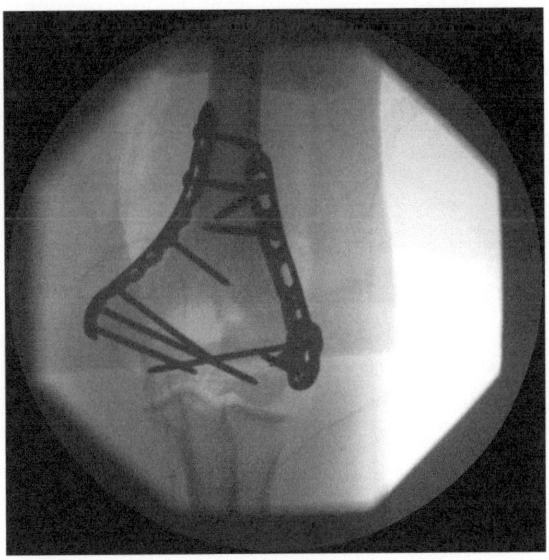

Fig. 16.23 Osteosynthesis of the distal humerus

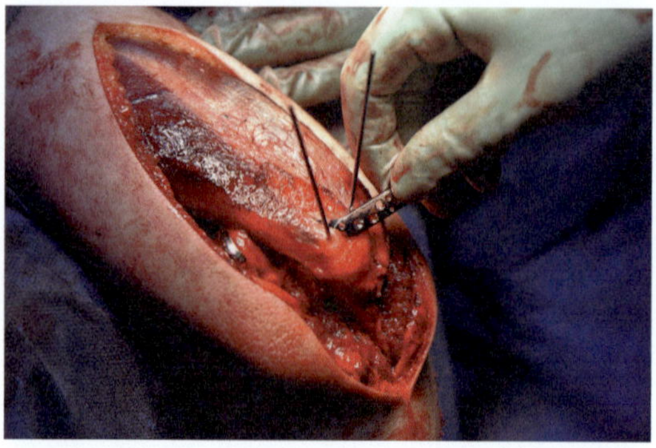

Fig. 16.24 Osteosynthesis of the olecranon osteotomy. In osteoporotic bone, we prefer an angular stable plate fixation

to the olecranon tip, by sliding it through a triceps tendon split (Fig. 16.24). A lag screw is used through the plate to obtain compression of the osteotomy.

Summary of Tips and Tricks-Pitfalls

- Obtain good quality intraoperative fluoroscopic views.
- Aim for anatomic reduction of the humerus. Comminuted articular surfaces should be supported by angular, stable, interdigitating 2.7 mm screws. Comminuted columns should be fixed by angular stable bridging plates. Simple fractures, both articular and metaphyseal, should be fixed by interfragmentary compression.
- Both 90° and 180° plate positions have their specific advantages and indications.
- Simple fractures can be treated using a dual window approach; complex fractures should be treated by olecranon osteotomy.
- In distal fractures, the ulnar nerve should be identified and in fractures with proximal extension the radial nerve. Try to protect the nerves by positioning a thin layer of soft tissues between the nerve and the implant.
- Fix an eventual osteotomy by plate and screw fixation, especially in osteoporotic bone.

References

1. O'Driscoll SW, Sanchez-Sotelo J, Torchia ME. Management of the smashed distal humerus. Orthop Clin North Am. 2002;33(1):19–33, vii
2. Shin SJ, Sohn HS, Do NH. A clinical comparison of two different double plating methods for intraarticular distal humerus fractures. J Shoulder Elb Surg. 2010;19(1):2–9.
3. Stoffel K, Cunneen S, Morgan R, Nicholls R, Stachowiak G. Comparative stability of perpendicular versus parallel double-locking plating systems in osteoporotic comminuted distal humerus fractures. J Orthop Res. 2008;26(6):778–84.
4. Penzkofer R, Hungerer S, Wipf F, von Oldenburg G, Augat P. Anatomical plate configuration affects mechanical performance in distal humerus fractures. Clin Biomech (Bristol, Avon). 2010;25(10):972–8.
5. O'Driscoll SW. The triceps-reflecting anconeus pedicle (TRAP) approach for distal humeral fractures and nonunions. Orthop Clin North Am. 2000;31(1):91–101.

17 Olecranon Fractures

Odysseas Paxinos, Theodoros H. Tosounidis, and Peter V. Giannoudis

Anatomical Fracture Location: Radiograph of Fracture Pattern

Olecranon fractures are common (about 10% of all upper extremity fractures) [1] and are one of the first fractures to be treated by junior surgeons, given the straightforward approach. However, loss of elbow extension and posttraumatic arthritis are common sequels [2], and good preoperative planning and proper surgical technique are necessary to avoid perioperative complications and long-term morbidity.

The ulnohumeral joint—in which the olecranon forms part of the concave side—allows for the flexion/extension movement of the elbow while being highly stable. The sigmoid notch is a saddle-shaped articular surface made of the olecranon proximally and the coronoid distally. The sigmoid notch is almost completely covered with cartilage (180°) except for the mid-portion that has a fatty cover and is devoid of cartilage. It articulates with the trochlea groove of the distal humerus that is also extensively covered by cartilage (320°). Stability of the elbow is mainly depended on the articular congruity with little additional support offered by the ligaments [1]. Resection of more of 60% of olecranon [3] and more of 40% of the coronoid [4] has been shown to destabilize the joint. Despite good congruency, the joint is not a rigid hinge one since there is some toggling of the axis of rotation (around 3–4°) due to the obliquity of the trochlear groove and the sigmoid notch. Although not a load-bearing joint, as much as three times the body weight may be transmitted across the elbow when lifting heavy weights. Noteworthy, restoration of joint congruency following a fracture is essential to avoid arthritis. Posttraumatic stiffness of the elbow is not rare, and the residual range of motion centres around 80° of flexion given that the capsule at this position has maximum expansion. Normal flexion-extension range of motion for the elbow is 0°–150°. For daily activities a range of 30°–130° is considered necessary with flexion deficits being more restricting [1].

The most commonly used classification of olecranon fractures is the Mayo that is based on the presence of displacement, instability and comminution. Type I is a stable joint with a minimally displaced fracture (less than 2 mm of gap between the fracture fragments), Type II is a stable joint with a displaced fracture, and Type III fractures

O. Paxinos, M.D., F.A.C.S
251 Hellenic Air Force Hospital, Athens, Greece

T.H. Tosounidis
Academic Department of Trauma and Orthopaedics, School of Medicine, University of Leeds, Leeds, UK

P.V. Giannoudis, M.D., F.R.C.S (✉)
Academic Department of Trauma and Orthopaedics, School of Medicine, University of Leeds, Leeds, UK

NIHR, Leeds, Musculoskeletal Biomedical Research Center, Chapel Allerton Hospital, Leeds, UK
e-mail: pgiannoudi@aol.com

P.V. Giannoudis (ed.), *Fracture Reduction and Fixation Techniques*,
https://doi.org/10.1007/978-3-319-68628-8_17

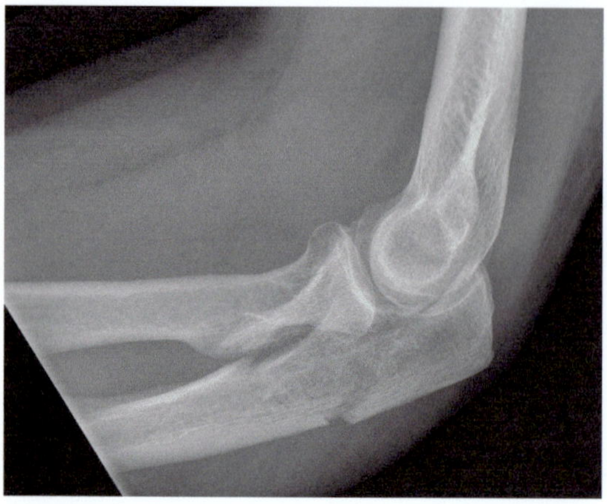

Fig. 17.1 A Type IIB olecranon fracture with concomitant coronoid fracture Type III

have associated instability of the joint. The Types II and III are further subdivided into subgroups A and B based on the presence of comminution. Coronoid fractures are also classified in three types according to the Regan-Morrey system. Based on the site of the fracture line visible in a lateral X-ray, Type I are tip fractures, Type II fractures with fragment less than 50% and Type III with a fragment more than 50% of the coronoid process (Fig. 17.1) [1].

Brief Preoperative Planning

It is necessary to define the type of fracture before surgery, since joint stability and fixation device effectiveness depend on fragment size and comminution. Fixation techniques include tension band wiring (TBW), conventional or locking plating systems, intramedullary nails and screws. Choice of implant should take into consideration the biomechanics of the fracture and of the fixation device. TBW and plates provide similar stability in simple fractures, while plates have been shown to be biomechanically more stable in comminuted fracture patterns. Bone graft may be needed to restore the geometry of the joint, and this should be taken into consideration when positioning and preparing the patient. When the olecranon fragment is very small and fixation is difficult (especially in elderly patients), one can plan for fragment resection and triceps reattachment since up to 60% of olecranon can be removed without loss of elbow function or stability [5]. Coronoid fractures in the presence of olecranon fractures should always be considered for fixation especially if the fragment is displaced and larger than simple tip fractures [4]. Since reduction and fixation of the coronoid will be performed through the fracture line, one needs to plan in advance the definitive fixation of the coronoid before reducing the olecranon fracture [1].

Patient Setup in Theatre

Olecranon fracture surgery can be accomplished in almost any surgical table. All possible patient positions (supine, lateral and even prone) have been described, but depending on surgeon preference and the availability of an assistant, the most commonly used positions are the supine and lateral decubitus. Both offer very good visualization of the fracture. Positioning the patient supine with the elbow flexed and the arm sited on the chest provides good visibility but requires an assistant from the other side. Although preferred in polytrauma patients, it may interfere with anaesthesia or chest expansion. In lateral decubitus the forearm hangs freely in front of the patient with the extremity resting over an arm support, negating the need for an assistant (Fig. 17.2).

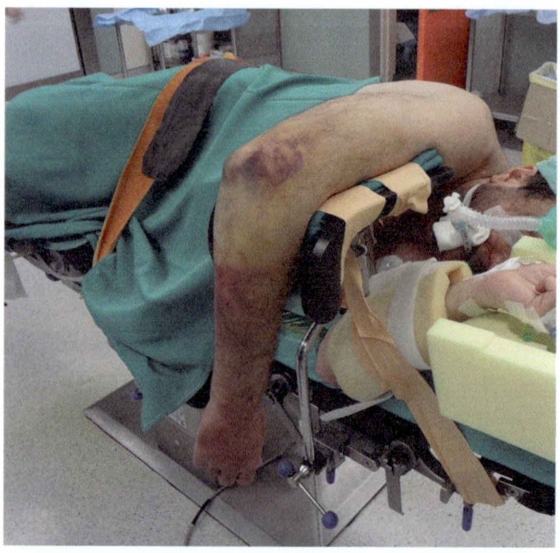

Fig. 17.2 Lateral decubitus position for elbow fracture fixation

Good AP and lateral fluoroscopic images are necessary to ensure anatomical fracture reduction and proper implant placement. The position of the image intensifier will depend on the positioning of the patient [1].

Closed Reduction Manoeuvres

Since the fracture is an intra-articular one, closed reduction should be only reserved for cases with significant soft tissue injury and for elderly patients [6]. In these cases, extending the elbow while pushing the olecranon tip with the thumb will reduce the fragment over the trochlea. Percutaneous K-wires may then hold the fragment in position supplemented by an external fixator until the soft tissues recover. In elderly patients the elbow may be immobilized in a splint until protected range of motion exercises begin.

Reduction Instruments

A hand surgery set and a small fracture fixation set will be sufficient to deal with most olecranon fractures. The surgeon will need K-wires in various sizes (usually 0.045 and 0.062 in.) as well as surgical wire 20G. Pointed reduction clamps are very useful and should be available in various sizes. Small-sized periosteal elevators will assist in mobilizing the impacted fragments, and 0.045 in. K-wires will provide provisional fixation. Vascular loops should be readily available in case the surgeon decides to explore and decompress the ulnar nerve.

Surgical Approach

Most surgeons prefer a straight midline incision either curving laterally over the olecranon or centred slightly medial to the middle line. Full-thickness flaps should be elevated until the olecranon is encountered and the fracture haematoma evacuated. The joint should be washed out to remove any bony or cartilaginous fragments and the trochlea inspected for defects (Fig. 17.3).

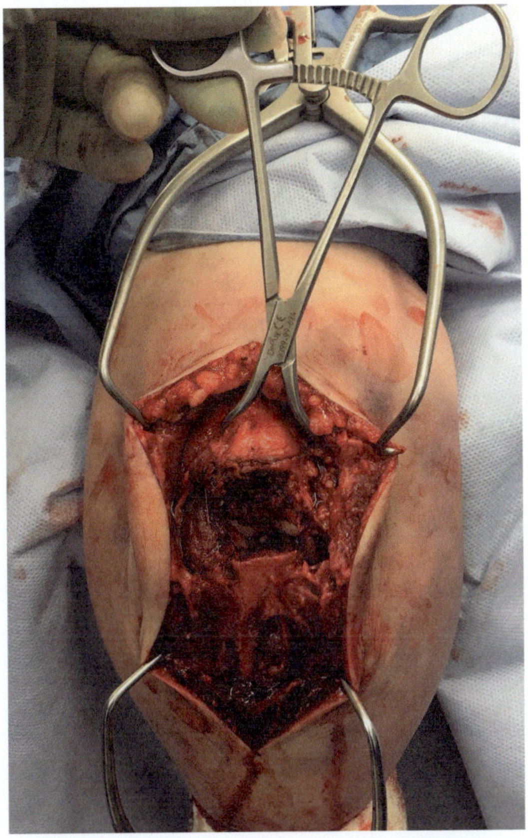

Fig. 17.3 Intraoperative inspection of the fracture line and joint surfaces

Depending on the preoperative planning and the intraoperative picture, the surgeon may decide to proceed medially and decompress the ulnar nerve. This can be easily identified proximally and followed distally. The nerve may be mobilized temporarily to allow reduction manoeuvres and implant positioning, but anterior nerve transport is not advisable. Final inspection of the fracture site will allow the surgeon to confirm that the preoperative plan developed and the fixation technique chosen are appropriate for the fracture pattern being stabilized [1].

Open Reduction Manoeuvres

The fracture is intra-articular and should always be anatomically reduced. This may be very easy to achieve in simple fracture patterns where

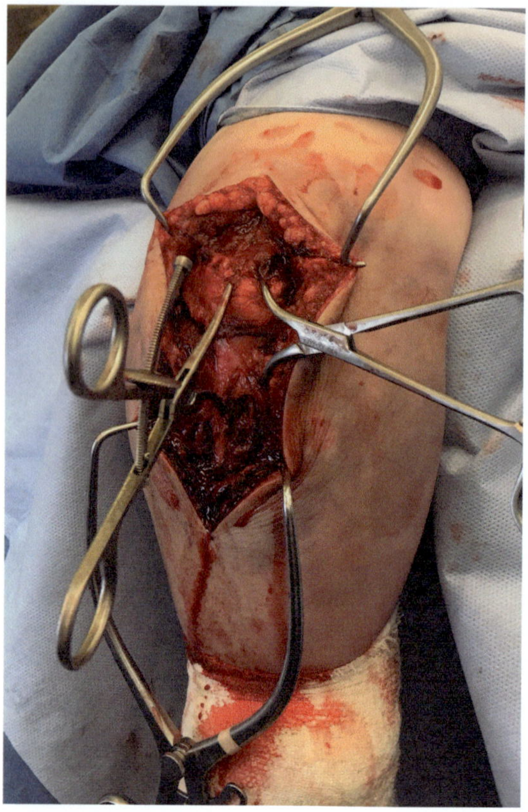

Fig. 17.4 Provisional fracture reduction with two pointed clamps

dorsal cortical apposition of the fragments restores joint congruity. In this case reduction can be provisionally held with either pointed reduction clamps or K-wires (Fig. 17.4). In complex fractures, one may have to use indirect reduction techniques utilizing the trochlea as a template to restore the sigmoid notch anatomy and then provisionally hold the fragments with K-wires. In cases with severe comminution, it may be easier to visualize through the major fracture line and in a stepwise manner reduce the smaller fragments and turn a multi-fragmentary fracture into a simple one. When there is a concomitant coronoid fracture that should be addressed first and held in place with guide wires, subsequently the coronoid fracture can be stabilized with the most appropriate method of fixation.

Implant Insertion

Type I and Type IIA Olecranon Fractures

In simple Type I and Type IIA olecranon fractures, one can use either tension band fixation with K-wires or plate and screws with equal stability and fusion rates. There is very little evidence to determine the best treatment for these fractures with confidence [7]. After fracture reduction and provisional fixation with pointed clamps, two parallel 0.045 in. Kirschner wires are inserted from the olecranon tip and directed to the anterior ulnar cortex distal to the coronoid [8]. However, fixation to the anterior cortex instead of intramedullary insertion has been shown to increase complications [2] (Fig. 17.5). After fluoroscopic confirmation of the position, the wires are withdrawn for 1 cm, and then a 20G or 22G surgical wire is looped around then and fixed in a figure of eight passing through 2.5 mm drill holes in the triangular-shaped part of the proximal dorsal ulna cortex. Alternatively, the K-wires can be inserted intramedullary towards the ulna styloid in a longer distance [8]. In order to avoid prominent hardware problems, it is better to pass the figure-of-eight wire as close to the

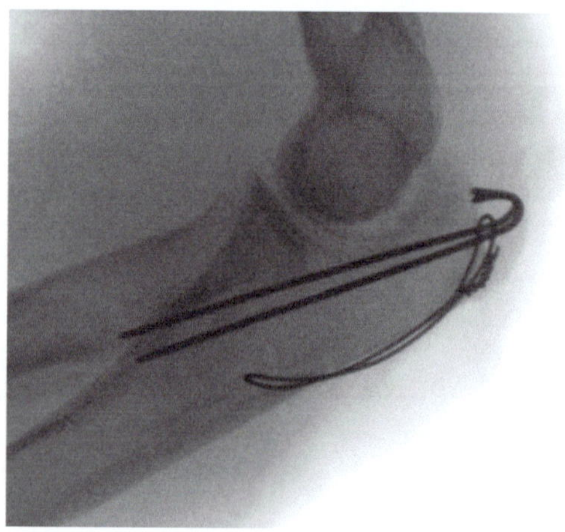

Fig. 17.5 Lateral fluoroscopic view of Type IIA olecranon fracture treated with a tension band construct with two K-wires and figure-of-eight wire loop

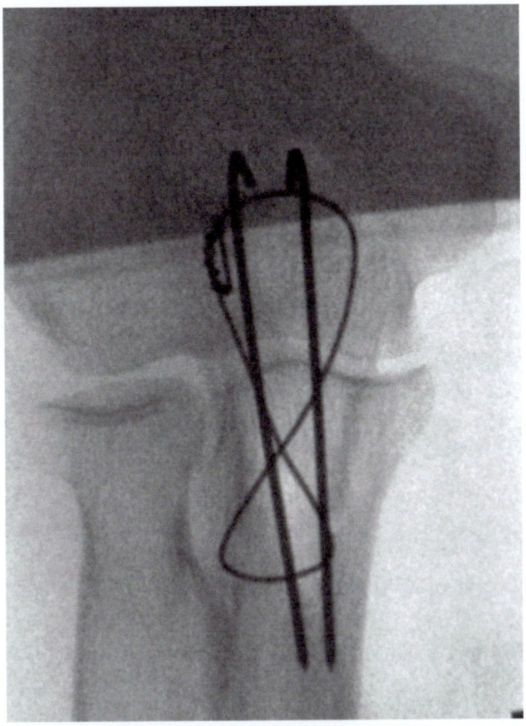

Fig. 17.6 AP intraoperative view of Type IIA olecranon fracture treated with tension band. Passing the figure-of-eight wire as close to the bone will decrease hardware problems

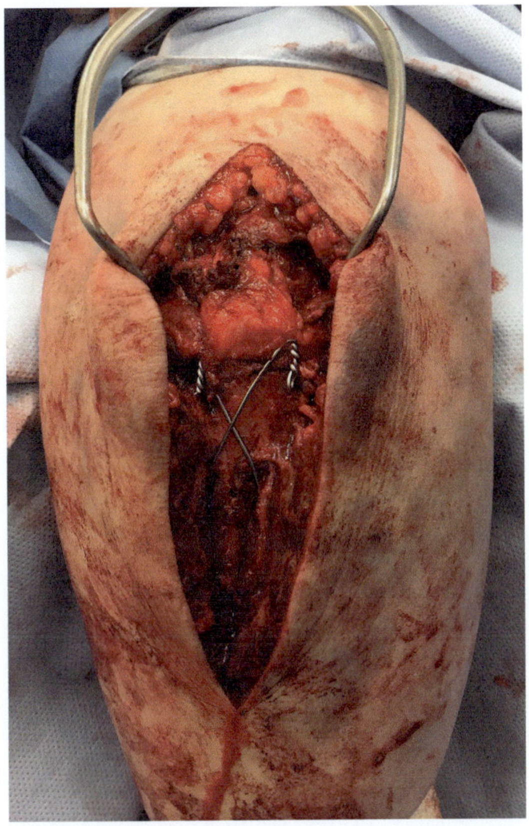

Fig. 17.7 Intraoperative picture of Type IIA olecranon fracture treated with tension band with two tightening knots

olecranon tip underneath the triceps tendon as possible (Fig. 17.6). Making two tightening twists instead of one seem to improve stability. The two K-wires are then cut and bent and impacted into the olecranon deep under the triceps tendon (Fig. 17.7). Instead of K-wires, intramedullary screws with or without figure-of-eight wire have been used with variable success. Although biomechanically inferior to K-wire tension band, they can be useful as low profile implants in non-comminuted fractures with good bone quality [8].

Type IIB and Type III Olecranon Fractures

Types IIB and III are better treated with plate fixation. If there is a concomitant large coronoid fracture (Type II or III), it should be reduced and fixed first with either simple partially threaded 4.0 mm lag screws or pullout wire [1]. A cannulated 3.5 screw will be easier to insert over the guide wire used to provisionally fix the coronoid fragment. The screw can be inserted either through the fracture line and buried in the bone or from the dorsal ulna cortex taking care not to interfere with the plate. After fixation of the coronoid, any other fragment is anatomically reduced using the trochlea as template before the major fracture line is closed and provisionally held in place. There are several plates marketed specifically for elbow fractures, although one can still use inexpensive 3.5 steel plates provided she/he respects the principles of fixation. The plate can

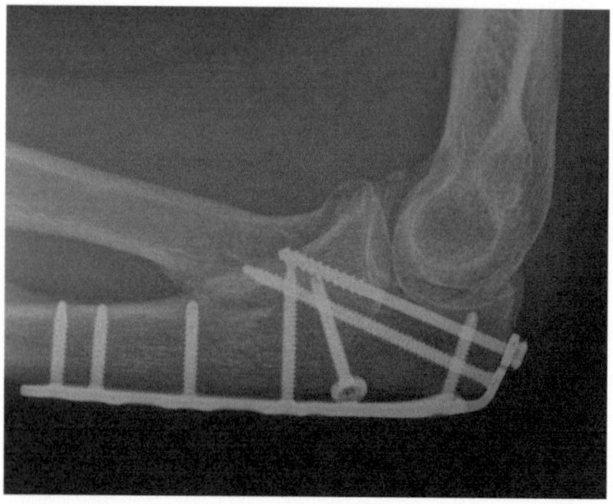

Fig. 17.8 Lateral X-ray of Type IIIB olecranon fracture treated with locking plate. The lag screw is directed to the coronoid fracture, while the two diagonal screws to the anterior cortex increase rigidity of the fixation

be positioned either dorsal or lateral since there is no biomechanical difference [9]. When using non-locking screws, it is important to bend the end of the plate over the olecranon tip as to allow for the insertion of one screw towards the coronoid. This configuration significantly improves the stability of the construct (Fig. 17.8). In osteopenic bones, one may choose locking plates for better purchase. When using locking plates, one should make sure the fragments are perfectly reduced since the plate will not provide interfragmentary compression. Hybrid plates may allow for both compression and locking screw insertion—however one needs to be familiar with the principles of absolute and relative stability to avoid implant failure and/or inadequate fracture reduction. Fluoroscopic imaging is important to avoid joint penetration. In elderly patients with severe comminution, one may opt either to treat conservatively or to excise the fragments and attach the triceps directly to the bone. Good results can be expected if the olecranon excised is less than 60% [10].

Summary of Tips and Tricks-Pitfalls

- The surgeon needs to respect the principles of intra-articular fracture fixation and aim for absolute stability in the articular part of the construct. Tension band with K-wires is only appropriate for stable Type I or IIA fractures. In elderly persons with comminution, one may consider conservative treatment or excision and reattachment of the triceps to the ulna.
- Reduction is essential before applying any fixation. In comminuted fractures the coronoid is reduced first and then all other fragments in a stepwise fashion before closing the main fracture line.
- When using K-wires through the anterior cortex, one should avoid over-penetration since neurovascular injury may occur. The correct length is estimated with the image intensifier, and the wires are pulled back 1 cm to cut and bend in over to avoid prominence into the anterior forearm when impacted in place. Alternatively, one may use long K-wire passing intramedullary into the ulna. Passing the figure-of-eight wire under the triceps mass will reduce the chance of prominent implant irritation and the need for wire removal.
- Plate fixation should be used whenever there is comminution. In osteoporotic bones, locking plates may be used. After fixation, in the lateral fluoroscopic view, the plate may be seen sitting away from the tip some millimetres despite having taking measures such as splitting the triceps insertion to improve apposition. This image should not raise concerns.

Conflict of Interest No benefits in any form have been received or will be received from a commercial party related directly or indirectly to the subject of this chapter.

References

1. Morrey BF, Sanchez-Sotelo J. The elbow and its disorders. 4th ed. Bone 2010:13-42.
2. Schneider MM, Nowak TE, Bastian L, et al. Tension band wiring in olecranon fractures: the myth of technical simplicity and osteosynthetical perfection. Int Orthop. 2014;38(4):847–55. https://doi.org/10.1007/s00264-013-2208-7.
3. Ferreira LM, Bell TH, Johnson JA, King GJW. The effect of triceps repair techniques following olecranon excision on elbow stability and extension

strength: an in vitro biomechanical study. J Orthop Trauma. 2011;25:420–4. https://doi.org/10.1097/BOT.0b013e3181fadd55.
4. Doornberg JN, Ring D. Coronoid fracture patterns. J Hand Surg Am. 2006;31(1):45–52. https://doi.org/10.1016/j.jhsa.2005.08.014.
5. Ikeda M, Fukushima Y, Kobayashi Y, Oka Y. Comminuted fractures of the olecranon. Management by bone graft from the iliac crest and multiple tension-band wiring. J Bone Jt Surg Br. 2001;83(6):805–8. https://doi.org/10.1302/0301-620X.83B6.11829.
6. Powell AJ, Farhan-Alanie OM, Bryceland JK, Nunn T. The treatment of olecranon fractures in adults. Musculoskelet Surg. 2017;101(1):1–9. https://doi.org/10.1007/s12306-016-0449-5.
7. Matar HE, Ali AA, Buckley S, Garlick NI, Atkinson HD. Surgical interventions for treating fractures of the olecranon in adults. Cochrane Database Syst Rev. 2014;11:CD010144. https://doi.org/10.1002/14651858.CD010144.pub2.
8. Huang T-W, C-C W, Fan K-F, Tseng I-C, Lee P-C, Chou Y-C. Tension band wiring for olecranon fractures: relative stability of kirschner wires in various configurations. J Trauma Inj Infect Crit Care. 2010;68(1):173–6. https://doi.org/10.1097/TA.0b013e3181ad554c.
9. King GJ, Lammens PN, Milne a D, Roth JH, J a J. Plate fixation of comminuted olecranon fractures: an in vitro biomechanical study. J Shoulder Elb Surg. 1996;5(6):437–41. https://doi.org/10.1016/S1058-2746(96)80015-2.
10. Iannuzzi N, Dahners L. Excision and advancement in the treatment of comminuted olecranon fractures. J Orthop Trauma. 2009;23(3):226–8.

18 Coronoid Fractures

Mark Philipson

Avulsion Fractures of the Coronoid

Indications for Surgery and Preoperative Planning

Small avulsion fractures of the tip of the coronoid are often found in association with elbow dislocations (Fig. 18.1). The avulsion fracture occurs as part of an injury to the anterior capsular attachments to the coronoid. Most can be successfully managed nonoperatively. When a coronoid avulsion exists together with an unstable radial head fracture and a medial collateral ligament rupture, then repairing the anterior capsule will confer additional stability to the elbow. In my practice, if I am reconstructing or replacing a radial head fracture and there is an associated avulsion of the tip of the coronoid, I will repair the anterior capsular avulsion injury. The additional stability gives me confidence to mobilise the elbow early.

A CT scan can be useful to confirm the presence of a coronoid avulsion and to assess an associated radial head fracture.

Patient Set-Up in Theatre

The patient is positioned supine with the arm on an armboard. I utilise a tourniquet. The surgeon sits on the cephalad side of the arm board. A C-arm can be positioned under the armboard.

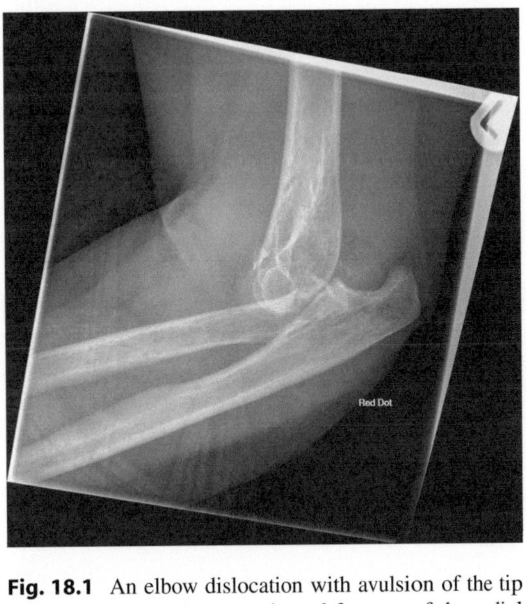

Fig. 18.1 An elbow dislocation with avulsion of the tip of the coronoid and a comminuted fracture of the radial head

M. Philipson
Leeds General Infirmary, Leeds, UK
e-mail: mrphilipson@hotmail.com

P.V. Giannoudis (ed.), *Fracture Reduction and Fixation Techniques*,
https://doi.org/10.1007/978-3-319-68628-8_18

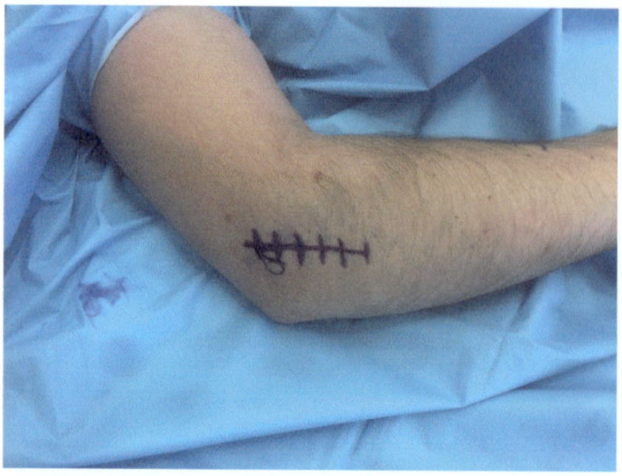

Fig. 18.2 The skin incision for an anterolateral approach to the elbow

Closed Reduction Manoeuvres

The ulnohumeral joint should be reduced with axial traction and flexion prior to making a skin incision.

Surgical Approach

A straight oblique incision is made starting just proximal to the lateral epicondyle and extending distally towards Lister's tubercle on the dorsum of the wrist for a distance of 5–10 cm (Fig. 18.2). This anterolateral approach is also known as a Kaplan interval approach. Invariably the lateral collateral ligament together with the extensor origin is avulsed from the lateral epicondyle. The forearm fascia is incised in line with the skin incision commencing just anterior to the lateral epicondyle. The surgeon will encounter a haematoma-filled wound cavity where the lateral collateral ligaments and extensor origin have been avulsed and the radiocapitellar joint is at the base of this wound. Reconstruction of a stable proximal radius by fixation or prosthetic replacement is essential. Fixation of the radial head is preferable to replacement if the surgeon is confident that union can be achieved. Prosthetic replacement has the advantage of giving a predictable stable reconstruction. It also makes access to the coronoid much easier if the radial head is excised. Even with an intact radial head, adequate access to the coronoid can be achieved with progressive release of brachioradialis and the anterior capsule from the humerus in a lateral to medial direction (Fig. 18.3). Obviously, it is important to minimise the release of anterior capsule from the humerus; otherwise, any benefit from repairing the anterior capsule to the coronoid is nullified.

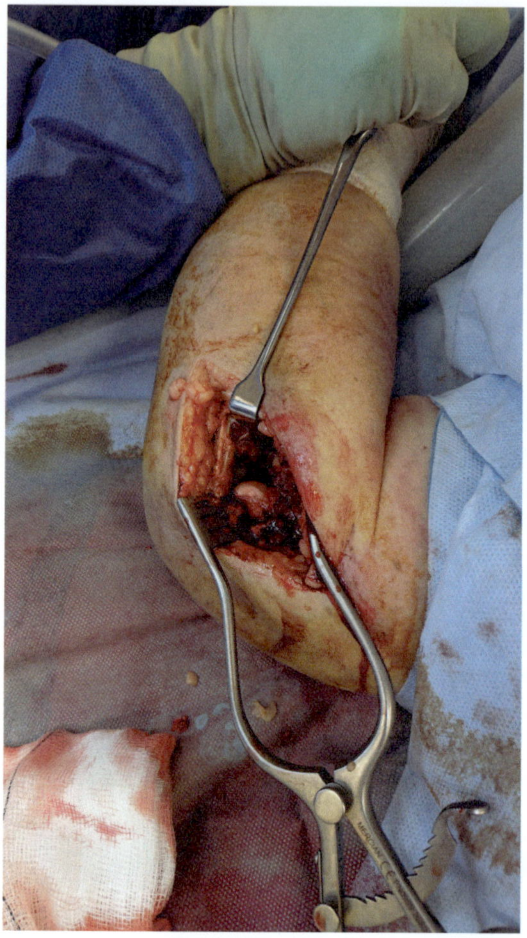

Fig. 18.3 An anterolateral approach has been used to access the coronoid tip. Note that the lateral epicondyle is denuded of all soft tissue attachments. This is the typical finding in cases of elbow dislocation

Open Reduction Manoeuvres

The challenge in this procedure is achieving adequate exposure of the coronoid without excessive release of anterior capsule from the humerus. Flex the elbow and place a single ring-handled spike with the tip over the medial aspect of the proximal ulna. This spike then retracts the brachioradialis, anterior capsule and brachialis medially. The anterior capsule and brachioradialis should then be released sequentially until adequate exposure of the fracture bed of the coronoid is achieved. An anchor double loaded with number 2 abrasion-resistant suture material is then implanted in the centre of the coronoid fracture bed. Both 5-mm threaded cuff anchors and 2.9-mm labral anchors can be used for this purpose. The torn anterior capsule is now located together with the avulsion fragment. The bony fragment can be trimmed or excised altogether with a pair of rongeurs. For each loop of suture, one limb is passed though the anterior capsule with several bites in the manner of a modified Mason-Allen suture; the other limb is passed with a single bite of capsule. The limb with a single bite will be used as a post when knot tying in order to pull the capsule down on to the coronoid. It is important to keep the suture bites near to the torn edge of the capsule to avoid over-tightening. The sutures should be left loose and untied (with some means of easily identifying which limbs are the posts) until reconstruction of the proximal radius is complete.

As the sutures are tied with a sliding locking knot, the anterior capsule and avulsion fragment are reduced onto the coronoid (Fig. 18.4).

Post-op Instructions

The aim is to achieve a repair that facilities immediate active movement. The patient wears a collar and cuff sling for comfort. Patient and physiotherapist are advised to avoid pushing extension past 30° in the first 6 weeks.

Tips, Tricks and Pitfalls

- A well-placed ring-handled spike with the elbow flexed gives better exposure of the coronoid than multiple retractors.
- Don't tie the sutures in the anterior capsule until reconstruction of the proximal radius is complete.
- Avoid overtightening the capsule as this will increase the risk of stiffness.

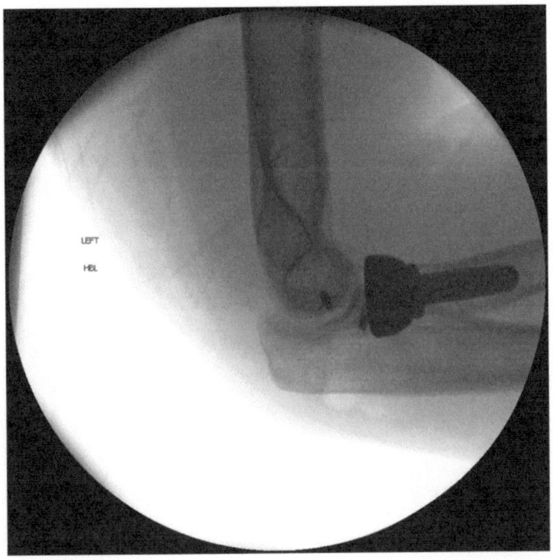

Fig. 18.4 The radial head has been replaced, and metallic anchors have been used to repair the coronoid avulsion and lateral collateral ligament injury

Fractures Through the Base of Coronoid

Indications for Surgery and Preoperative Planning

Fractures involving more than just the tip of the coronoid are uncommon. Frequently they are part of a complex unstable elbow injury. Fixation is necessary if there is clinical or radiographic evidence of instability (Fig. 18.5).

A CT scan is very useful for understanding the morphology of the fracture and planning fixation. This is especially true when there is an associated complex fracture of the olecranon.

Patient Set-Up in Theatre

The patient is positioned supine with the arm on an armboard. An arm tourniquet is used. The surgeon sits on the caudal side of the armboard. A C-arm can be positioned under the armboard. In many cases simultaneous fixation of the olecranon will be necessary. In these cases the olecranon is fixed with the patient supine with the arm bent over a cushion on the patient's chest. The

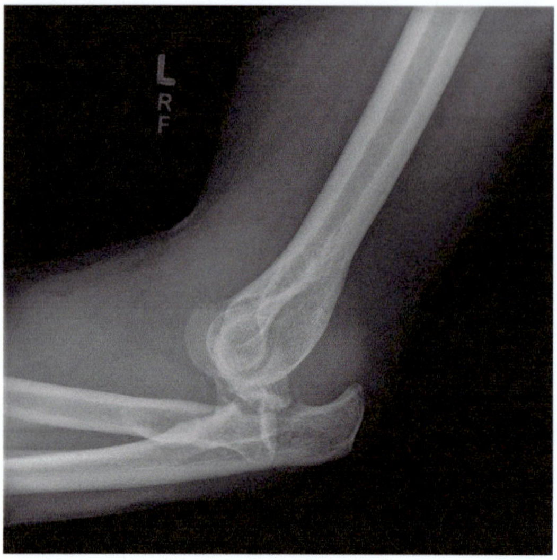

Fig. 18.5 An elbow dislocation with a fracture through the base of the coronoid. This is a grossly unstable injury (Figure courtesy of Mr. S Vollans, Leeds Teaching hospitals)

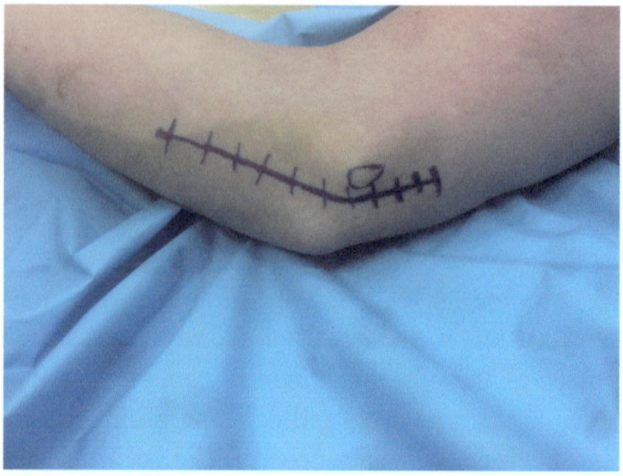

Fig. 18.6 The skin incision for a medial approach to the coronoid

arm can then be moved down on to an armboard for the coronoid fixation. All image intensifier images can be obtained with the arm swung outwards on to the armboard.

Closed Reduction Manoeuvres

The ulnohumeral joint should be reduced with axial traction and flexion prior to making a skin incision.

Surgical Approach

For isolated fractures of the coronoid, the incision starts 5 cm proximal to the medial epicondyle then passes in line with the ulnar nerve just behind the medial epicondyle and extends 5–10 cm distal to the medial epicondyle (Fig. 18.6). If exposure of the olecranon is also required then I utilise a single midline posterior incision curved medially around the olecranon. In cases where access to the radiocapitellar joint is required but not the olecranon, I will utilise separate anterolateral and posteromedial incisions.

In cases of high-energy trauma, there may be an obvious defect in the muscular envelope over the medial aspect of the proximal ulna. The surgeon should be flexible and utilise such a defect for the exposure of the coronoid. Otherwise I approach the coronoid via the floor of the ulnar nerve between the two heads of flexor carpi ulnaris (FCU). The ulnar nerve is mobilised and transposed anteriorly so as to avoid any kinks or tension on the nerve. The two heads of FCU are then separated to expose the proximal ulna.

Open Reduction Manoeuvres

A traction suture in the anterior capsule is used to aid reduction of the coronoid fragment. Limited access does not normally allow application of reduction forceps.

I recommend the use of a pre-contoured locking plate specifically designed for the coronoid with an anterior paddle which sits over the coronoid fragment to act as a buttress and resist anterior displacement. I utilise the Biomet ALP plate (Fig. 18.7).

Postoperative Instructions

The aim is to achieve a reconstruction that facilitates immediate active elbow movement once the skin wound has settled. The patient is provided

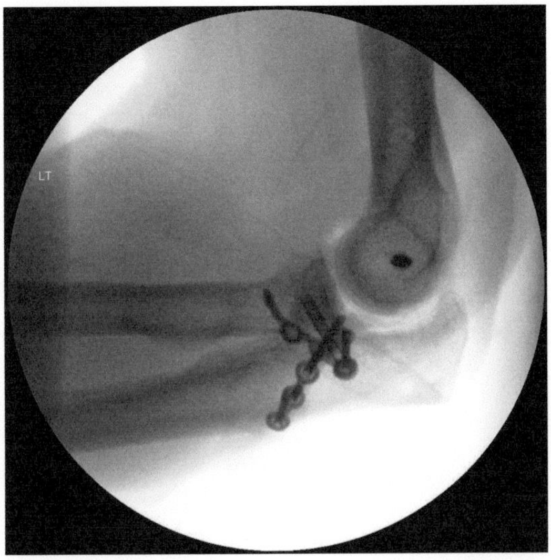

Fig. 18.7 The base of coronoid fracture has been fixed with a pre-contoured plate and a cannulated screw (Figure courtesy of Mr. S Vollans, Leeds Teaching hospitals)

with a collar and cuff sling for comfort. Patient and physiotherapist are advised to avoid pushing extension past 30° in the first 6 weeks.

Tips, Tricks and Pitfalls

- Utilise a pre-contoured plate designed for the coronoid.
- Avoid the temptation to fix the coronoid with screws alone.
- Any associated radial head fracture must be securely reconstructed.

Further Reading

Chan K, Faber KJ, King GJ, Athwal GS. Selected anteromedial coronoid fractures can be treated nonoperatively. J Shoulder Elb Surg. 2016;25(8):1251–7.

Han SH, Yoon HK, Rhee SY, Lee JK. Anterior approach for fixation of isolated type III coronoid process fracture. Eur J Orthop Surg Traumatol. 2013;23(4):395–405.

Hartzler RU, Llusa-Perez M, Steinmann SP, Morrey BF, Sanchez-Sotelo J. Transverse coronoid fracture: when does it have to be fixed? Clin Orthop Relat Res. 2014;472(7):2068–74.

Ring D, Horst TA. Coronoid Fractures. J Orthop Trauma. 2015;29(10):437–40.

Rhyou IH, Lee JH, Kim KC, Ahn KB, Moon SC, Kim HJ, Lee JH. What injury mechanism and patterns of ligament status are associated with isolated coronoid,isolated radial head, and combined fractures? Clin Orthop Relat Res. 2017;475(9):2308–15.

Wang P, Zhuang Y, Li Z, Wei W, Fu Y, Wei X, Zhang K. Lasso plate - an original implant for fixation of type I and II Regan-Morrey coronoid fractures. Orthop Traumatol Surg Res. 2017;103(3):447–51.

Yoon RS, Tyagi V, Cantlon MB, Riesgo AM, Liporace FA. Complex coronoid and proximal ulna fractures are we getting better at fixing these? Injury. 2016;47(10):2053–9.

Radial Head and Neck Fracture

19

Austin Hill and David Ring

Fracture Location and Pattern

Fractures of the radial head not associated with other ligament injuries or fractures are typically stable (intact periosteum, impacted, not mobile) and usually involve the anterolateral aspect of the radial head or the neck of radius [1].

Fractures associated with other ligament injuries (e.g. elbow dislocation or interosseous ligament of the forearm) or fractures (e.g. fracture of the proximal ulna) are usually displaced and unstable and may involve the entire head of the radius [1]. Unstable fractures may have limited periosteal connections. For unstable fracture, the overall injury pattern helps determine what to do with the radial head [2]. For instance, in the setting of elbow dislocation with fractures of the radial head and coronoid (the terrible triad lesion), restoration of radiocapitellar contact is so important that tenuous or incomplete repair of a radial head fracture is risky and surgeons should have a low threshold to resect the radial head and insert a prosthesis [3, 4]. In contrast, many extra-articular posterior Monteggia injuries have a stable ulnohumeral joint, making preservation of radiocapitellar contact less important [5]. In this setting, if the radial head fracture does not hinder forearm rotation or cause crepitation, it may not benefit from specific treatment. And if it does, resection without replacement is an option.

For unstable fractures, it can be useful to obtain a computed tomography scan, make 3D reconstructions, and subtract the distal humerus to get a good look at the fracture [6]. It is intuitive to think that partial articular fractures will have fewer fragments, but a recent study suggests that there are more and small fragments, making them more difficult to repair than a fracture of the entire head of the radius (Fig. 19.1) [7]. A CT scan can also be used for radial neck fractures to

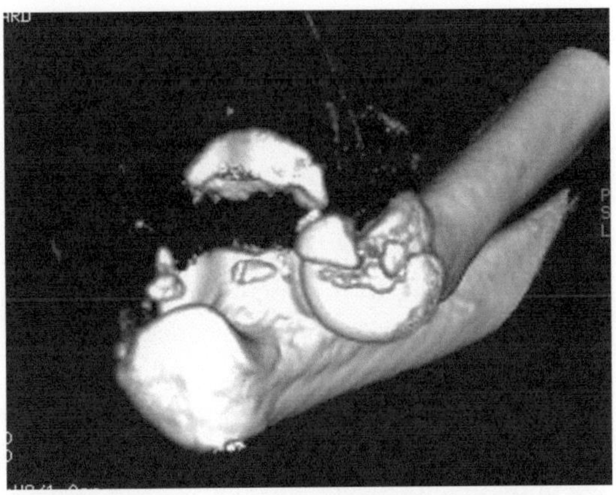

Fig. 19.1 A 3D CT scan with the distal humerus subtracted shows a partial articular fracture of the radial head as part of a terrible triad pattern injury. The radial head is fragmented, with numerous small fragments. This radial head should be replaced with a prosthesis

A. Hill, M.D. • D. Ring, M.D., Ph.D. (✉)
Department of Surgery and Perioperative Care, Dell Medical School—The University of Texas at Austin, Austin, TX, USA
e-mail: david.ring@austin.utexas.edu

P.V. Giannoudis (ed.), *Fracture Reduction and Fixation Techniques*,
https://doi.org/10.1007/978-3-319-68628-8_19

get a sense of how impacted/angulated it is and the potential bone defect that might exist after the fracture is reduced.

Brief Preoperative Planning

When the surgeon understands the injury pattern and has radiographs and 3D-CT with the distal humerus subtracted, there are very few surprises at surgery [2].

For impacted partial articular fractures of the articular surface and impacted radial neck fractures, it can be useful to have a broad (1 cm or greater) bone tamp; the tamp can be used to realign the fracture without disrupting any bent but intact metaphyseal bone or intact periosteum. The surgeon should be prepared for a substantial defect and consider obtaining autogenous cancellous bone graft from the proximal ulna, distal radius, or iliac crest or a graft alternative. For most of these fractures, a few small screws are sufficient for fixation. Countersunk screws with a head are fine for the nonarticular part of the head. Headless screws are used for the unusual fracture that involves a part of the radial head that articulates with the lesser sigmoid notch of the ulna in the proximal radioulnar joint [8].

For unstable fractures, small Kirschner wires and bone clamps can assist with reduction. Some unstable fractures with no bone defect can be treated with screws alone. Even fractures of the radial neck or whole-head articular fractures can be fixed with screws alone if there is no metaphyseal bone defect—a few long screws cross obliquely from the articular margin across the fracture to the radial neck distal to the fracture [9]. If there is a bone defect, a plate and screws are needed.

For unstable, fragmented fractures, the surgeon should be prepared to replace the radial head with a prosthesis or craft a spacer prosthesis out of methyl methacrylate bone cement [10].

Patient Set-Up in Theatre

For most radial head fractures, the patient lies supine on a standard operating table with the arm supported on a hand table (Fig. 19.2). A sterile tourniquet makes it easier to access the elbow and manipulate the arm. When the fracture of the radial head is associated with a fracture of the olecranon or proximal ulna, a lateral decubitus position with the arm supported on a bolster is preferred.

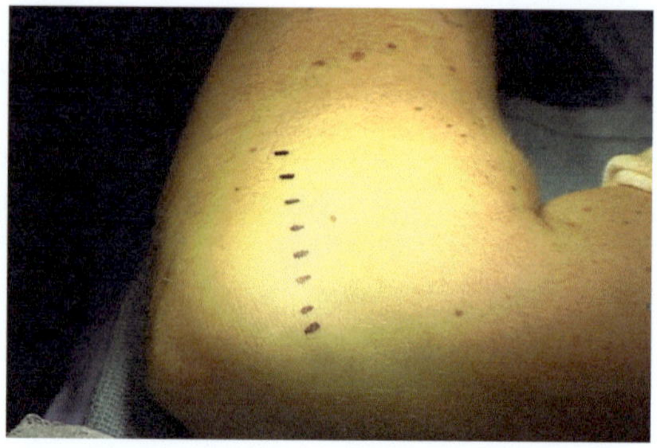

Fig. 19.2 The patient lies supine with the arm supported on a hand table. A sterile tourniquet provides good access to and mobility of the arm. A lateral skin incision is an option. A posterior skin incision could also be used

Closed Reduction Manoeuvres

There is no point in attempting closed reduction of a radial head fracture.

Surgical Approach

The skin incision can be lateral or posterior depending on associated injuries and surgeon and patient preferences. The preferred muscle interval to expose a fracture of the radial head is between the extensor carpi radialis brevis and extensor digitorum communis (eponym Kaplan) or slightly posterior. It is not possible to distinguish the interval. Rather the common extensor muscle mass is split at the 50:50 anterior posterior division of the capitellum. This can be done by feel or by elevating the origin of the extensor carpi radialis brevis from the supracondylar ridge and looking into the joint as the split is extended distally [11]. The annular ligament is split in this interval. The supinator muscle is separated using blunt dissection with small scissors and elevated distally using a blunt elevator keeping the periosteum in place if possible.

This anterior exposure may not provide access to some posterior displaced, unstable articular fragments. In that case the anconeus can be split to retrieve this fragment and bring it to the anterior part of the elbow.

Open Reduction Manoeuvres

If the fracture does not move and there is intact periosteum, it is considered impacted. It is helpful to try to maintain as much of the inherent stability of this type of fracture as possible. A tip for doing this is to place a bone tamp on the nonarticular part of the radial head or neck and use a small mallet with as little force as needed and gradually push the fracture back into position with many small blows (Fig. 19.3 (a,b)). Done well and with a little luck, the fracture will be repositioned and maintain some inherent stability.

For unstable fractures, it can help to skewer the fragments with small (0.8–1.1 mm) Kirschner wires. It can also be helpful to use a dental pick to align and hold fragments along with a small pointed tenaculum forceps (Fig. 19.4). The wires can then be used to help place and position the fragment while another wire is drilled across to hole the fragment in place. Once all the fragments are aligned, the decision is made whether or not to apply bone graft or bone graft substitute. Screws or a plate and screws are then applied.

If at any point there are missing, deformed, or small fragments that are important to the stability of the elbow, the radial head is resected and a prosthesis inserted.

Implant Insertion

The screws or plate should be applied within a 90 degree arc centred directly lateral with the forearm in neutral rotation. There is a little more room anterior than posterior for the implants [12].

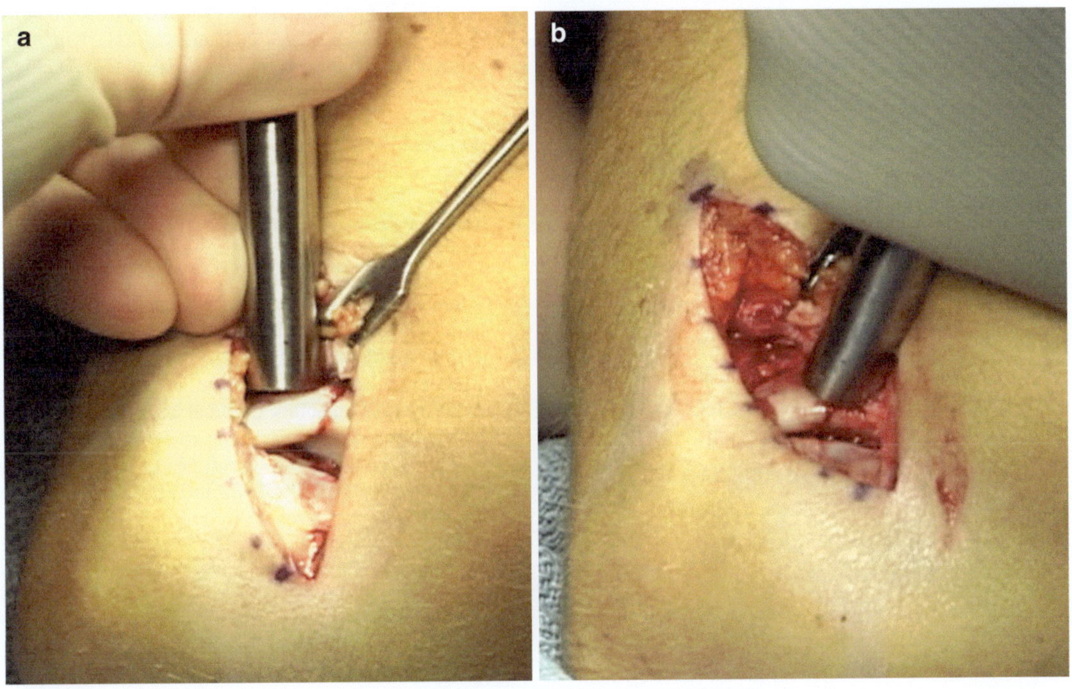

Fig. 19.3 A stable isolated partial articular fracture of the radial head. (**a**) A bone tamp is used to realign the fracture. (**b**) Stability and periosteal attachments are maintained

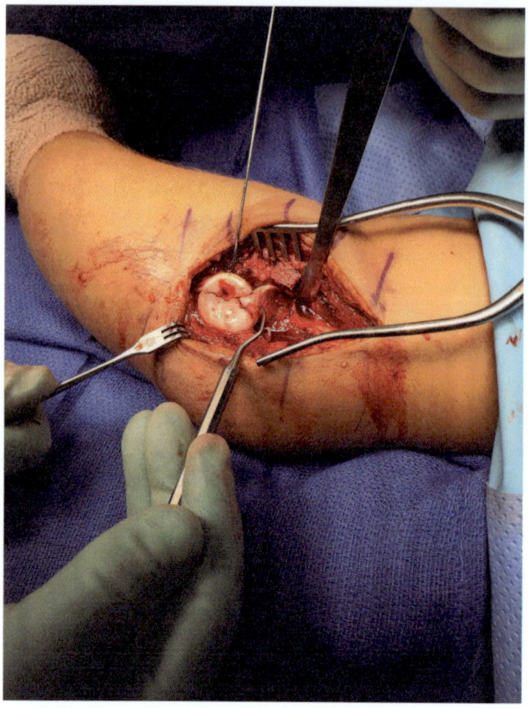

Fig. 19.4 A dental pick, Kirschner wires, and tenaculum clamps can help reduce complex fractures of the entire head of the radius

Summary of Tips, Tricks, and Pitfalls

- Most stable, isolated fractures do not benefit from fixation. It should be the unusual substantially impacted fracture that is considered for surgery [1].
- Most unstable, displaced fractures are part of an unstable elbow or forearm injury, are fragmented, create small fragments and metaphyseal impaction, and are difficult to fix. A radial head prosthesis might be a better option here [13].
- Anticipate avulsion of the lateral collateral ligament from the lateral epicondyle with an elbow fracture dislocation. It will make exposure much easier. Use drill holes through the lateral epicondyle or suture anchors to reattach the lateral collateral ligament complex.
- Consequently, it is difficult to become familiar with these reduction techniques. Based on preoperative evaluation, if you think it may be possible to repair the fracture, consider doing the surgery with a colleague that has substantial experience with open reduction and internal fixation of the radial head.
- The pitfalls are to fix a fracture tenuously and have it collapse, place implants on the articular surface of the proximal radioulnar joint or too long and into the joint, or to harm the posterior interosseous nerve. It is wise to avoid placing a retractor over the anterior part of the radial neck to avoid injuring the posterior interosseous nerve.

References

1. Duckworth AD, McQueen MM, Ring D. Fractures of the radial head. Bone Joint J. 2013;95-B(2):151–9. https://doi.org/10.1302/0301-620X.95B2.29877. Review. PubMed PMID:23365021
2. Doornberg JN, Guitton TG, Ring D. Science of Variation Group.. Diagnosis of elbow fracture patterns on radiographs: interobserver reliability and diagnostic accuracy. Clin Orthop Relat Res. 2013;471(4):1373–8. https://doi.org/10.1007/s11999-012-2742-4. Epub 2012 Dec 18. PubMed PMID: 23247817; PubMed Central PMCID: PMC3586040
3. Pugh DM, Wild LM, Schemitsch EH, King GJ, McKee MD. Standard surgical protocol to treat elbow dislocations with radial head and coronoid fractures. J Bone Joint Surg Am. 2004;86-A(6):1122–30. PubMed PMID: 15173283
4. Ring D, Jupiter JB, Zilberfarb J. Posterior dislocation of the elbow with fractures of the radial head and coronoid. J Bone Joint Surg Am. 2002;84-A(4):547–51. PubMed PMID: 11940613
5. O'Driscoll SW, Jupiter JB, Cohen MS, Ring D, McKee MD. Difficult elbow fractures: pearls and pitfalls. Instr Course Lect. 2003;52:113–34. Review. PubMed PMID: 12690844
6. Guitton TG, Ring D, Science of Variation Group. Interobserver reliability of radial head fracture classification: two-dimensional compared with three-dimensional CT. J Bone Joint Surg Am. 2011;93(21):2015–21. https://doi.org/10.2106/JBJS.J.00711. PubMed PMID: 22048097
7. Guitton TG, van der Werf HJ, Ring D. Quantitative three-dimensional computed tomography measurement of radial head fractures. J Shoulder Elb Surg. 2010;19(7):973–7. https://doi.org/10.1016/j.jse.2010.03.013. Epub 2010 Jun 20. PubMed PMID:20566295
8. van Leeuwen DH, Guitton TG, Lambers K, Ring D. Quantitative measurement of radial head fracture location. J Shoulder Elb Surg. 2012;21(8):1013–7. https://doi.org/10.1016/j.jse.2011.08.056. Epub 2011 Nov 9. PubMed PMID: 22071412

9. Smith AM, Morrey BF, Steinmann SP. Low profile fixation of radial head and neck fractures: surgical technique and clinical experience. J Orthop Trauma. 2007;21(10):718–24. PubMed PMID: 17986889
10. Clembosky G, Boretto JG. Open reduction and internal fixation versus prosthetic replacement for complex fractures of the radial head. J Hand Surg Am. 2009;34(6):1120–3. https://doi.org/10.1016/j.jhsa.2008.12.031. Epub 2009 May 28. PubMed PMID: 19481361
11. Hotchkiss RN. Displaced fractures of the radial head: internal fixation or excision? J Am Acad Orthop Surg. 1997;5(1):1–10. PubMed PMID: 10797202
12. Smith GR, Hotchkiss RN. Radial head and neck fractures: anatomic guidelines for proper placement of internal fixation. J Shoulder Elb Surg. 1996;5(2 Pt 1):113–7. PubMed PMID: 8742874
13. Ring D, Quintero J, Jupiter JB. Open reduction and internal fixation of fractures of the radial head. J Bone Joint Surg Am. 2002;84-A(10):1811–5. PubMed PMID: 12377912

Check for updates

20 Monteggia Fracture and Monteggia-Like Lesion – Treatment Strategies and Intraoperative Reduction Techniques

Dorothee Gühring and Ulrich Stöckle

Anatomy

Fractures of the proximal ulna in combination with a dislocation of the proximal radioulnar joint (PRUJ) and the radiohumeral joint (dislocation of the head of the radial bone) are named "Monteggia fractures" after the individual who first described such fractures, Giovanni Monteggia [1]. The dislocation mechanism that takes place in the context of a Monteggia injury often results in a concomitant fracture of the neck or head of the radial bone and/or a fracture of the coronoid process. These complex injuries are summarized by the term "Monteggia-like lesion" (Fig. 20.1).

Preoperative Planning

Conventional diagnostic X-rays of the elbow in two planes provide an overview of the extent of injury and serve the purpose of evaluating the joint components in relation to one another. In addition to conventional diagnostic X-rays, computed tomography is to be regarded as standard for substantiated preoperative planning (Fig. 20.2).

Since a Monteggia injury is a dislocation fracture, a timely and anatomical reconstruction of the ulna fracture should be aimed for. Often, Monteggia injuries are fractures with significant closed or open soft tissue damage which requires emergency intervention. If open reconstruction is not possible due to the severity of soft tissue injury, the elbow joint should be temporarily stabilized using an external fixation device (Fig. 20.3).

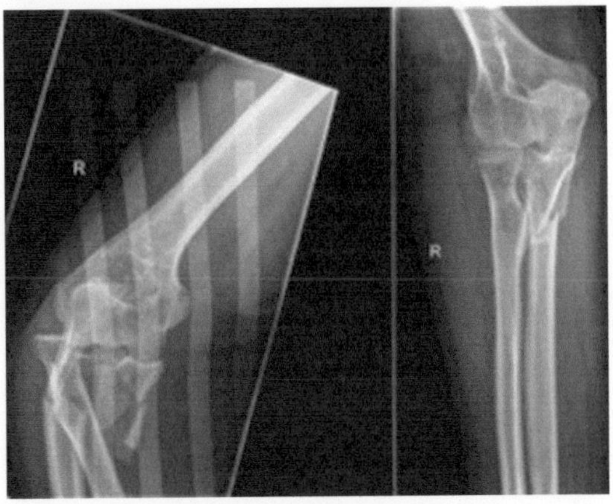

Fig. 20.1 Monteggia-like lesion. Fracture of the proximal ulna in combination with a fracture of the radial head and the coronoid process

D. Gühring
Klinik im Kronprinzenbau, Reutlingen, Germany

U. Stöckle (✉)
Trauma and Reconstructive Surgery, BG Unfallklinik, Tübingen, Germany
e-mail: ustoeckle@bgu-tuebingen.de

P.V. Giannoudis (ed.), *Fracture Reduction and Fixation Techniques*, https://doi.org/10.1007/978-3-319-68628-8_20

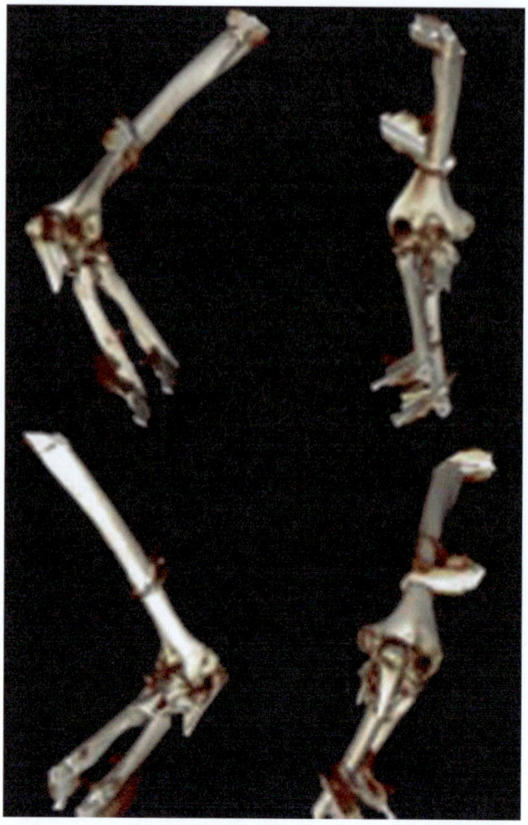

Fig. 20.2 Computed tomography of the Monteggia-like lesion. Three dimensional imaging

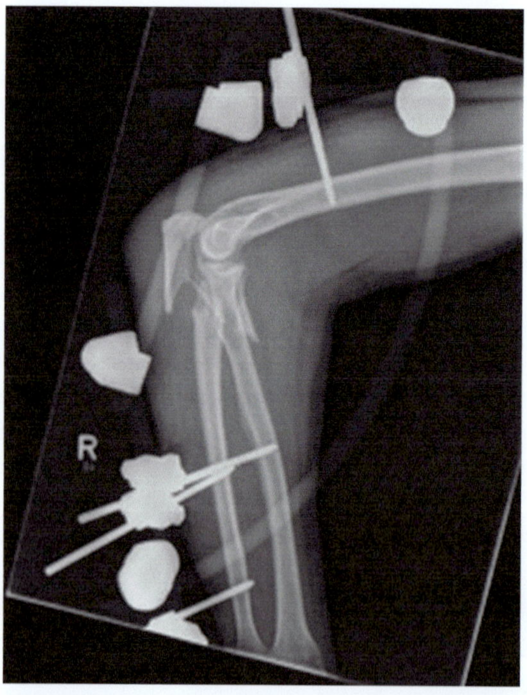

Fig. 20.3 External fixation device

General Considerations

Monteggia Lesion

In Monteggia fracture dislocations, anatomical reduction with correct length and stable fixation of the ulna are mandatory, in order to ensure stable relocation of the radial head. Once operative fixation of the ulna has been completed, the surgeon must ensure the stability of the reduced radial head, preferably under image intensification. Anatomic reduction and fixation of the ulna is achieved first, through a standard posterior approach.

Check the position of the radial head, which reduces spontaneously in most of these cases (>90%). The surgeon must determine the position of forearm rotation in which the radial head is most stable. This is very often in full supination after the radial head has dislocated anterolaterally. The stable rotational position of the forearm is that which will be used when postoperative splintage is applied.

If the radial head does not reduce correctly or if it dislocates on forearm movement (pronation/supination and flexion/extension), this may be due to either malreduction of the ulnar shaft or there may be interposed soft tissue. If ulnar reduction is confirmed and radial head dislocation persists, access the radial head via a short lateral approach or an extension into a Speed and Boyd approach (<10%).

In cases of persisting radial head instability after anatomical fixation of the ulna, interposed annular ligament or the torn joint capsule is usually the cause and should be extracted from the joint and sutured.

Monteggia-Like Lesion

C3 fractures, with extensive comminution of coronoid and radial head. are characteristic of posterior olecranon fracture dislocation. Lateral collateral ligaments are typically disrupted. Restoration of elbow stability requires repair of the proximal ulna; radial head ORIF, or replacement; and lateral collateral ligament repair. A coronoid fragment, if present, may be reduced and fixed through the olecranon fracture and/or a medial extension of the usual posterior approach. Radial fracture repair or replacement follows. Then the remainder of the proximal ulna must be reduced and fixed in correct length. While it may be possible to reduce the multifragmentary ulna fracture anatomically, occasionally length can be determined better from the radius, after fixation or replacement. Stability of the elbow must be confirmed at the conclusion of reduction and fixation. If instability remains, supplementary external fixation may be necessary.

Patient Set-Up in Theater

Prone Position

The patient lies prone with the arm on a radiolucent support, or on a padded post (Fig. 20.4). Either of them gives maximum freedom to approach the elbow. The forearm should be in a position so that it can be flexed beyond 100 degrees. A small padded table can be placed under the forearm to support the elbow in extension when necessary. A tourniquet at the proximal arm is optional.

Posterior Approach

A number of fracture patterns of the proximal forearm can be addressed using this approach (Fig. 20.5). The more complex the fracture configuration, the more extensile the approach needs to be.

The ulna is a subcutaneous bone. Start the incision a few centimeters proximal to the tip of the olecranon, as needed for access to the injured area. Curve slightly radially around the tip of the olecranon, and go distally for a few centimeters, as needed to provide access to the injured area (Fig. 20.6).

Elevation of the lateral flap provides access to the lateral structures of the elbow. In the proximal portion, dissect and elevate the subcutaneous tissue. Over the olecranon, remove the olecranon

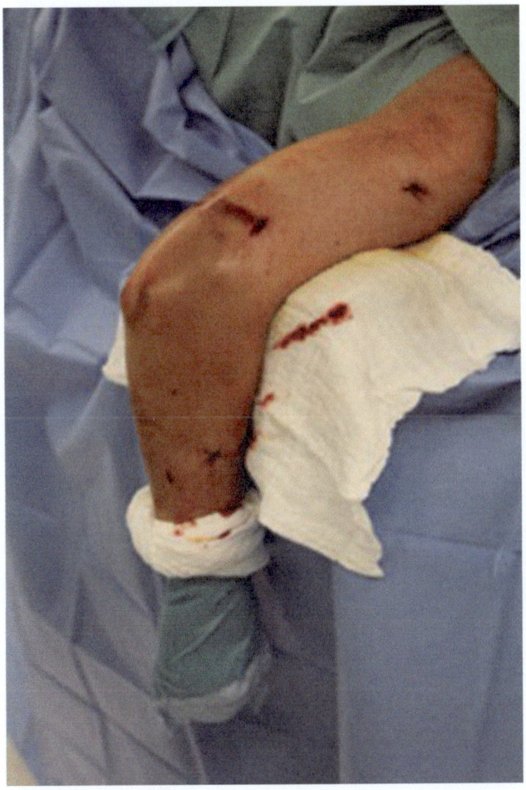

Fig. 20.4 Prone position with the arm on a padded post

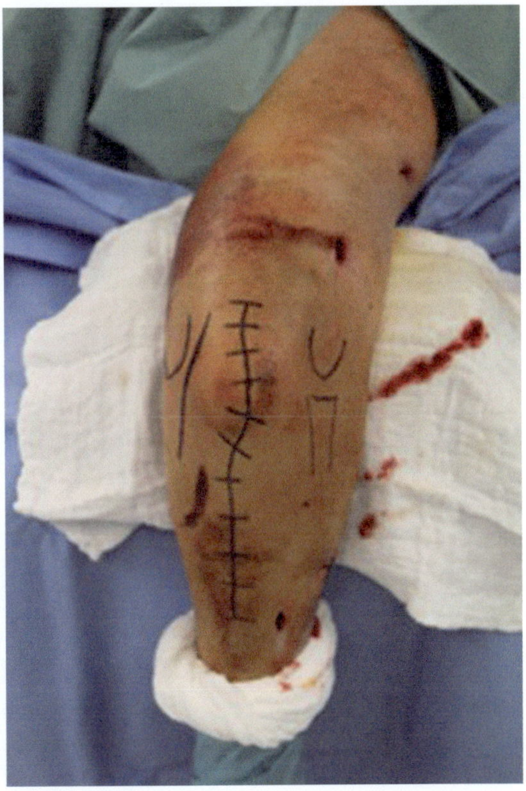

Fig. 20.5 Skin incision of the posterior approach

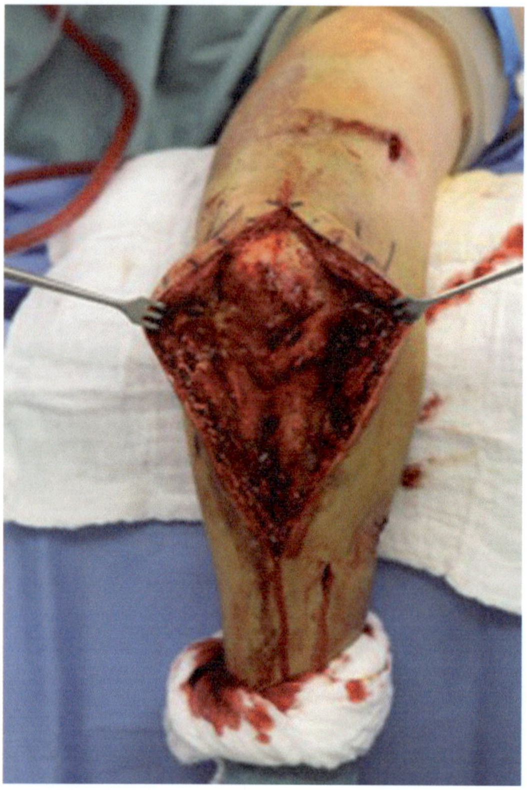

Fig. 20.6 Posterior approach after skin incision

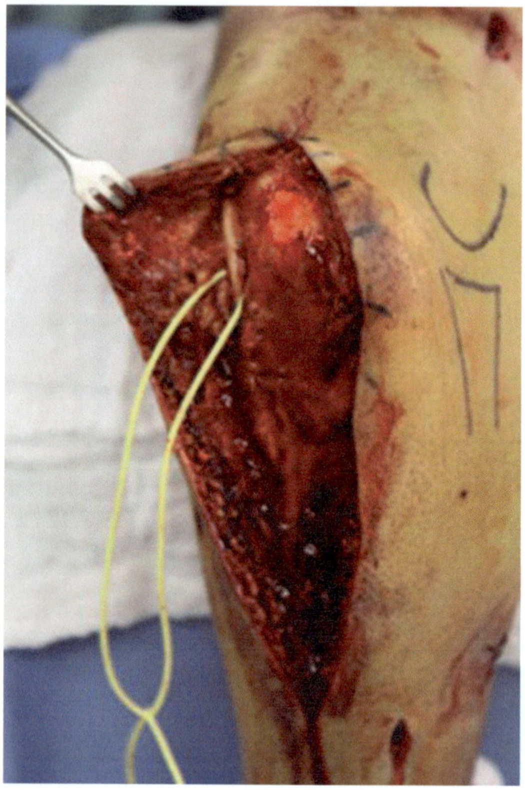

Fig. 20.7 Ulnar nerve

bursa and incise the triceps aponeurosis exposing the bone. Behind the medial humeral epicondyle, identify and protect the ulnar nerve (Fig. 20.7).

Detach the flexor carpi ulnaris muscle on the medial side and the anconeus muscle on the lateral side as far as necessary to expose the involved articular surfaces and for an anatomical reduction and stable fixation. Some coronoid fractures can be addressed through the proximal ulna fracture or the lateral extension of this approach, particularly with the elbow dislocated, and/or with displacement of a proximal radius fracture. The decision to detach the anconeus muscle from the ulna depends on the necessity to address a fracture of the radial head, or neck, or a fracture of the proximal ulna involving the sigmoid notch (Fig. 20.8).

In a combined, simple proximal ulnar and radial fracture, it may not be necessary to detach the anconeus. The proximal radial fracture may be approached by dissecting and elevating the subcutaneous tissues laterally exposing the septum between the anconeus and the extensor carpi ulnaris muscle.

ORIF

Radial Head

Radial fracture repair or replacement usually follows reduction and fixation of the coronoid process. Exposure of both fractures is a good initial step (Fig. 20.9).

The radial head is completely covered with articular cartilage. The implant is applied to the radial head in a location that causes the least compromise of full pronation and supination. Release the annular ligament as necessary to see the radius. Expose the fracture with minimal soft tissue dissection off the bone. Remove hematoma and irrigate. Directly reduce the joint fragments

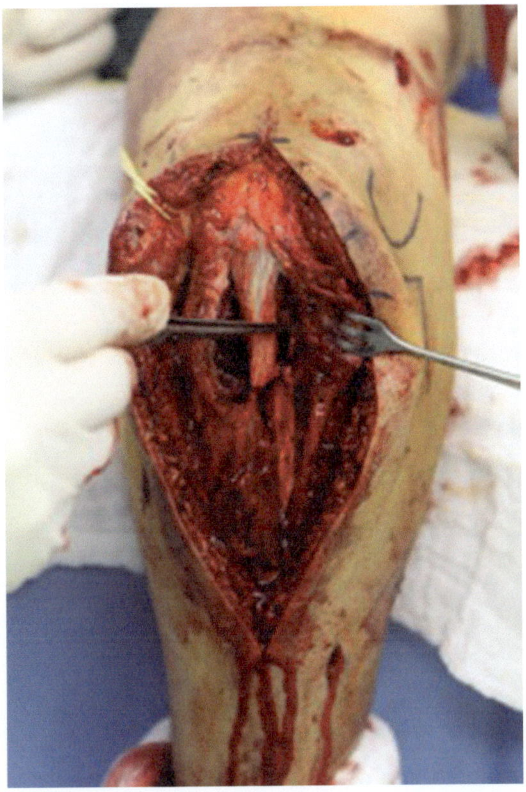

Fig. 20.8 Detach of the anconeus muscle

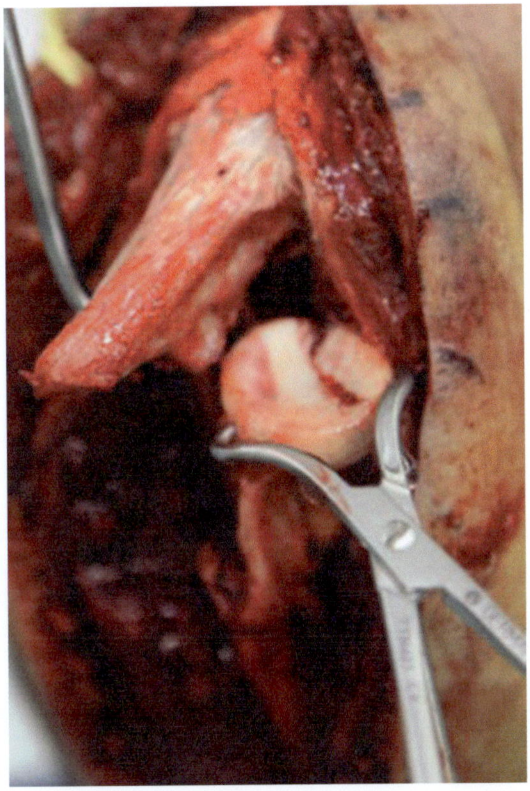

Fig. 20.9 Exposure of the radial head

with the help of small pointed reduction forceps and provisionally fix them with two K-wires (Fig. 20.10).

If joint depression is encountered, the depressed joint fragment is elevated, and the underlying defect may be bone grafted with bone from the lateral humeral condyle.

Insert two horizontal lag screws (1.5 or 2.0 mm) into the proximal fragment (Fig. 20.11). Control reduction with direct visualization of articular surface, and confirm with C-arm fluoroscopy (Fig. 20.12). Repair the annular ligament using non-absorbable sutures.

Proximal Ulna

Absolute stability is desirable for articular fractures. However, this may not be possible in multifragmentary fractures of the proximal ulna. Every effort should still be directed at anatomical reduction and absolutely stable fixation of the major articular surface fragments, particularly the coronoid process. Compression will deform the articular surface, so it no longer fits the trochlea. In this situation, the fracture must be bridged without compression to preserve size and shape of the olecranon fossa. Small interfragmentary screws or K-wires may improve stability.

Bridge Plating

A bridge plate is analogous to locked intramedullary nail fixation of a comminuted shaft fracture. In multifragmentary fractures of the olecranon, anatomical reconstruction of the articular surface itself is the primary goal. Intermediate, nonarticular fragments do not need to be reduced anatomically. Cancellous bone graft can be used to support the articular fragments and fill defects. Directly manipulate only the articular fragments.

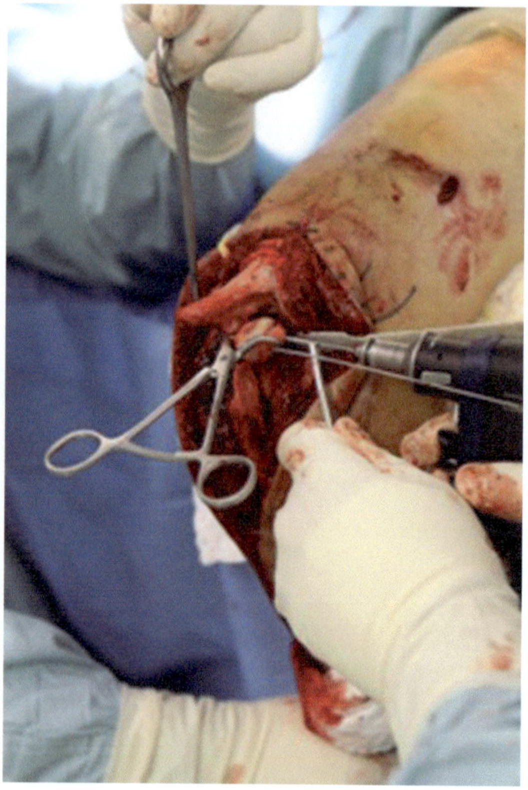

Fig. 20.10 Reduction of the joint fragments with forceps and K-wire

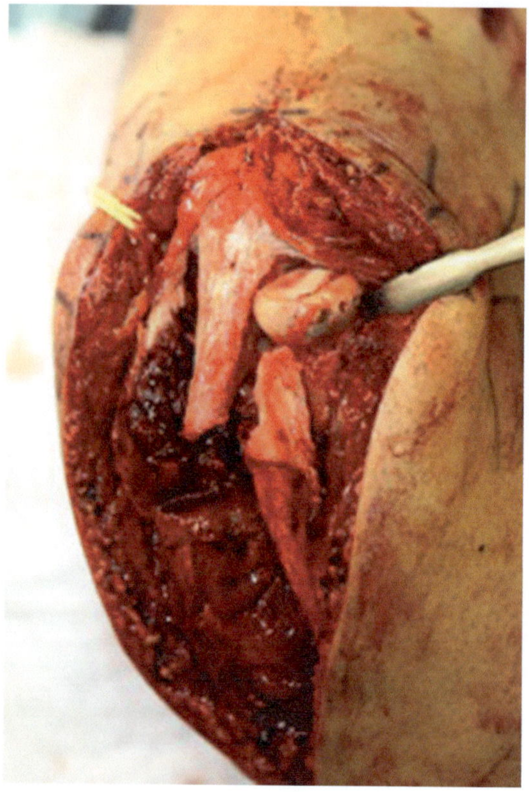

Fig. 20.11 2.0 mm lag screws

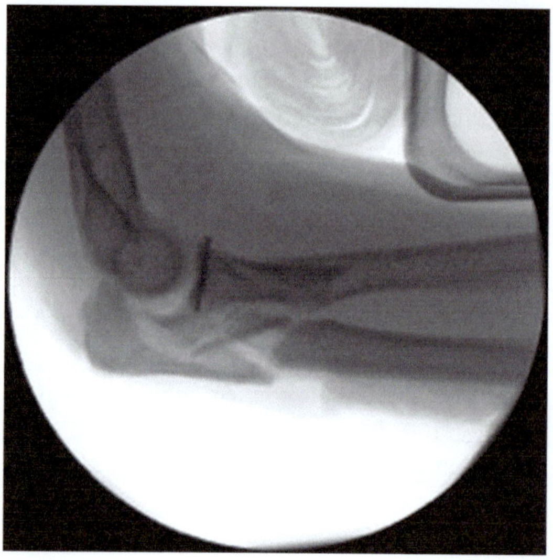

Fig. 20.12 C-arm fluoroscopic control of the radial head

Excessive manipulation of intermediate fragments risks disturbing their blood supply. If the soft tissue attachments are preserved, and the fragments are relatively well aligned, healing is predictable. Alignment of the main fragments can usually be achieved indirectly utilizing traction and soft tissue tension. Mechanical stability, provided by the bridging plate, is adequate for indirect healing (callus formation). Correct length of the ulna is the key for the treatment of Monteggia-like lesions.

Through the posterior incision, release the joint capsule medially and laterally at the fracture site. With direct visualization, manipulate and anatomically reduce the articular fragments. Use the distal humerus as a template for reduction. Provisionally fix the fragments with 1.0 mm K-wires (Fig. 20.13).

Reduce the proximal part of the olecranon with pointed reduction forceps, and temporarily hold the reduction with one or two K-wires. Insert all K-wires in a position where they do not interfere with the planned plate and screws.

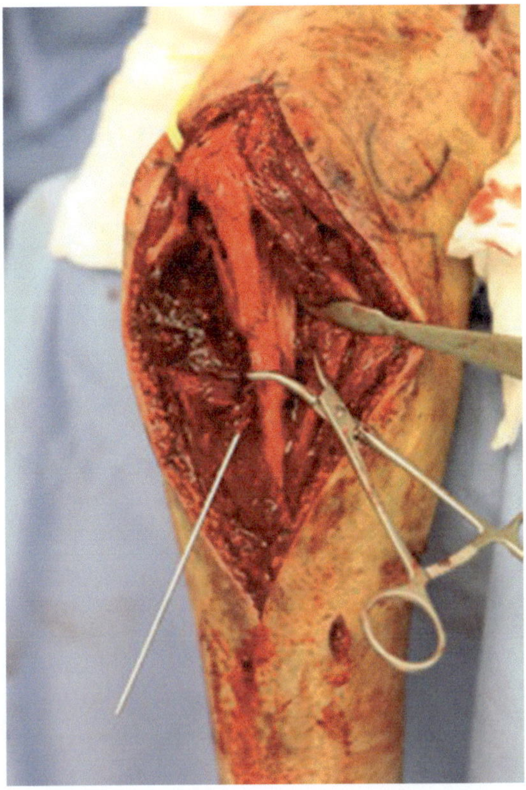

Fig. 20.13 Provisionally reduction with K-wires and forceps

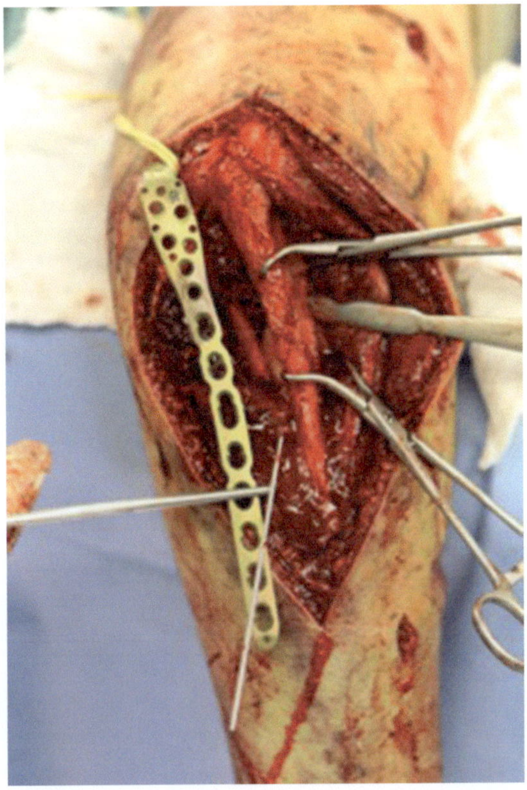

Fig. 20.14 Preshaped olecranon LCP with locking head screws

Control reduction with direct visualization of the sigmoid notch and the posterior cortex of the olecranon, and confirm with C-arm fluoroscopic.

Implant Choice

A 3.5 dynamic compression plate (DCP), reconstruction plate, limited contact dynamic compression plate (LC-DCP), or locking plate (LCP) can be used. The reconstruction plate is the least durable and should be used cautiously as a bridged plate. Choose the length of the plate so that at least three screws can be inserted in the most proximal fragment and three in the diaphysis. If the fracture is very proximal or in osteoporotic bone, a preshaped olecranon LCP with locking head screws is preferred to allow best possible fixation (Fig. 20.14). To achieve close bone plate contact, split the triceps attachment before positioning the plate (Fig. 20.15).

Anchor the plate with three screws to the proximal olecranon. Make sure that the screws do not protrude into the joint. Whenever possible, insert the screws bicortically, aiming the drill to the lateral or to the medial cortex. Insert three bicortical screws in the distal fragment and in a divergent pattern. Make sure to maintain contour and size of the olecranon's articulation (Fig. 20.16).

Reduction of a large coronoid component of multifragmentary proximal ulna fractures can often be done through the fracture site. Provisional or definitive fixation can be placed at that time, but sometimes it helps to use a screw through a posterior plate for its fixation, as shown here. Insert this as a lag screw, as perpendicularly as possible to the fracture plane at the base of the coronoid. Smaller diameter screws may be better (Fig. 20.17).

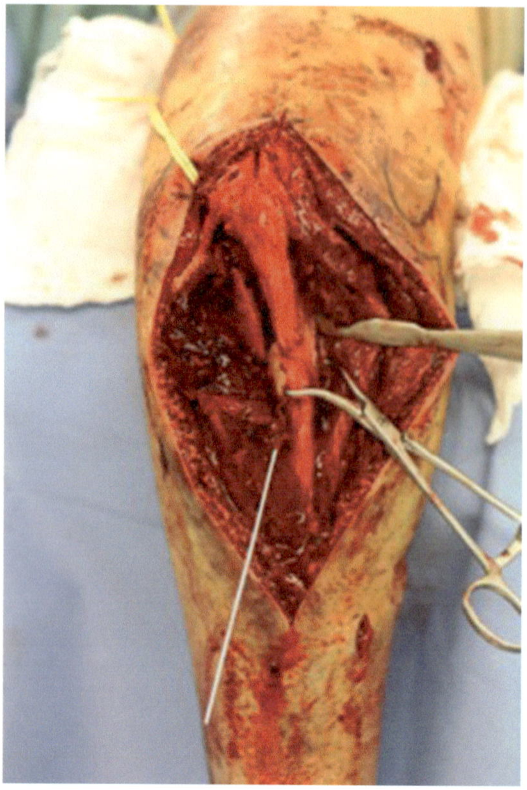

Fig. 20.15 Triceps split

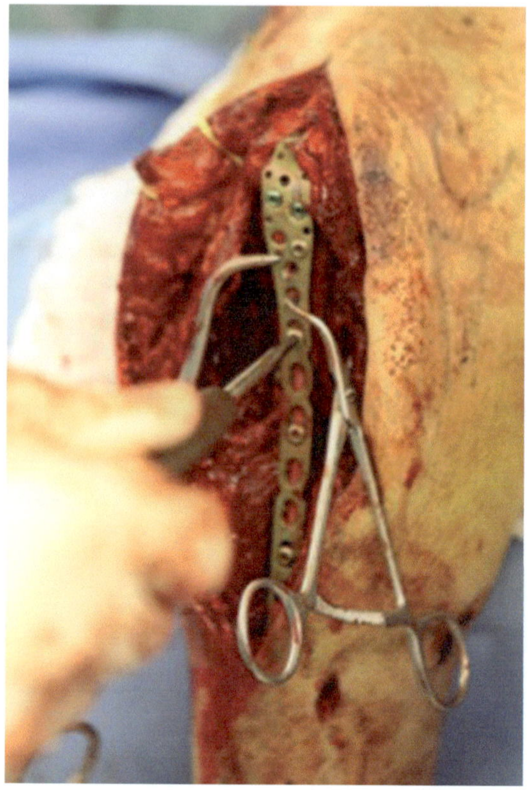

Fig. 20.17 Reduction of the coronoid process with a lag screw through the plate

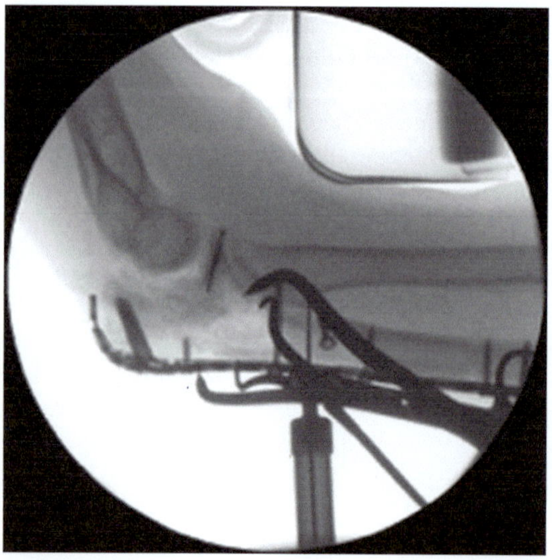

Fig. 20.16 C-arm fluoroscopic control of the plate installed

Control reduction with direct visualization of the sigmoid notch and the posterior cortex of the olecranon, and confirm with C-arm fluoroscopic control (Fig. 20.18).

Aftercare

Finally, after fixing both radius and ulna, assess the range of motion in pronation, supination, flexion, and extension. Fixation should be stable, and crepitus or restricted motion should be absent (Fig. 20.19). Radiocapitellar and ulnohumeral joints should remain located through a full range of motion. Postoperative treatment with a removable splint in supination for three weeks is then recommended to allow controlled mobilization of the elbow. Also X-rays are taken in two planes after six and twelve weeks (Fig. 20.20).

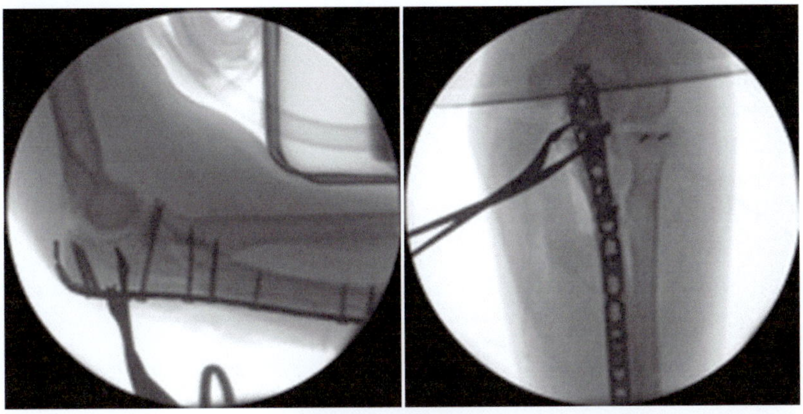

Fig. 20.18 C-arm fluoroscopic control of the coronoid process

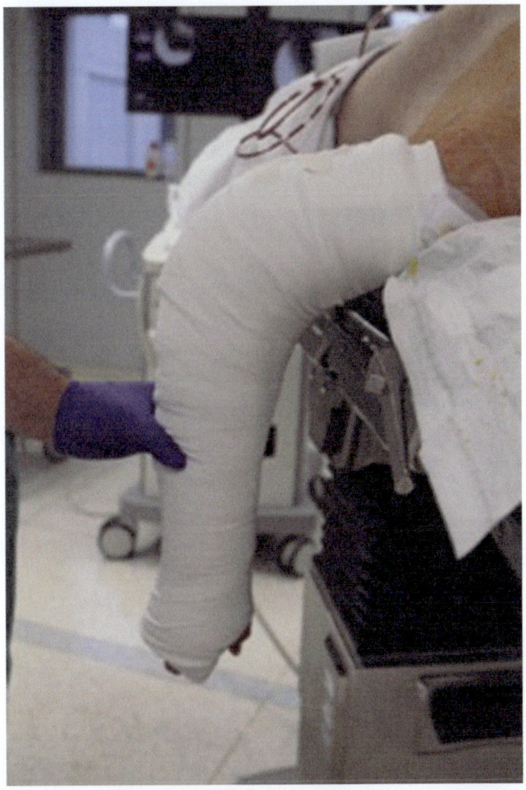

Fig. 20.19 Close contact casting in operation theater

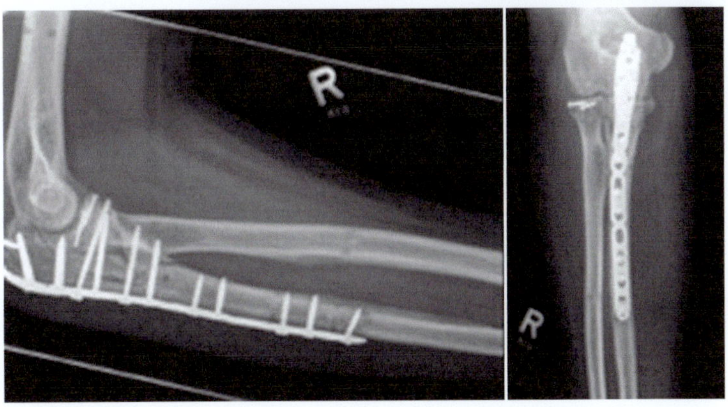

Fig. 20.20 Postoperative X-ray of the elbow in two planes

Reference

1. Monteggia GB. Instituzioni chirurgiche. Milano: Maspero; 1814.

Further Reading

Guitton TG, Ring D, Kloen P. Long-term evaluation of surgically treated anterior monteggia fractures in skeletally mature patients. J Hand Surg Am. 2009;34(9):1618–24.

Konrad GG, Kundel K, Kreuz PC, Oberst M, Sudkamp NP. Monteggia fractures in adults: long-term results and prognostic factors. J Bone Joint Surg Br. 2007; 89(3):354–60.

Ring D. Monteggia fractures. Orthop Clin North Am. 2013; 44(1):59–66.

Wong JC, Getz CL, Abboud JA. Adult monteggia and olecranon fracture dislocations of the elbow. Hand Clin. 2015;31(4):565–80.

21 Forearm Fractures

Katharina Sommer and Ingo Marzi

Anatomical Fracture Location: Radiograph of Fracture Pattern

Usually fractures of the forearm are associated with high-energy loads. Both bones ulna and radius can be involved. In a case of dislocation of one of the two bones, the other bone should be suspected to be fractured as well, though this might not be visible on the radiograph. As consequence, the adjacent joints, elbow, and wrist need to be visualized by X-ray in these cases [1].

Important for later rotational function is the anatomical reconstruction of both the radius and the ulna [2, 3]. Failure in restoration of the physiological bowing of the radius with an axis deviation that measures more than 5° will result in loss of forearm rotation and grip strength. The best picture to understand the forearm is to look at it like a joint. Therefore, every fracture needs an evaluation of the distal and proximal radioulnar joint. First of all, knowledge of the anatomical variations of these joints is essential for correct reduction (Figs. 21.1 and 21.2).

The forearm is a two-bone structure that is stabilized by the interosseous membrane. This membrane is a complex structure that allows smooth forearm rotation [4]. It is also important for load transfer between the radius and ulna from the distal to the proximal portion. The force distribution at the elbow is 43% ulnar and 57% radial, whereas at the wrist the radius bears 80% and the ulna only 20% of the load [5]. It consists of membranous portions, which are soft and thin, and different stronger bands. The most homogenous and robust structure of these bands is the central band. Its fibers are orientated at an angle of 21° to the longitudinal axis of the ulna. It originates from the proximal third of the radius and inserts at the distal third of the ulna. Accessory bands are highly variable in number, thickness, and location. Their fibers display the same orientation as those of the central band. Posttraumatic fibrosis of the interosseous membrane may result in restricted forearm rotation [6] (Fig. 21.2).

Most commonly, fracture pattern of the forearm is grouped by the AO classification. It divides the diaphyseal fractures into three main types. The simple fractures are classified A, the wedge fractures B, and the complex fractures C. It also distinguishes whether the radius, the ulna,

K. Sommer • I. Marzi (✉)
Department of Trauma, Hand and Reconstructive Surgery, Goethe University of Frankfurt, Frankfurt, Germany
e-mail: marzi@trauma.uni-frankfurt.de

P.V. Giannoudis (ed.), *Fracture Reduction and Fixation Techniques*,
https://doi.org/10.1007/978-3-319-68628-8_21

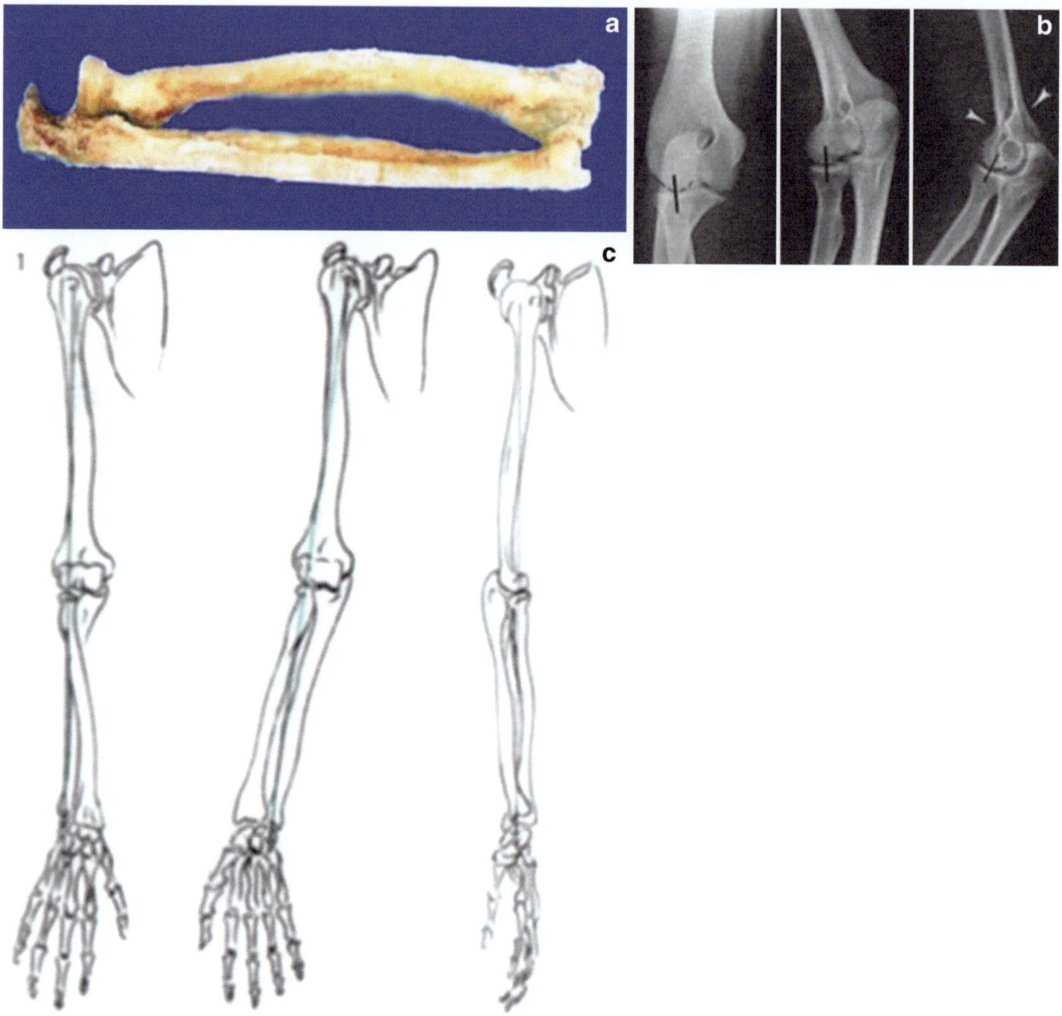

Fig. 21.1 (**a**) Normal appearance of the "forearm joint," (**b**) correct projection of the radius head to the capitellum at the elbow, (**c**) alignment of the bones of the forearm in pronation, supination, and neutral position

or both bones are broken. The knowledge about the muscle forces of the forearm is helpful to understand direction of dislocation of the fracture (Fig. 21.3).

A particular injury to the forearm is the Essex-Lopresti lesion that comprises a fracture of the radial head with a dislocation of the distal radio-ulnar joint [7]. This is the result of an approximation of the radius as the interosseous membrane is torn. Though the injury occurs seldom, it should be considered in radial head fractures with pain in the ulnar-sided wrist, DRUJ instability, or loss of forearm rotation [8]. Radiographs typically show a significant positive ulnar variance for more than 7 mm. MR imaging may allow the visualization of this rare injury in these cases.

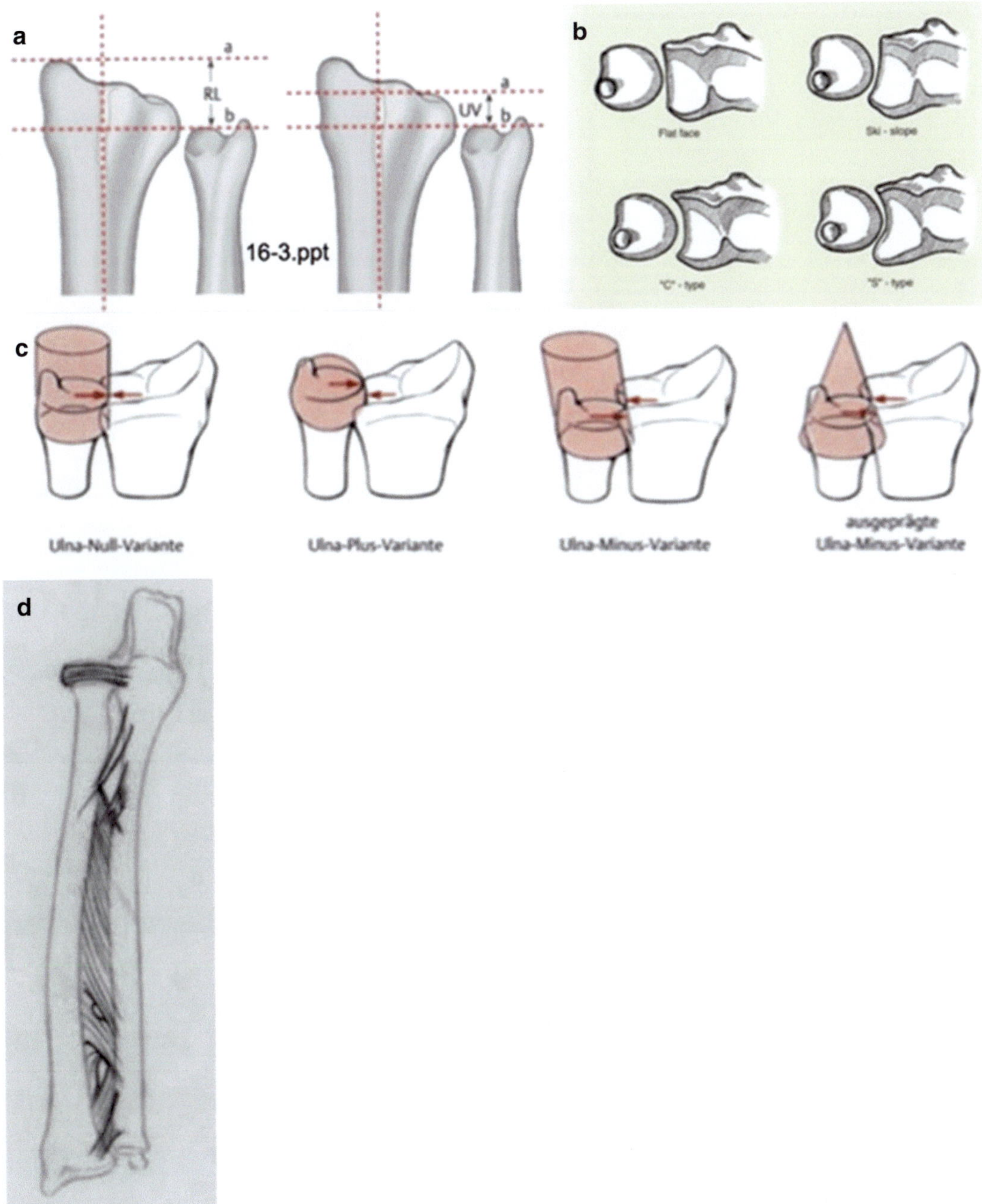

Fig. 21.2 (**a**) Normal relation of the radial (8–18 mm) and ulnar (−4 – +4 mm) length, (**b**) normal variation of the sigmoid notch, (**c**) normal variation of the position of the distal radioulnar joint in the frontal plane, (**d**) interosseous membrane

Fig. 21.3 (**a**) AO fracture classification of forearm fractures, (**b**) fracture dislocation

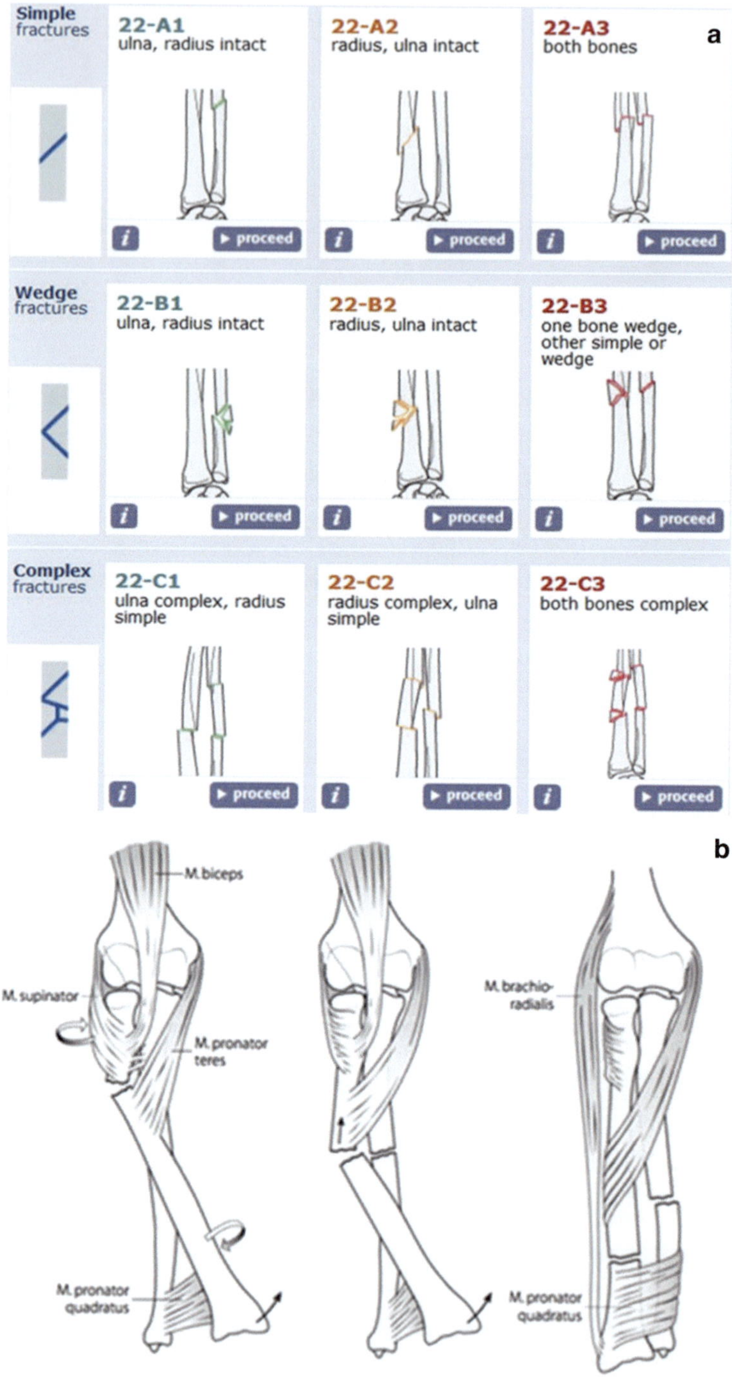

Brief Preoperative Planning

Fractures of the diaphyseal forearm in adults usually require surgical treatment to restore normal biomechanics. There are only rare cases of minimally displaced or stable reduced ulna fractures that do not involve the distal or proximal radio-ulnar joint and can be treated by cast immobilization (AO Classification A1.2 fractures) [9]. Casting may also be considered in patients with a

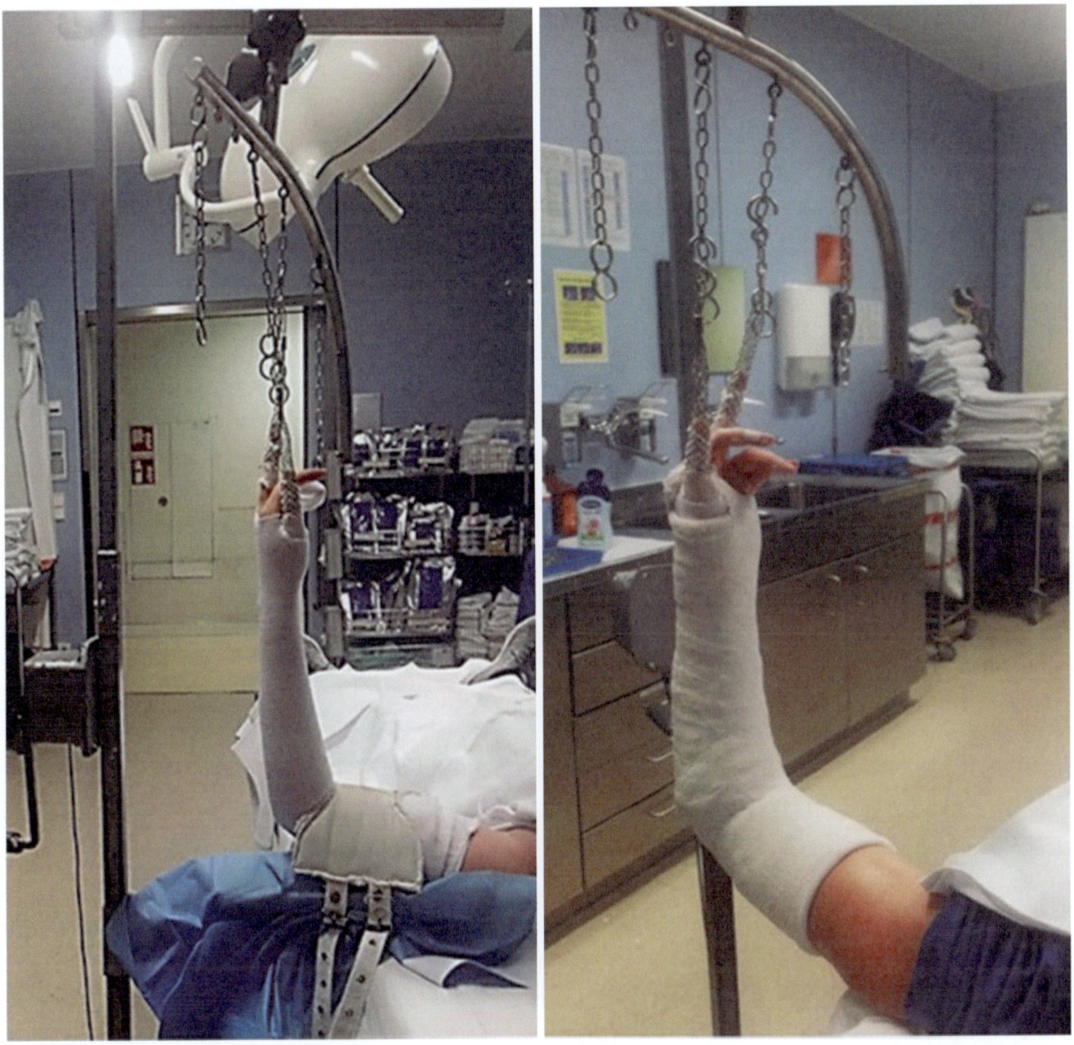

Fig. 21.4 Closed reduction by hanging traction and circular casting

significant disease limiting surgery in severe soft tissue damage resulting in compromised functional outcome.

For casting, both wrist and elbow joint have to be immobilized with the elbow in 90° flexed position. It should end proximal to the palmar flexor crease and spare the thumb to allow full range of motion of all fingers. Right after trauma the cast should be split to avoid compartment syndrome due to progressive swelling. It can be closed after swelling has subsided (Fig. 21.4).

In children, fractures with an angle less than 10° can be treated conservatively by casting [10]. Only in very young children, even a dislocation up to 20° can be tolerated [11]. A long arm cast as described above achieves the immobilization. After 2–5 days wedging of the circular cast can be performed to improve fracture positioning. This has to be done thoroughly in a very well-adapted cast, but the effects of wedging are critically discussed. In all other children, elastic stable intramedullary nailing is the primary choice of treatment [12] (Fig. 21.5).

Most of the times, fractures of the diaphyseal forearm are unstable and need surgical treatment. Furthermore, conservatively treated fractures tend to fail bone healing, and angulation results in an impairment of rotation or joint

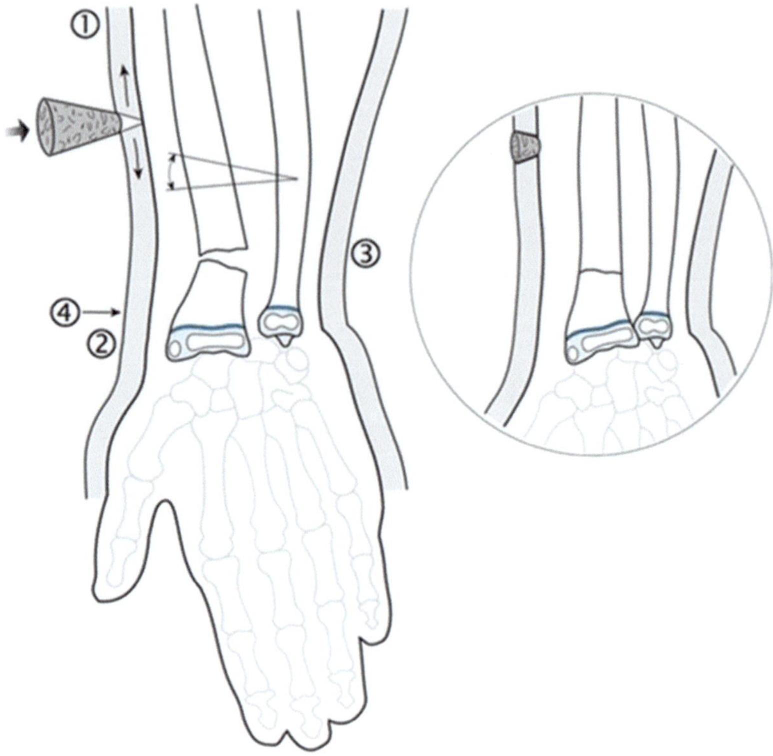

Fig. 21.5 Reduction by wedging of the circular cast

incongruence. If possible, plate osteosynthesis should be favored in most of the cases. Intramedullary rigid nailing lacks rotational stability, thus resulting in nonunion of the bone as well as synostosis and has not been established in adults [6, 13]. However, if such a method is chosen, a sugar tongue splint or a similar brace can add stability and improve healing allowing elbow and wrist movement at the same time. Hybrid treatment with plating of the radius and intramedullary elastic nailing of the ulna can be considered but is not a standard procedure. In case of absent other options, external fixation is possible, but usually results are not satisfactory, and it has the risk for radial nerve injury.

Plate osteosynthesis of the radius and ulna may be performed as compression osteosynthesis or as indirect bridging in the sense of a biological osteosynthesis. Most commonly used is a LCP (Locking Compression Plate). In case of an oblique fracture, a lag screw should be inserted either through the plate or independently. By doing so the plate is used as a neutralization plate. If in transverse fractures a lag screw is not possible, the plate can be used as a compression plate. These two options are only possible in simple fractures as complex and compound fractures may not be compressed. In these cases, a bridging of the fracture site leaving the partially vascularized fragments untouched should be done. Preoperatively, length of the needed implant should be determined with the aid of the radiograph. At least three bicortical screws are needed in each of the main fragments. The advantage of the LCP implant is that it can be used as both an internal fixator as well as for compression of the fragments. As plating of the forearm needs an open access to the bone, open reduction is used most of the times in adults. Nevertheless, a biological osteosynthesis that preserves blood supply to the fracture side should be sought (Fig. 21.6).

In case of severe soft tissue injury, loss of bone, and infection, an external fixator is an alternative for plate osteosynthesis. Defect after infection or bone loss due to the trauma can be bridged

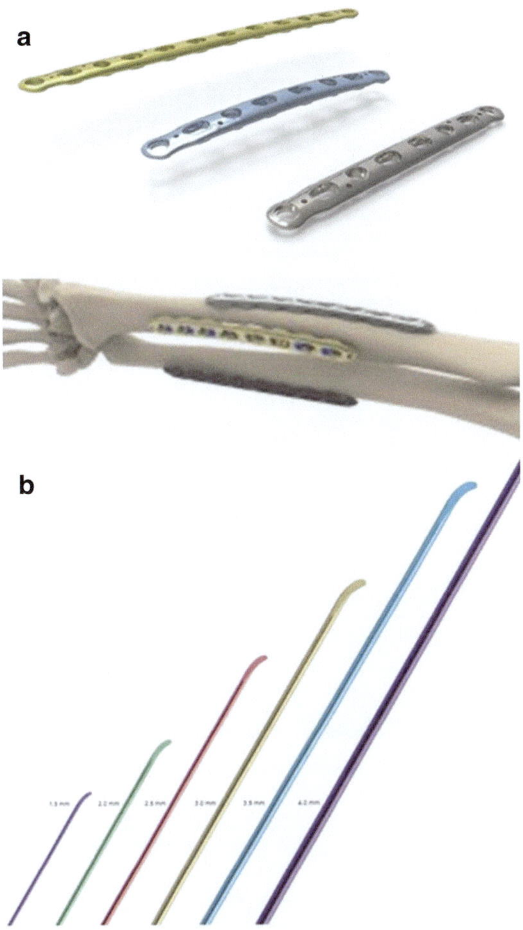

Fig. 21.6 (**a**) LCP for radius and ulna, (**b**) intramedullary nails

using bone cement and later replaced by bone grafting, thus applying the Masquelet technique (Fig. 21.7) [14].

Patient Setup in Theater

For surgery, the patient is placed in a supine position with the fractured arm on a hand table. Alternatively, the arm may be placed across the torso of the patient or in an overhead arm gutter. If using a Henry approach, the arm is put in supine position (Fig. 21.8). A non-sterile pneumatic tourniquet is applied to the forearm above the elbow to improve intraoperative reduction of bleeding and enhancement of intraoperative

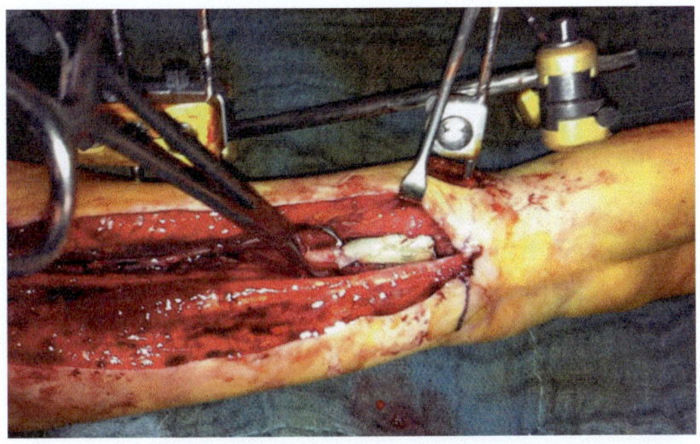

Fig. 21.7 Bridging of a radial defect with a cement spacer

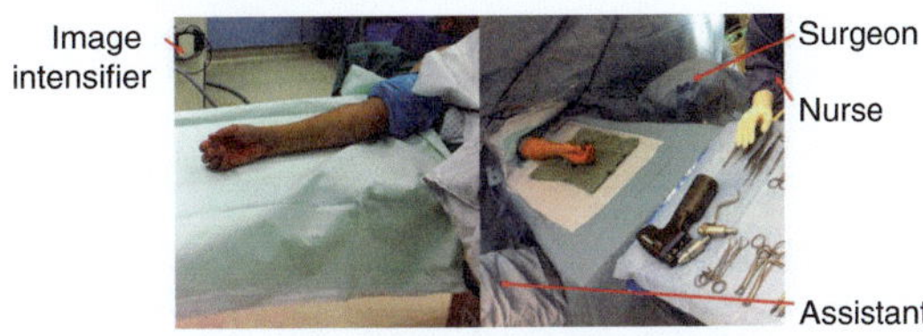

Fig. 21.8 Patient setup in operation theater

view. For optimal intraoperative positioning of the arm, it is favorable to drape up to the mid part of the upper arm. The surgeon sits on a stool that can be adjusted in height either on the radial or the ulnar side of the forearm depending on the fracture. The assistant is positioned on the opposite side of the arm. The image intensifier is placed on the distal side opposite of the surgeon. In cases of intramedullary nailing, a counter device at the elbow might be helpful for distraction (Figs. 21.9 and 21.10).

Closed Reduction Maneuvers

For closed reduction, the arm can be suspended in Chinese finger traps in a supine position with the elbow bent 90°. If conservative treatment is sought, the cast can be molded into the groove between the radius and ulna to help separate the two bones.

In the operation theater, manual longitudinal traction and rotation often suffice for fracture reduction. When performing intramedullary nailing, it is advisable first to push both the ulnar and the radial nail right up to the side of the fracture. Then reduction is performed by traction and rotation, and both nails are moved beyond the fracture in an alternating way (Figs. 21.10 and 21.11). Traction can also be exerted horizontally during surgery by a special traction table with a hypomochlion put in the 90° flexed elbow (Fig. 21.9). If the fracture is more distal, hyperextension of the distal fragment in traction before flexion helps in reduction (Fig. 21.12). In certain cases, the reduction of the second forearm bone might be very difficult, if one side is fixed.

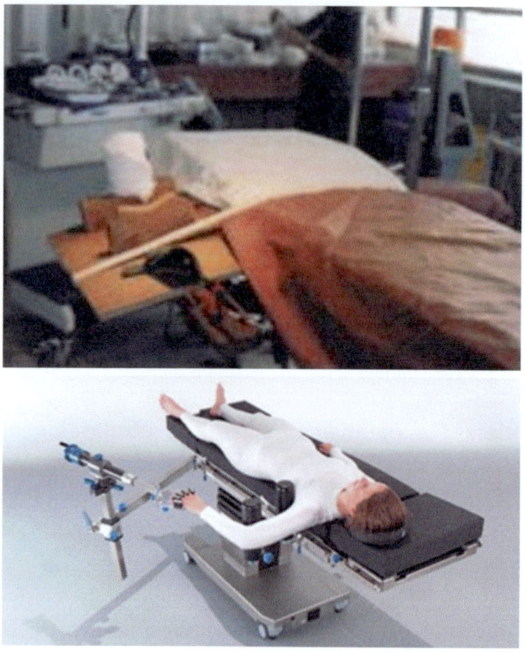

Fig. 21.9 Traction table for the forearm for intramedullary nailing [15]

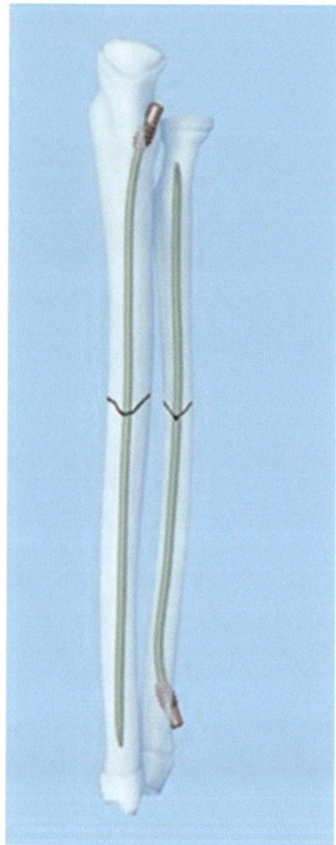

Fig. 21.10 Insertion point for intramedullary nails on the radius and the ulna

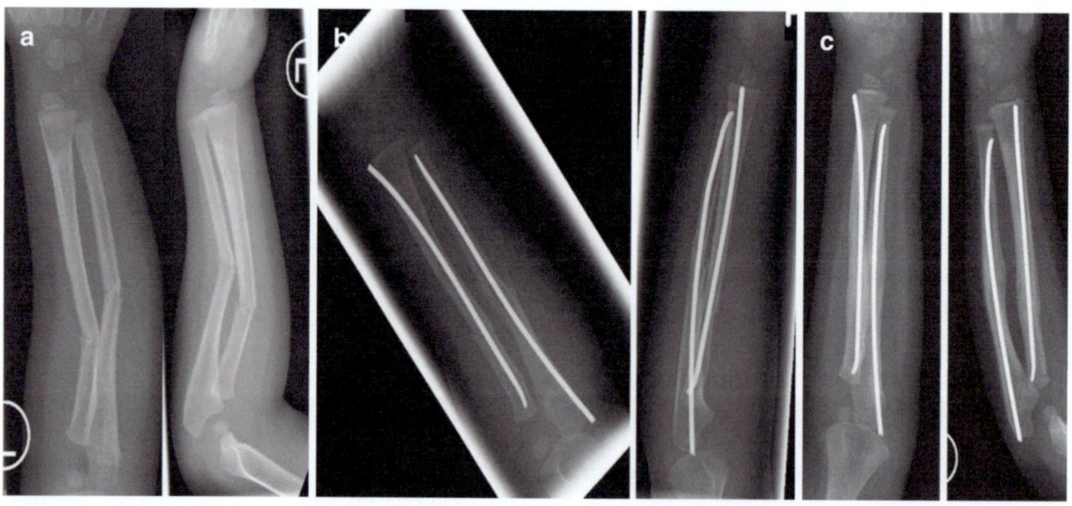

Fig. 21.11 Intramedullary nailing of a complete forearm fracture in a child (**a**) before surgery, (**b**) after surgery, and (**c**) after bone consolidation

Reduction Instruments

Open reduction can be helped by placing reduction forceps on each main fragment. Beyond that, a small bone lever can be used to set the fragments in place. Another way for reduction in oblique fractures is to place a reduction forceps in the area of the fracture and twist it, thereby lengthening and compressing the fracture. A pointed or a blunt reduction forceps is usually used to maintain fracture reduction (Fig. 21.13). In forearm fractures the plate itself is very helpful for fracture reduction. Especially in commuted fractures, new anatomic plates address the form of the radial bone very well. Thus, the plates can temporarily be fixed with reduction clamps after achieving anatomic reduction.

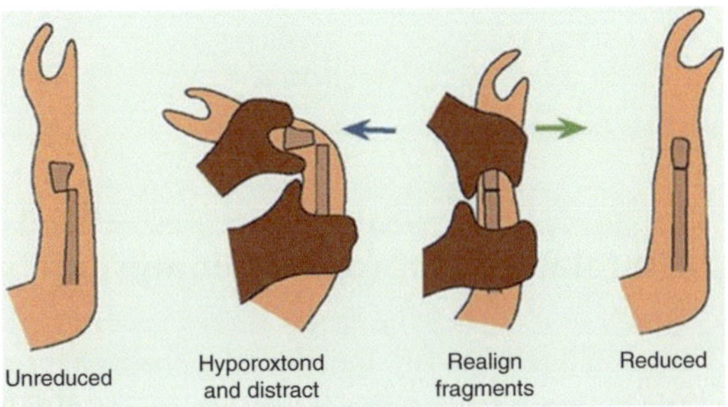

Fig. 21.12 Closed reduction technique with hyperextension and traction before reduction by flexion

Surgical Approach

If both bones need to be taken care of, a separate approach to the radius as well as to the ulna is chosen as a single approach increases the risk for synostosis. The interval between the two skin incisions should at least be 5 cm in order to avoid skin necrosis.

Overview of the different approaches can be seen at Table 21.1.

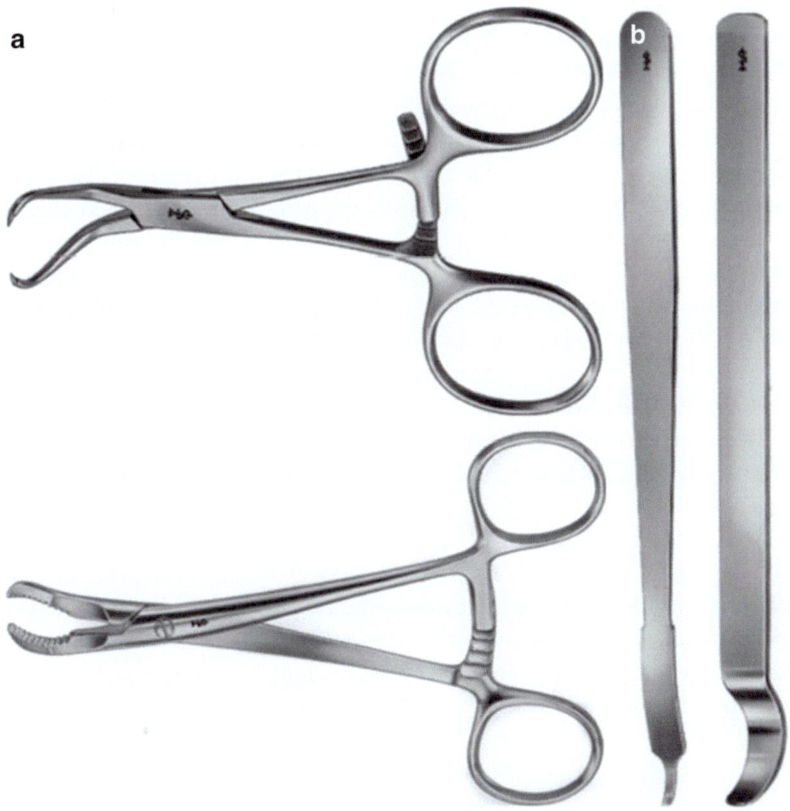

Fig. 21.13 (**a**) Pointed and blunt reduction forceps, (**b**) pointed and blunt bone lever

Table 21.1 Summary of approaches to the forearm

Approach	Henry	Thompson	Lateral to the ulna	Intramedullary nailing	Kocher	Boyd	Kaplan	Medial to elbow
Access to	Radius (volar side)	Radius (dorsolateral side)	Ulna	–	Lateral capsule, lateral ligaments, distal humerus, proximal radius	Lateral ulna ligaments	Capitulum humeri, radial head	Processus coronoideus, medial capsule and ligaments
Structures at risk	Deep and superficial branch of the radial nerve	Dorsal interosseous nerve	Dorsal branch of ulna nerve	Superficial radial nerve			Motoric branch of radial nerve	Ulna nerve

Anterior Approach (Henry)

For this approach the forearm is laid out in full supination. The surgeon sits on the ulnar side of the arm. The incision runs proximally from the biceps tendon distally to the radial styloid process. The fascia is opened between the interval of the brachioradialis muscle that is mobilized to the radial side. The flexor carpi radialis muscle is retracted ulnar. The lateral recurrent branches of the radial artery are to be ligated. The superficial branch of the radial nerve needs to be carefully dissected to avoid accidental injury. Then the supinator muscle needs to be freed from the periosteum to be retracted to the radial side. For further distal dissection, the underlying pronator teres muscle is gently to be stripped from the bone radially to expose the radial shaft. Care must be taken not to completely strip off the flexor pollicis longus muscle.

If dissection is in the distal part of the forearm, care has to be taken not to injure the deep (m. supinator) and superficial (m. brachioradialis) branch of the radial nerve by lever traction. In the proximal part, the lateral cutaneous nerve of the forearm is to be preserved. However, the radial bone at the palmar side between the radial tuberosity is flat and therefore provides a good orientation for reduction – especially to avoid malrotation (Fig. 21.14).

Posterolateral Approach (Thompson)

The skin incision for the dorsal approach is a straight line between the lateral epicondyle and the Lister's tubercle. The arm is lightly pronated. The deep dissection lies between the extensor digitorum communis muscle and the radial forearm extensors (especially the extensor carpi radialis brevis). The underlying abductor pollicis longus and extensor pollicis brevis muscles are partially freed and retracted radially. For distal exposure, these two muscles can be detached proximally. For proximal exposure, the distal third of the supinator muscle can be stripped from the radius. The proximal part of the muscle may not be touched as the dorsal interosseous nerve lies within (Fig. 21.15).

Lateral Approach to the Ulna

The forearm is fully pronated. The surgeon sits on the lateral side of the arm. The skin incision runs the whole way 1 cm dorsally to the edge of the ulna. The fascia is separated between the extensor carpi ulnaris muscle that is carefully pushed from ulna and the flexor carpi ulnaris muscle. The dorsal branch of the ulna nerve is to be gently dissected at the very distal part of the ulna (Fig. 21.16).

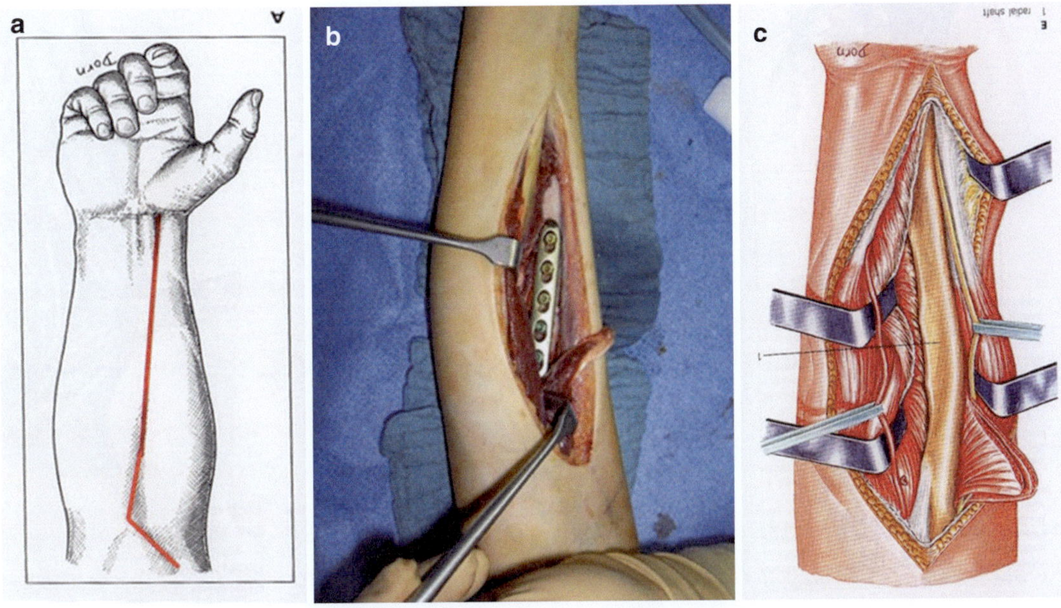

Fig. 21.14 Henry approach. (**a**) Skin incision, (**b**) intraoperative photograph, (**c**) anatomical picture

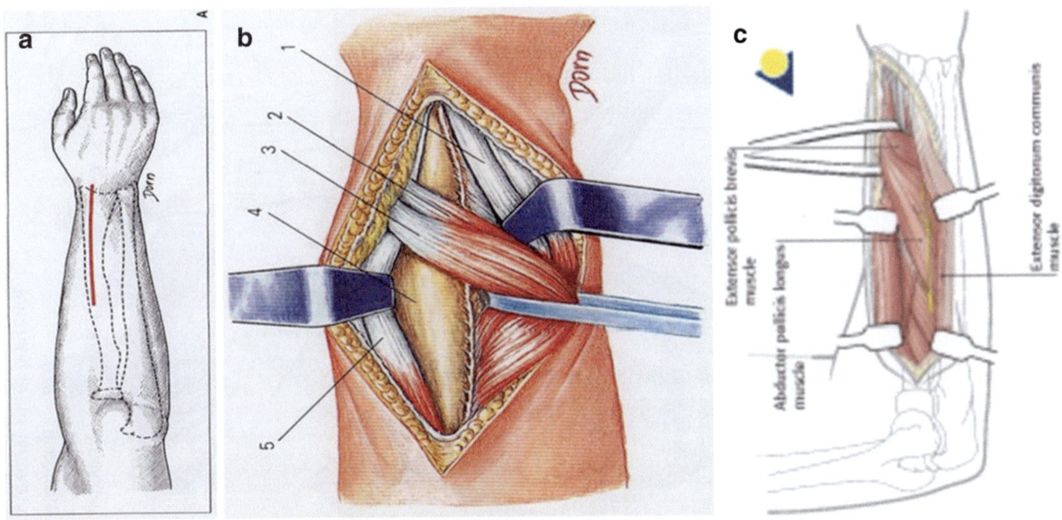

Fig. 21.15 Thomson approach. (**a**) Skin incision, (**b+c**) anatomical picture showing the abductor pollicis longus and extensor pollicis brevis crossing the radius

Approach for Intramedullary Nailing

For intramedullary nailing a small incision is made at the dorso-radial side of the ulna about 3 cm distal to the ulna apophysis. The incision for the radius is either on the distal radial side or on the dorsal side in the area of the Lister's tubercle. If the radial incision is used, care has to be taken not to injure the superficial radial nerve. Thus, after skin incision, preparation is performed with blunt instruments.

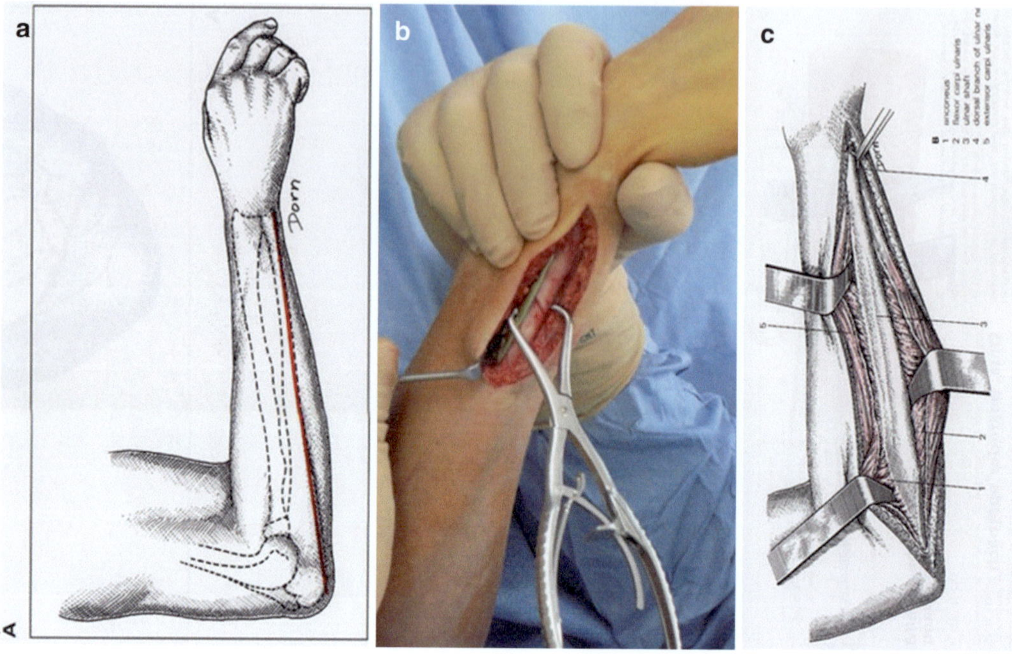

Fig. 21.16 Lateral approach to the ulna. (**a**) Skin incision, (**b**) intraoperative photograph, (**c**) anatomical picture

This technique is usually only used in children when elastic stable intramedullary nailing is performed.

Lateral Approach to the Elbow (Kocher)

The typical Kocher approach is chosen for the treatment of injuries of the lateral capsule and ligaments as well as the distal humerus and the proximal radius. The dorsolateral portion of the joint capsule can be reached through the gap between the anconeus and extensor carpi ulnaris muscle in order to stabilize the ligament for example (Fig. 21.17).

Lateral Approach to the Elbow (Boyd)

In case of injuries to the lateral ulna ligaments, the approach needs to be modified to exhibit the more dorsally localized ligaments that originate lower to the lateral epicondyle and distend to the olecranon. For this purpose, the anconeus muscle and the distal part of the triceps muscle are mobilized dorsally. Finally, the extensor muscles as well as the extensor carpi ulnaris muscle are dissected to the ventral side and lifted up (Fig. 21.17).

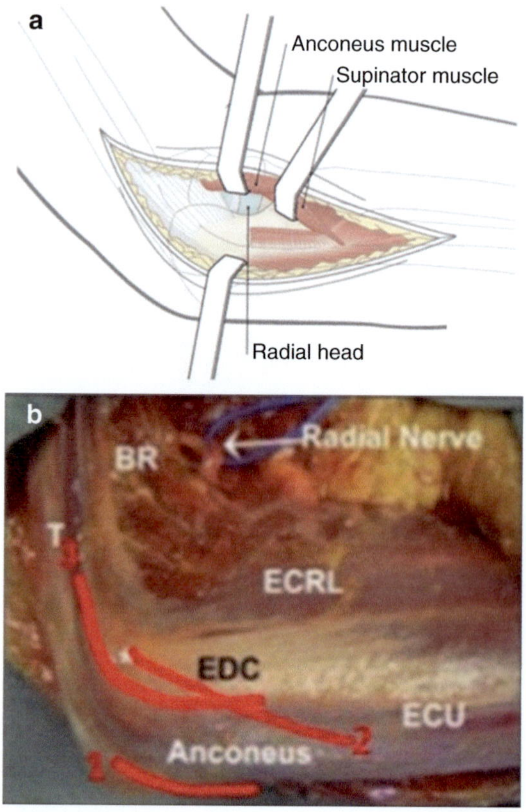

Fig. 21.17 (**a**) Skin incision and dissection for Boyd's approach, (**b**) anatomical view of dissection plane for (1) Boyd, (2) Kocher, and (3) Kaplan

Anterolateral Approach (Kaplan)

This approach gives access to the capitulum humeri as well as the radial head. The entrance is between the extensor carpi ulnaris and the extensor digitorum muscles. For this approach, it is generally important to take care of the deep motoric branch of the radial nerve (Fig. 21.17).

Medial Approach

The medial approach is needed for the treatment of the distal medial humerus, the coronoid process, and the medial structures of the capsule and ligaments. It is most important in this approach to mobilize the ulnar nerve sufficiently. In the distal part of the upper arm, the intermuscular septum is identified and excised if need. Afterward, the pronator muscle and part of the flexor communis muscles are separated, and the muscles to the distal side are split. Now the capsule and the brachialis muscle are visible. Incision of the capsule enables the view into the medial joint, especially the coronoid process. Detachment of the distal part of the triceps muscle from the distal medial column of the humerus allows display of the medial complex of the capsule and ligaments (Fig. 21.18).

Open Reduction Maneuvers

In case of a whole forearm fracture, the bone with the simpler fracture should be approached first and fixed preliminary as this helps in correct alignment and rotation of the forearm. Then osteosynthesis of the other bone is performed. Sometimes fixation of the first bone hinders reposition of the other. Thus loosening of the first osteosynthesis might be needed in order to anatomically reduce the other bone. If fracture pattern is similar in both bones, the ulna usually is taken care of first before osteosynthesis of the radius because the ulna is less curved and anatomical reduction is easier to achieve.

Manual Traction

Usually rotation and alignment of the bones can be achieved by traction and rotation of the forearm. The reduction result can be maintained either by applying a reduction forceps on the fracture side or by fixing the plate as a template with two clamps on the bone in comminuted fractures. A small bench or a roll can assist in reposition as a hypomochlion (Fig. 21.19a).

Temporal External Fixation

In case that reduction cannot be achieved or maintained directly, an external fixator can be applied to temporarily fix length and rotation. Care has to be taken that the pins do not interfere with the positioning of the plate (Fig. 21.19b).

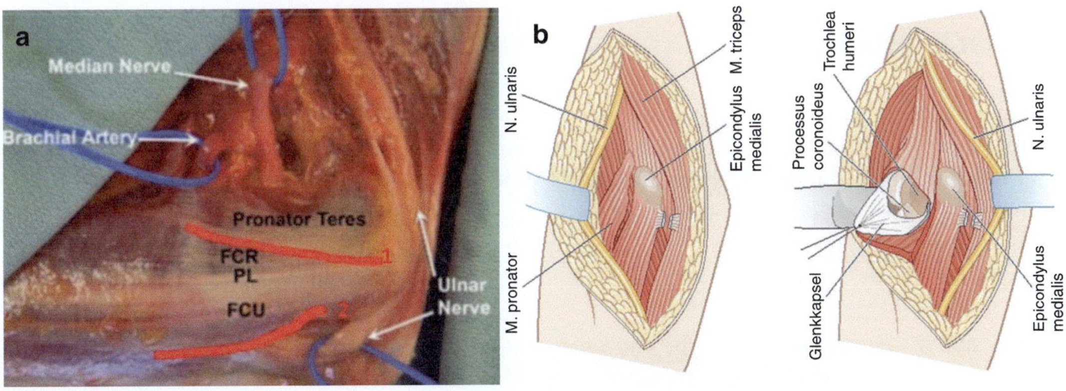

Fig. 21.18 Medial approach to the elbow. (**a**) Anatomical view for (1) Hotchkiss, (2) approach between the two heads of the flexor carpi ulnaris muscle, (**b**) deep dissection for Hotchkiss approach "over the top"

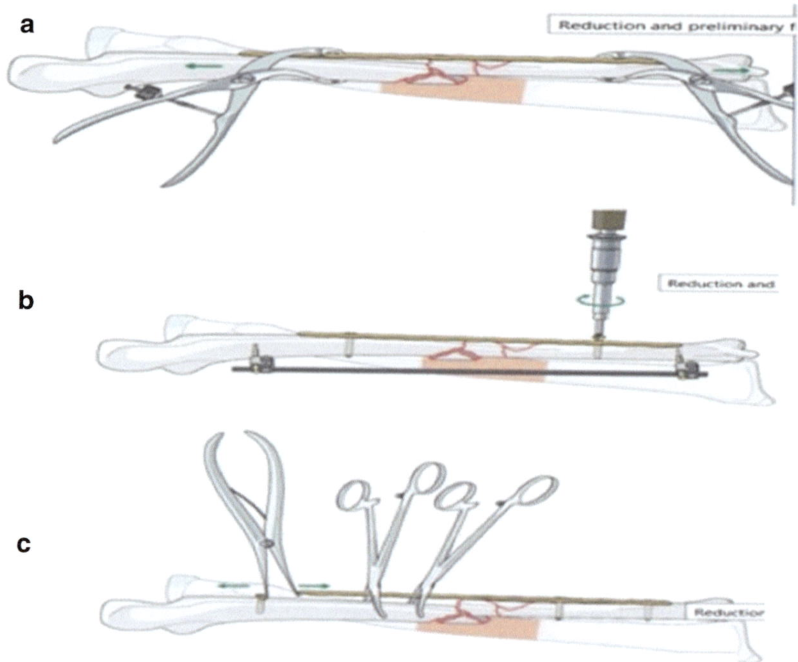

Fig. 21.19 (**a**) Fracture reduction by plate fixation as a template, (**b**) temporal external fixation, (**c**) plate distraction

Plate Distraction

For this technique, the plate is fixed to one of the main fragments, firstly with two bicortical screws in the desired position. Secondly, a screw is applied distant to the plate on the other main fragment. The plate is held loosely in place with blunt reduction forceps still allowing a sliding motion along the shaft of the bone. A laminar spreader is put between the separate screw and the plate. By opening distraction is achieved up to the desired length. Lastly, the plate is fixed to the other main fragment (Fig. 21.19c).

Implant Insertion

If available, a 3.5 mm LC-DCP is the implant of choice in adults. If needed, the plate can be bent with bending irons or pliers. Correct bending of the plate supports the reconstruction of the curved form of the radius in the middle of the shaft where it bents away from the ulna (Figs. 21.20–21.22).

The size of the implant should be chosen so that there are at least three bicortical screws in the proximal and distal main fragment. In case of revision surgery, even four bicortical screws might be needed. Only in simple fractures, two bicortical screws may be possible to reduce soft tissue damage.

If possible, e.g., in oblique fractures, a lag screw is to be inserted separately or through a plate hole. It is also possible in wedge fractures to fix the wedge fragment to one of the main fragments by lag screw fixation.

On the ulna the plate should be positioned dorsally underneath the extensor carpi radialis muscle if possible. The position under the flexor carpi radialis muscle and the interval in between is also feasible if dorsal positioning is impractical.

On the radius the plate can be positioned volar or dorsal as required by fracture pattern. As the Henry approach ensures extensile exposure, a volar position is usually chosen in complex fractures.

In multilevel fractures, correct alignment can be helped by treating each fracture individually. Thus, double plating on one bone is a good option for correct reduction. For this, plates need to be placed in an overlapping fashion to avoid stress fractures in the plane between the two plates (Fig. 21.23).

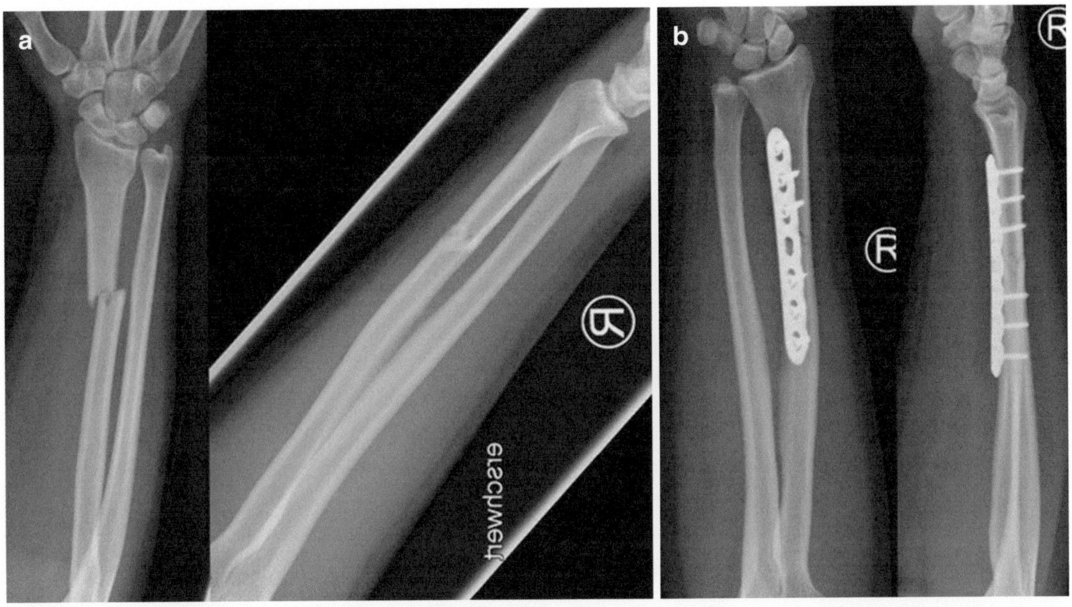

Fig. 21.20 Fracture treatment of the radial shaft by plate osteosynthesis. (**a**) Before operative care, (**b**) after osteosynthesis by plate

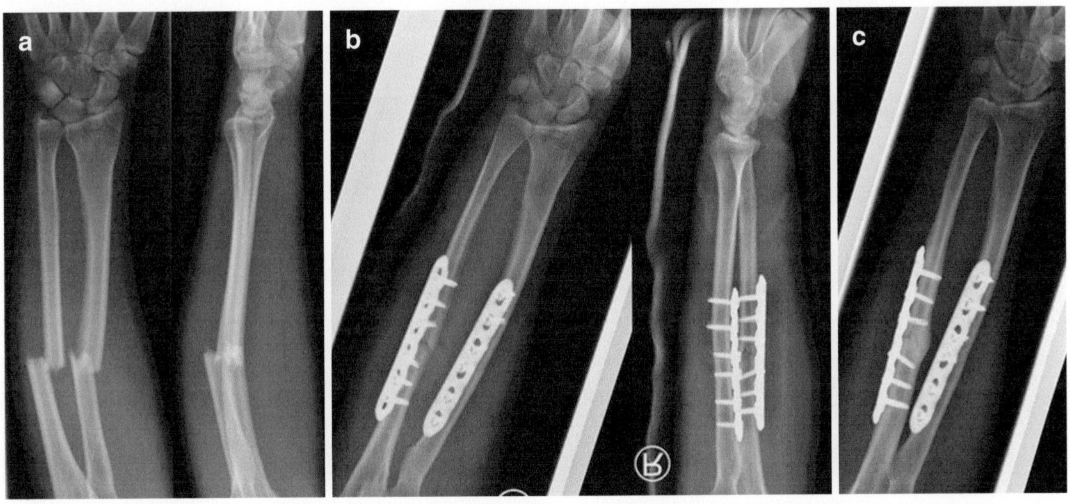

Fig. 21.21 Fracture treatment of the radial shaft by plate osteosynthesis. (**a**) Before operative care, (**b**) after osteosynthesis by double plate, (**c**) after consolidation of the bone with primary bone healing on the radius and secondary bone healing of the ulna; notice the callus formation

For correct implant positioning and verification of correct alignment of the bones, exact radiographs AP and laterally are essential. Correct alignment can also be judged by thickness of the bone cortex. In case of inhomogeneous thickness or steps in caliber, an incorrect reduction is likely (Fig. 21.24).

After successful osteosynthesis, the DRUJ should be assessed for possible instability ruling out an Essex-Lopresti injury. Furthermore, rotation should be checked to verify that full range of motion is possible that is achieved by anatomical reduction. In addition, the rotation in the DRUJ has to be checked as well.

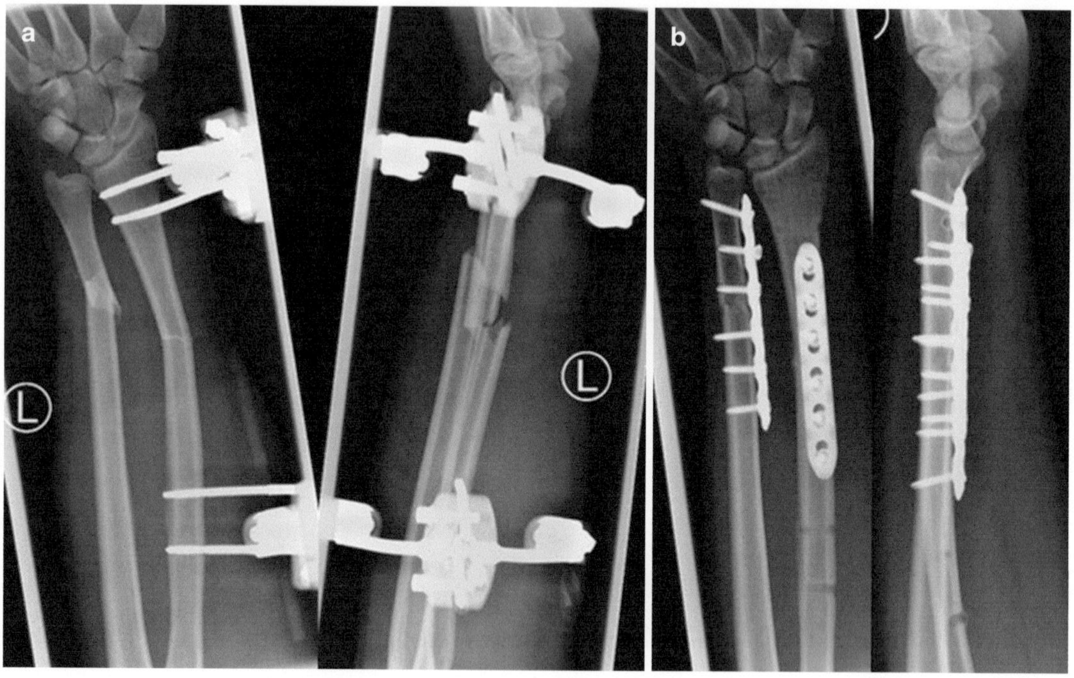

Fig. 21.22 (**a**) Temporary reduction of the complete forearm fracture by external fixation in case of severe tissue damage, (**b**) definitive treatment by plate osteosynthesis is carried out in an interval; notice ulna plating is performed on the volar side due to sever tissue damage

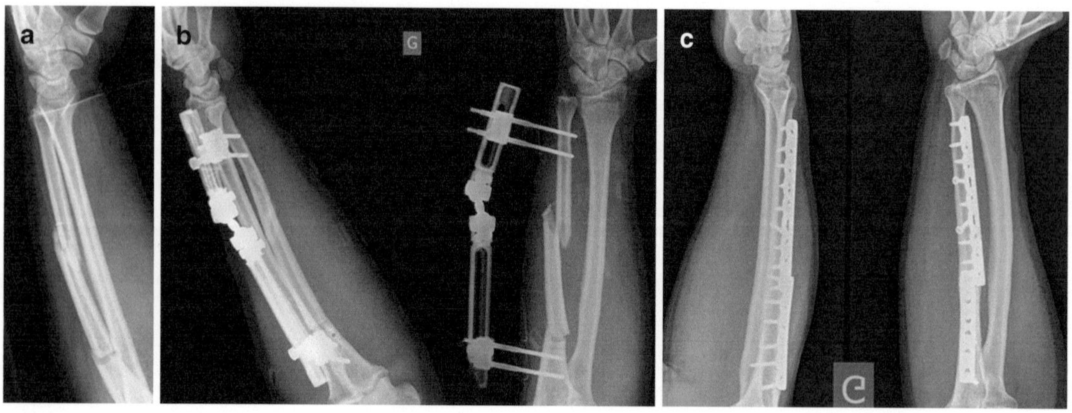

Fig. 21.23 Treatment of a multilevel fracture of the ulna, (**a**) radiograph before surgery, (**b**) after temporary external fixation, (**c**) definitive treatment with two plates

After ORIF treatment early rehabilitation with free range of motion without weight bearing should be the aim. In case of a healing fracture in the radiograph, pain depending full weight bearing should be performed after 6 weeks [16].

In Essex-Lopresti injury, rotation of the forearm should be avoided for the first 4 weeks after surgery. Thus, a splint or orthosis is required for aftercare. Passive and active flexion and extension of the elbow should be performed out of the cast during this time. After 4 weeks, the patient can start with gentle forearm rotation that can be extended to passive exercises after 6 weeks. Weight bearing can be

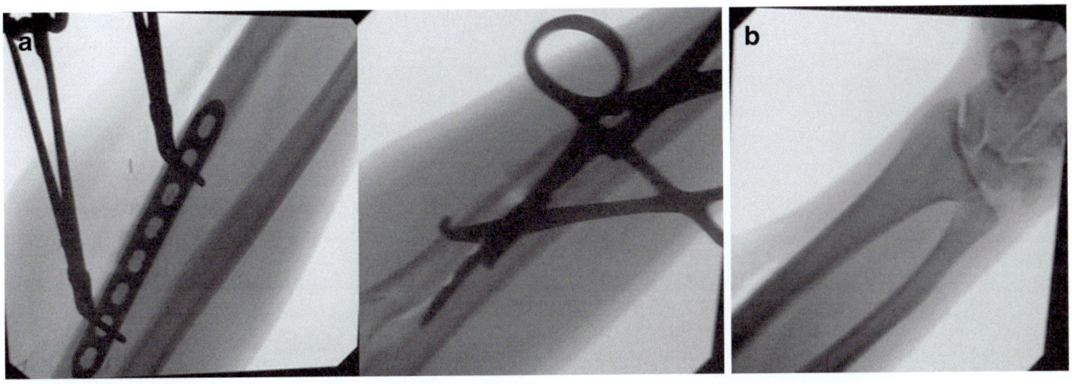

Fig. 21.24 Intraoperative assessment of (**a**) plate position and fracture reduction, (**b**) evaluation of correct alignment in the distal radioulnar joint

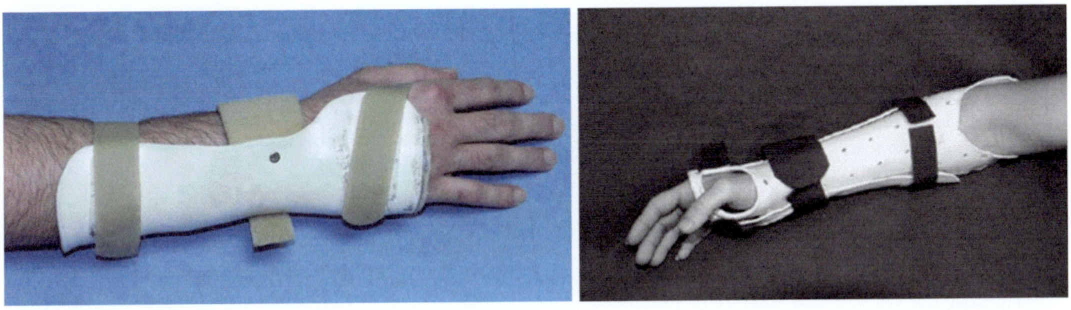

Fig. 21.25 Splint for immobilization of the distal radioulnar joint

initiated 8 weeks after surgery progressing as tolerated (Fig. 21.25).

In children, ESIN (elastic stable intramedullary nailing) is be performed retrograde in the radius and antegrade in the ulna [17]. The ulna is addressed by a small incision dorso-ulnar in the metaphyseal area of the ulna, and the prebent elastic nail is inserted antegrade. The approach to the radius is in the distal radial metaphysis, but there, the superficial branch of the radial nerve should be seen and protected. The nail is inserted retrograde up to the proximal radial neck under X-ray observation. Diameter of the elastic nails is 2 or 2.5 mm in general. Other approaches such as radius from dorsal or ulna from distal are not recommended due to higher complication rates.

Implants in adults can be removed after 18 months with secure bone consolidation. In children intramedullary nails are usually removed after 4–6 month. In younger children, removal might be performed earlier due to faster growth.

Summary of Tips and Tricks-Pitfalls

- If both bones are fractured, the simpler fracture should be approached first and anatomically fixed.
- Correct reduction and implant position have to be checked at the end of the surgery by image intensifier including elbow and wrist joints [18].
- The forearm needs to be tested for complete rotational ability with the elbow bent at 90° as well as instability of the DRUJ.
- After surgery be careful to watch for signs of compartment syndrome [19].

References

1. Pandey S, Pandey A. Chapter-27 fracture of forearm bones (Radius and Ulna). Fundamentals of orthopedics & trauma. 1st ed. Bengaluru: Jaypee Brothers Medical Publishers (P) Ltd; 2015. p. 479–88.
2. Yasutomi T, Nakatsuchi Y, Koike H, Uchiyama S. Mechanism of limitation of pronation/supination of the forearm in geometric models of deformities of the forearm bones. Clin Biomech. 2002;17:456–63.
3. LaStayo PC, Lee MJ. The forearm complex: anatomy, biomechanics and clinical considerations. J Hand Ther. 2006;19:137–44.
4. Skahen JR, Palmer AK, Werner FW, Fortino MD. The interosseous membrane of the forearm: anatomy and function. J Hand Surg Am. 1997;22:981–5.
5. Shaaban H, Giakas G, Bolton M, Williams R, Wicks P, Scheker LR, et al. The load-bearing characteristics of the forearm: pattern of axial and bending force transmitted through ulna and radius. J Hand Surg Br. 2006;31:274–9.
6. Bauer G, Arand M, Mutschler W. Post-traumatic radioulnar synostosis after forearm fracture osteosynthesis. Arch Orthop Trauma Surg. 1991;110(3):142–5.
7. Sabo MT, Watts AC. Longitudinal instability of the forearm: anatomy, biomechanics, and treatment considerations. Shoulder Elbow, vol. 4. London: SAGE Publications; 2012. p. 119–26.
8. Green JB, Zelouf DS. Forearm instability. J Hand Surg Am. 2009;34:953–61.
9. Fisher H. Splint for fracture of the forearm. Lancet. 1883;122:722.
10. Laurer H, Sander A, Wutzler S, Walcher F, Marzi I. Therapy principles of distal fractures of the forearm in childhood. Chirurg. 2009;80:1042–52.
11. Högström H, Nllsson BE, Wlllner S. Correction with growth following diaphyseal forearm fracture. Acta Orthop Scand. 2009;47:299–303.
12. Lascombes P, Prevot J, Ligier JN, Metaizeau JP, Poncelet T. Elastic Stable Intramedullary Nailing in Forearm Shaft Fractures in Children: 85 Cases. J Pediatr Orthop. 1990;10:167.
13. Dhariwal Q, Inamdar P, Arora P, Shyam A. Stacked flexible nailing for radius ulna fractures: revival of a lost technique. J Orthop Case Rep. 2017;7:106–8.
14. Masquelet AC, Fitoussi F, Begue T. Reconstruction of the long bones by the induced membrane and spongy autograft. Ann Chir Plast Esthet. 2000;45:346–53.
15. Yaligod V. Forearm fracture table for closed nailing of fractures of shafts of forearm bones in adults. J Evol Med Dent Sci. 2013;2:7347–56.
16. Matsuura Y, Rokkaku T, Suzuki T, Thoreson AR, An K-N, Kuniyoshi K. Evaluation of bone atrophy after treatment of forearm fracture using nonlinear finite element analysis: a comparative study of locking plates and conventional plates. J Hand Surg Am. 2017;42:659.e1–9.
17. Weinberg A-M, Castellani C, Amerstorfer F. Elastic stable intramedullary nailing (ESIN) of forearm fractures. Orthop Traumatol. 2008;20:285–96.
18. Damle A. Chapter-15 bow fracture of forearm. Tips & tricks in orthopedic surgery. 1st ed. Bengaluru: Jaypee Brothers Medical Publishers (P) Ltd; 2015. p. 108–12.
19. Royle SG. Compartment syndrome following forearm fracture in children. Injury. 1990;21:73–6.

22 Galeazzi Fracture

Theodoros H. Tosounidis and Paul J. Harwood

Anatomical Fracture Location: Radiograph of Fracture Pattern

Galeazzi fracture or otherwise known as "fracture of necessity" is a fracture of the distal radius with disruption of the distal radioulnar joint (DRUJ). It is called fracture of necessity because in adults its management necessitates the surgical treatment with anatomic reduction and stable fixation of both the radial fracture and the DRUJ. It is well established that non-surgical management of this highly unstable fracture results in malunions with significant functional deficit and unsatisfactory results [1]. The fracture of the radius that involves the distal third of the bone is the result of the axial loading of the forearm in either supination or rotation. A short oblique fracture with apex anterior (volar) [2] (Fig. 22.1a, b) or apex posterior (dorsal) [3] (Fig. 22.2a, b) angulation of the radius occurs, respectively. The torsional mechanism of the injury results to concomitant disruption of the DRUJ and injury to its primary stabiliser (triangular fibrocartilage complex—TFCC) [4].

T.H. Tosounidis (✉) • P.J. Harwood
Academic Department of Trauma and Orthopaedic Surgery, University of Leeds, Leeds, UK
e-mail: ttosounidis@yahoo.com

The above translates into the characteristic radiographic appearance of the Galeazzi fracture, i.e. a short oblique distal third ulnar fracture and a subluxation/dislocation of the DRUJ. Most of the times, the latter is obvious on the anteroposterior and true lateral radiographs of the wrist, but when this is not the case, indirect radiographic signs of DRUJ injury include the fracture of the ulnar styloid and the shortening of the radius more than 5 mm. A contralateral wrist radiograph for comparison is always helpful in equivocal cases [5].

Brief Preoperative Planning

Anatomic reduction and stable fixation are the goals of surgical management of Galeazzi fracture. This mandates for open reduction and internal fixation. Indirect and minimally reduction and fixation techniques yield suboptimal result and should be avoided. Standard open reduction and internal fixation techniques with meticulous soft tissue handling should be employed.

Preoperative planning should take into account the reduction and fixation of the radius as well as the potential reduction and fixation of the DRUJ.

Fixation of radius: 3.5 mm and dynamic compression plates with 3.5 mm cortical screws (Fig. 22.2a). 2.7 mm and 3.5 mm cortical screws.

DRUJ fixation: 1.6 mm k-wires.

P.V. Giannoudis (ed.), *Fracture Reduction and Fixation Techniques*,
https://doi.org/10.1007/978-3-319-68628-8_22

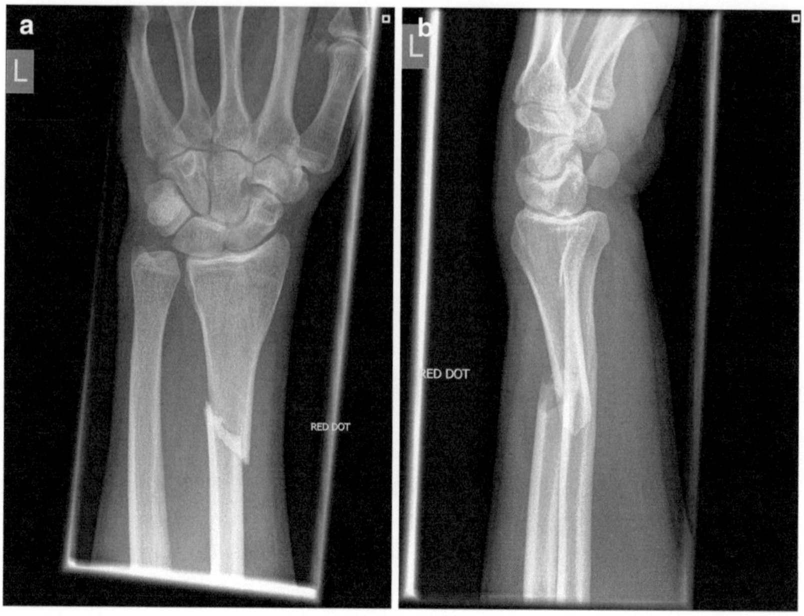

Fig. 22.1 AP and lateral radiographs demonstrating an apex anterior (**a**, **b**) Galeazzi fracture

Fixation of the ulnar styloid and or TFCC: 1 mm cerclage wires and 1 mm k-wires, cannulated mini fragment screws.

Patient Setup in Theatre

General anaesthesia is preferred over regional due to potential masking of postoperative compartment syndrome when the latter is used.

The patient is positioned supine on a standard table, and the affected arm is placed on a radiolucent hand table. The table is placed in such a way that unobstructed intraoperative imaging can be performed. This usually requires rotation of the table 45° or 90° so that the affected extremity is placed at the centre of the operating theatre. A tourniquet is placed, and the affected extremity is prepped and draped following the administration of intravenous antibiotics. The image intensifier is brought from the top or the side of the patient.

Closed Reduction Manoeuvres

Closed reduction manoeuvres are not used for Galeazzi fractures.

Reduction Instruments

For the radius, reduction tools that can be used are the following: small Hohmann retractors, small periosteal elevators, Howarth elevator, pointed reduction clamps, blunt/serrated bone holding forceps/clamps (small "crocodile" clamps) and articulated tension device.

DRUJ reduction is performed manually.

For the reduction of the ulnar styloid, a pointed reduction clamp or a stay suture (e.g. No 1 Vicryl) is needed.

Surgical Approach

The volar approach to the radius is the workhorse for the surgical treatment of Galeazzi fractures. This can either be a flexor carpi radialis (FCR) sheath or the classic Henry's approach. The latter is used when the radial fracture is more proximal. For the FCR approach, the volar sheath of the FCR tendon is identified after the skin incision which is centred over the short oblique radial fracture and measures 10–12 cm (Figs. 22.3 and 22.4). Then the FCR tendon is retracted ulnarly (Fig. 22.5). The dorsal (deep) sheath of the

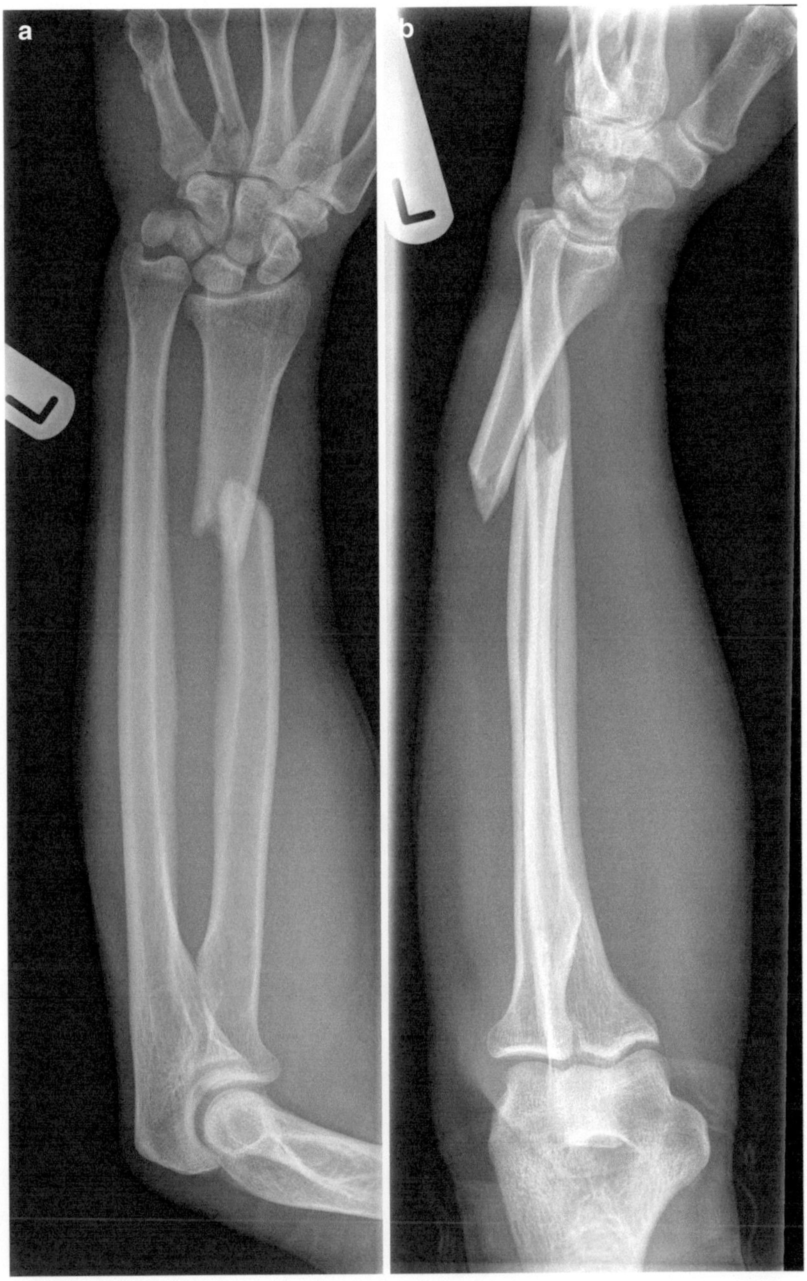

Fig. 22.2 AP and lateral radiographs demonstrating an apex posterior (**a**, **b**) Galeazzi fracture

investing fascia is identified and incised (Fig. 22.6). The flexor pollicis longus tendon is identified and retracted ulnarly (Fig. 22.7). This manoeuvre protects the median nerve. The fracture of the radius is then visible (Fig. 22.8).

The dorsal and direct radial approaches to the radius are not indicated for the surgical fixation of the Galeazzi fractures. The former has been associated with soft tissue complications (irritation/attrition of tendon with risk of postoperative rupture), whilst the latter is technically more challenging since it requires mobilisation of the brachioradialis tendon and the sensory branch of the radial nerve.

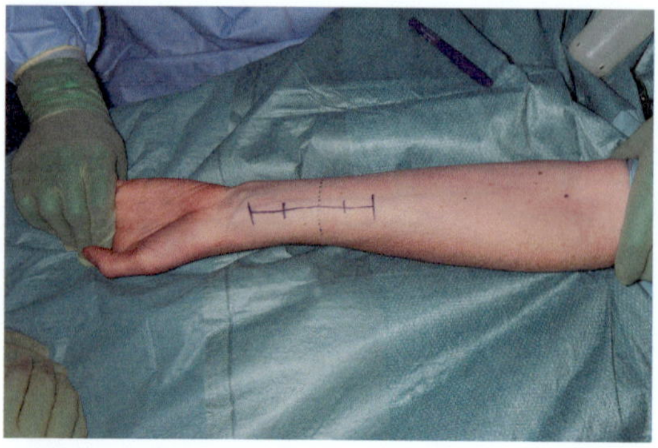

Fig. 22.3 Marking of the incision centred over the radius fracture in line with the FCR

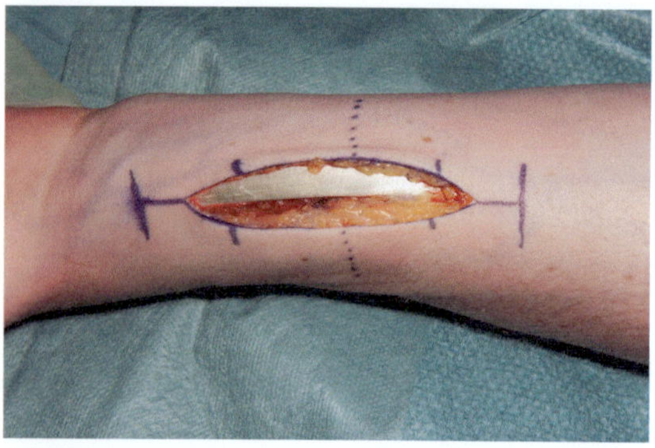

Fig. 22.4 The FCR tendon is identified, and the investing sheath is dissected

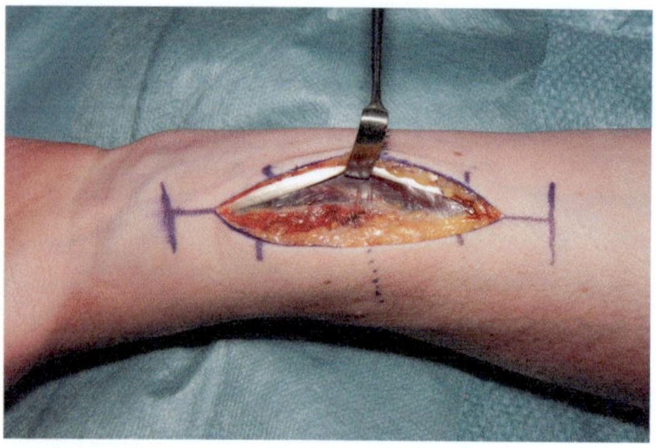

Fig. 22.5 The FCR tendon is retracted ulnarly

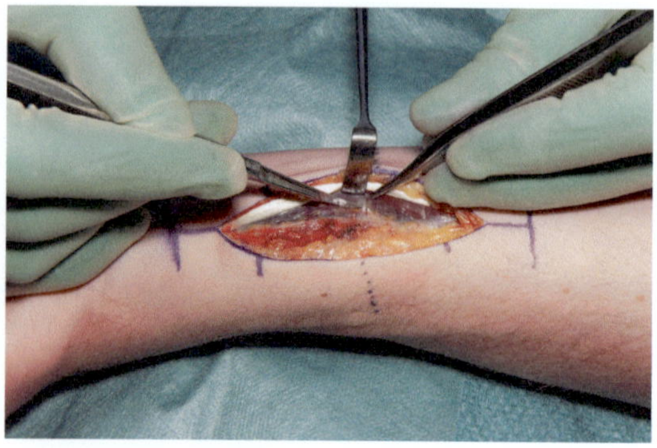

Fig. 22.6 The dorsal (deep) sheath of the investing fascia is identified and incised

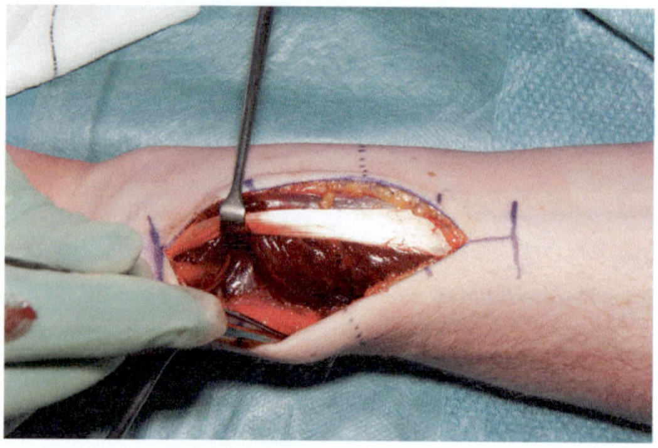

Fig. 22.7 The flexor pollicis longus tendon is identified and retracted ulnarly

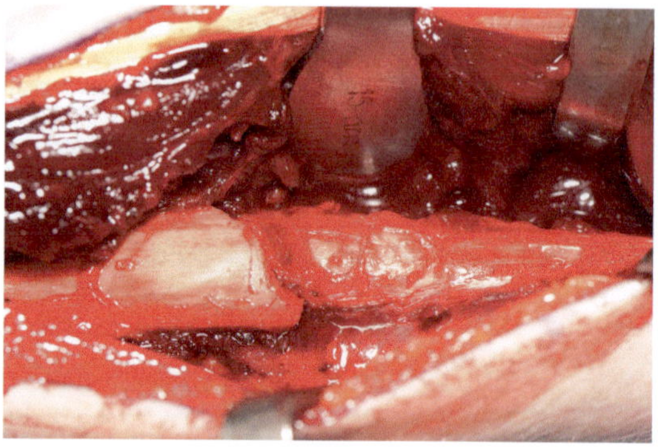

Fig. 22.8 Identification of the radius fracture. Note its short oblique configuration

Open Reduction Manoeuvres

The fracture is identified, and it is debrided from soft tissue debris and hematoma. A dental pick is an instrument quite useful for manipulation of fracture fragments whilst minimising the soft tissue damage. The facture can also be manipulated with pointed reduction forceps, and debridement is performed using a small curette (Fig. 22.9). Minimal dissection of the periosteum (especially in areas of infolded periosteum) is performed along the edges of the fracture. The fracture fragments are exposed sufficiently enough without

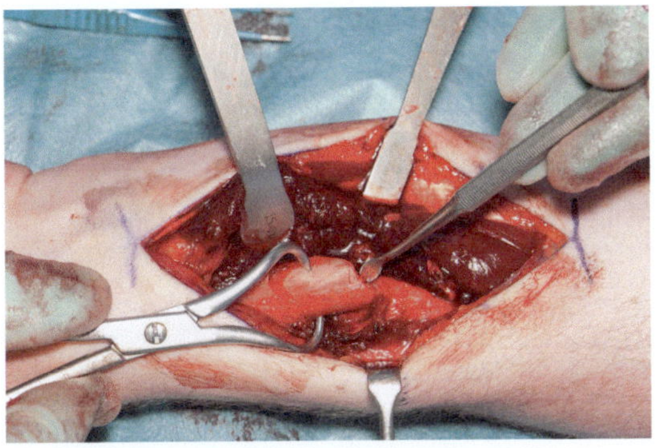

Fig. 22.9 The facture is manipulated with pointed reduction forceps, and debridement is performed using a small curette

stripping the periosteum and violating the surrounding soft tissue envelope.

Open Reduction and Fixation

The fracture fragments are mobilised using small serrated reduction clamps (Fig. 22.10). The fracture is then provisionally stabilised with a pointed or serrated clamp. Galeazzi fractures have usually short oblique configuration, and a Howarth's elevator or a small Hohmann retractor can be used to lever the fracture with intrafocal manipulation. Combinations of longitudinal traction along with twisting of the fragments represent useful manoeuvres in fracture reduction. The surgeon should keep in mind that the fracture was produced by a torsional moment to the bone, and reversing the mechanism of injury helps reducing the fracture. Pure traction or pure rotation of the fracture fragments is not enough for reduction.

At that stage the fracture is inspected, and the plan for anatomic reduction is confirmed. This means that the preoperative radiographs and the intraoperative fracture configuration are correlated, and the plan for anatomic reduction and fixation either with a lag screw and neutralisation plate or with plate used as a reduction tool is confirmed. When a lag screw is utilised, the correct entry point and the trajectory of the screw are of paramount importance. In order to achieve the above, the three-dimensional configuration of the fracture has to be taken into account. Most of the times, a 3.5 mm lag screw is sufficient, but in short oblique fractures, a 2.7 mm lag screw is sometimes useful in achieving the compression without propagation of the fracture ends (Fig. 22.11a–c). At that stage intraoperative fluoroscopic confirmation is obtained with particular attention paid at the DRUJ. Good quality true AP and lateral wrist views are obtained.

A neutralisation plate is then applied taking into account the natural bent of the radius which has "two concavities", one facing volarly and one facing ulnarly (Figs. 22.12, 22.13 and 22.14). Bending the plate on the sagittal plane allows for proper sitting of the plate on the bone. An 8 hole 3.5 mm DCP is usually sufficient to support a short oblique fracture, but occasionally a longer plate is necessary. Three bicortical screws proximally and three screws distally are needed for adequate fixation. In the vast majority of cases, the use of locking plates is neither needed nor advocated. Fluoroscopic confirmation is again obtained.

When lagging of the fracture is not possible due to the configuration of the fragment (transverse, short oblique <30°), then the DCP plate should be applied in compression mode after provisional stabilisation of the fracture. In short oblique fractures, this can be done by initially fixing the plate in one of the bone fragments in such a way that an obtuse angle (axilla) between the plate and the bone can be created. This is followed by re-apposition of the other fragment and eccentrically loading the screws and thus compressing the gap providing absolute

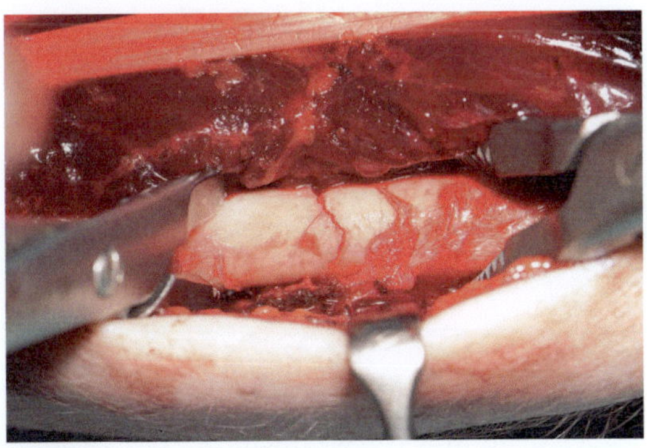

Fig. 22.10 Small serrated clamps are used to manipulate and reduce the fracture fragments

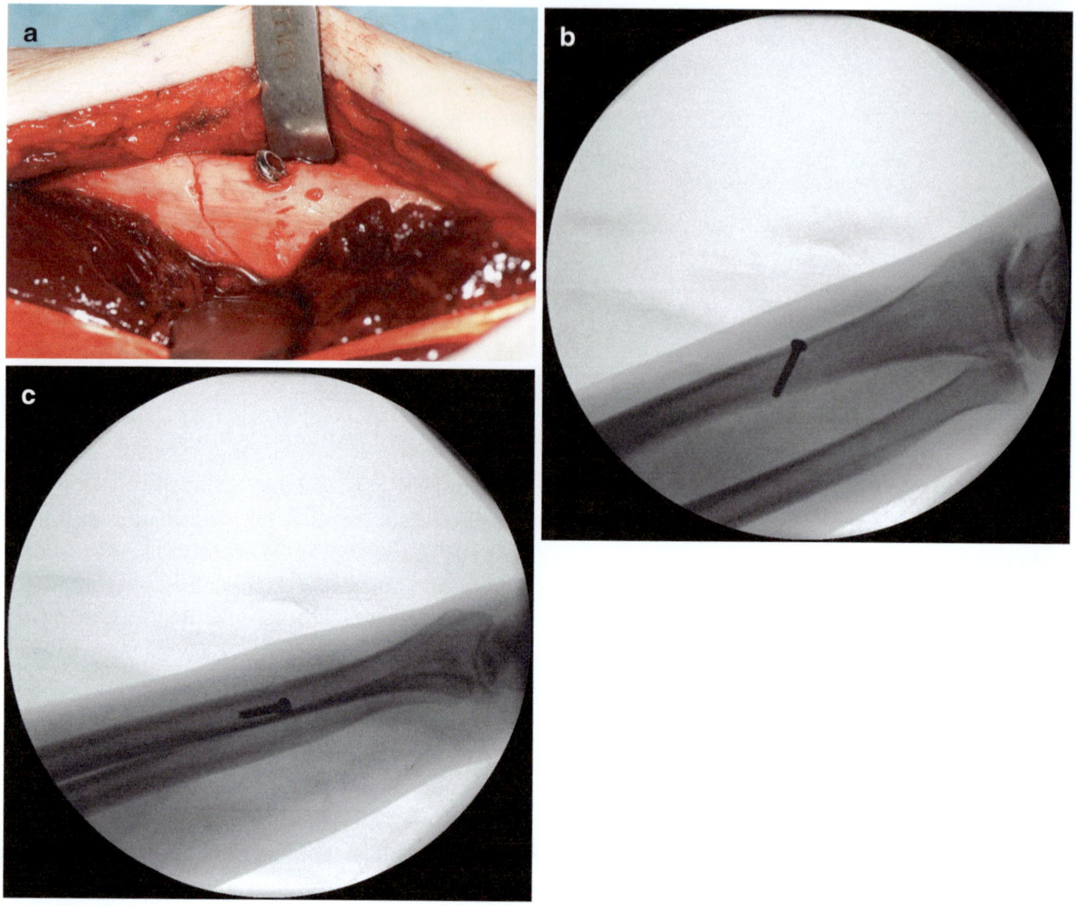

Fig. 22.11 Intraoperative picture (**a**) and fluoroscopic images (**b**, **c**) showing the lag screw fixation of the radius

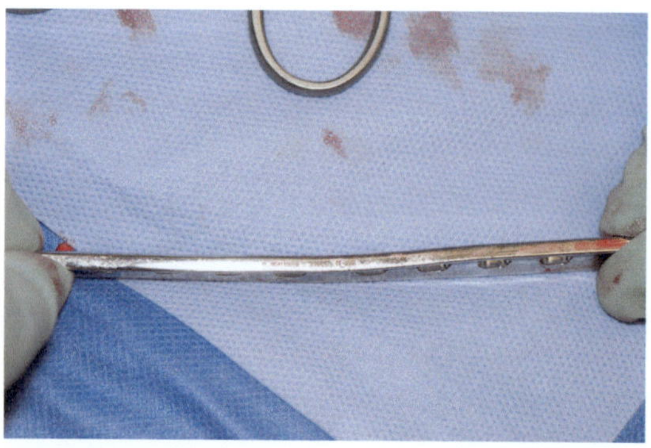

Fig. 22.12 Picture showing the bent applied to a straight DCP plate in order to accommodate the volar concavity of the radius

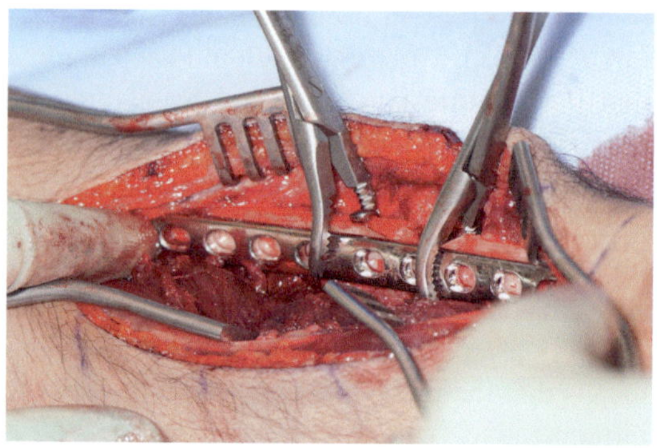

Fig. 22.13 Plate holed with clamps in the reduced radius

stability. In transverse fractures, the plate is fixed to one fragment, and then the other fragment is reduced onto the plate. Maintenance of the reduction using serrated clamps is needed in this situation.

After the fixation of the radius, the DRUJ is checked and classified as reduced/stable, reduced/unstable or irreducible [5] (Fig. 22.15).

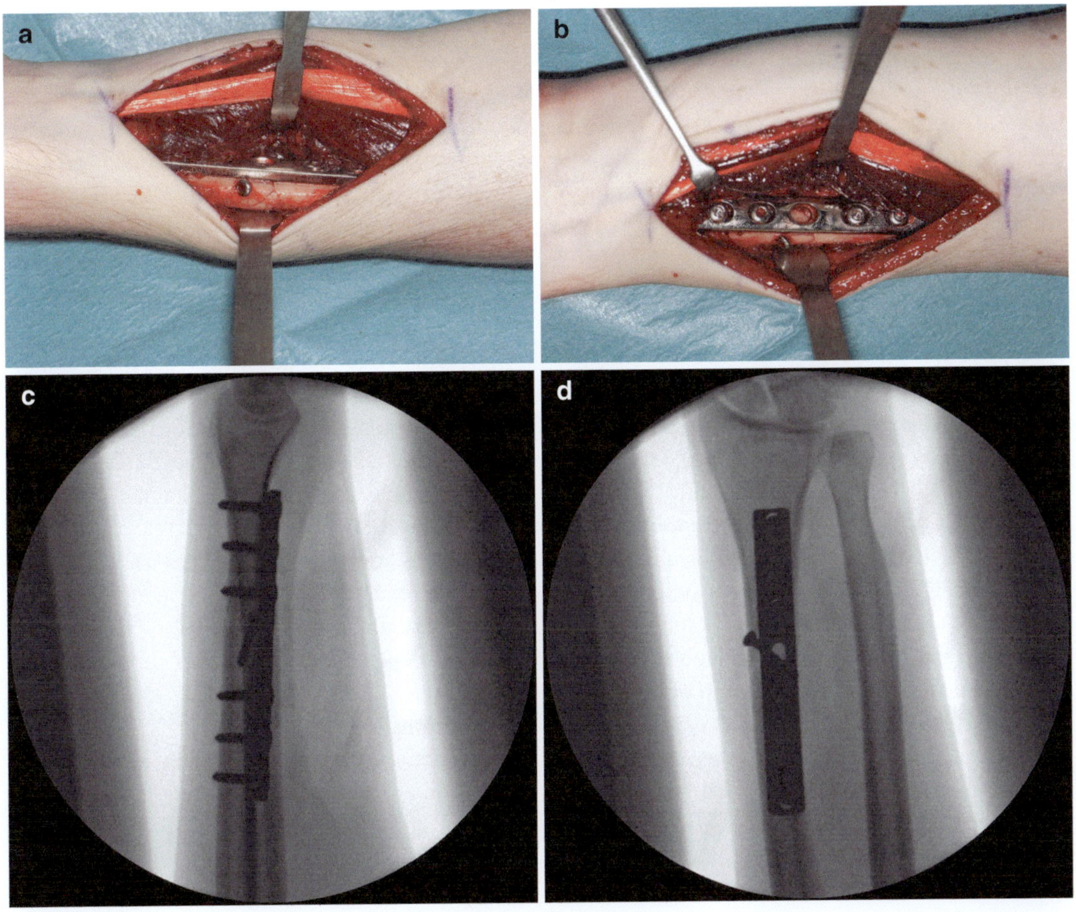

Fig. 22.14 Lateral (**a**, **c**) and AP (**b**, **d**) intraoperative pictures and fluoroscopic images showing the lag screw and the neutralisation plate

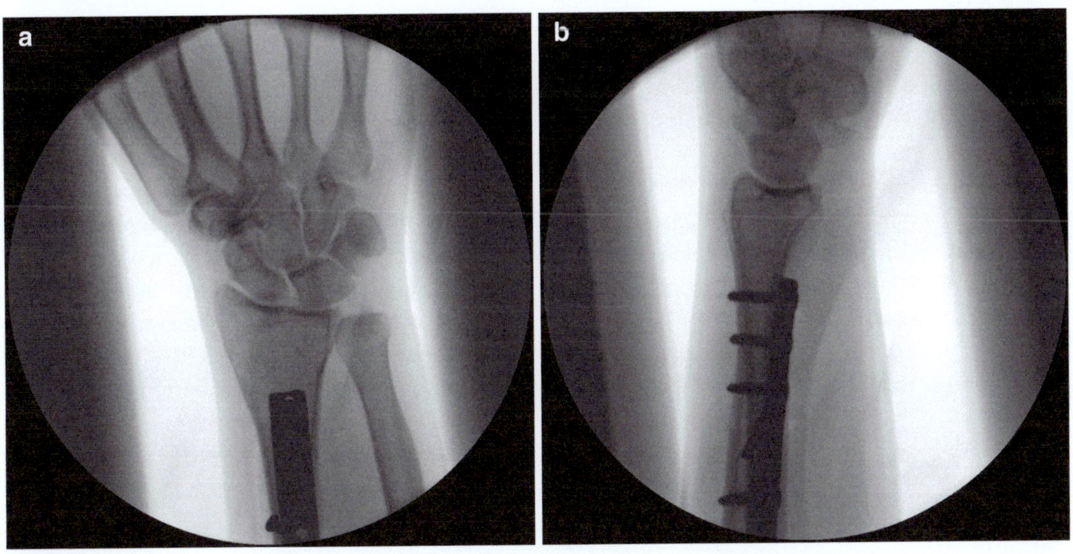

Fig. 22.15 Lateral (**a**) and AP (**b**) fluoroscopic images showing a reduced DRUJ

Reduction and stability are tested both clinically and fluoroscopically. Intraoperative true AP and lateral fluoroscopic views are obtained without excessive forcing the wrist. If undue force is applied, the DRUJ can be potentially reduced even with existing soft tissue interposition. After its reduction, the stability of the DRUJ is tested, and in supination and pronation, instability is defined when gross translation of the ulna in relation to the sigmoid notch is observed.

- If reduced/stable status is observed, then no further intervention is required.
- If the DRUJ is in reduced/unstable state, then the TFCC should be explored and repaired. This is performed through a dorsal approach to the DRUJ. The TFCC is usually avulsed from its ulnar attachment and is repaired with anchor and bone sutures through drill holes. In these situations, transfixation of the ulna to the radius is advocated using two 1.6 mm k-wires, which are driven from the ulnar border of the distal ulna to the radial border of the radius. The k-wires should be parallel to each other, should not be placed to the DRUJ (the most distal one should be placed just proximal to DRUJ) and should be left protruding to the medial border of the ulna and the lateral border of the radius (making easier their later retrieval). In the case that the DRUJ is stable only in supination and not in pronation, consideration could be given to the immobilisation of the arm initially in long arm cast and later in a brace for 4–6 weeks without application of transfixation k-wires. If there is an ulnar styloid fracture, this is reduced and fixed with cannulated screws or more commonly with k-wires using a tension band technique.
- If the DRUJ is irreducible, then exploration of the joint is required. Commonly the reduction is prohibited by the interposition of the extensor carpi ulnaris tendon or small fracture fragments. After the reduction via a dorsal approach to the wrist, the joint is again tested for stability, and the aforementioned steps are performed.

Summary of Tips and Tricks-Pitfalls

- Obtain good quality intraoperative fluoroscopic views.
- Aim for anatomic reduction of the radius that facilitates anatomic reduction of the DRUJ. This can be achieved either by a lagging screw and neutralisation plate (Fig. 22.16a, b) or by a compression plate (Fig. 22.16c, d).
- Open reduction necessitates manoeuvring of both fracture fragments.
- Use small serrated reduction forceps/clamps without causing soft tissue and periosteal stripping.
- Reduction of the radius is achieved by combination of traction and rotation.
- Test the reduction and stability of the DRUJ after fixation of the ulna.
- Irreducible DRUJ necessitates open reduction via a posterior approach
- Reduced but not stable DRUJ should be managed with fixation of the TFCC and transfixation k-wires. Make k-wires tetracortical to facilitate their retrieval in case they break.
- Reduced and stable DRUJ does not require any further surgical intervention. Protective splint and early forearm range of motion are advocated.
- After fixation of the reduced/unstable and irreducible DRUJ conditions, the arm should be immobilised in an above-the-elbow cast with the forearm in supination from 4 to 6 weeks. The transfixation k-wires should be kept in place for the same period of time.

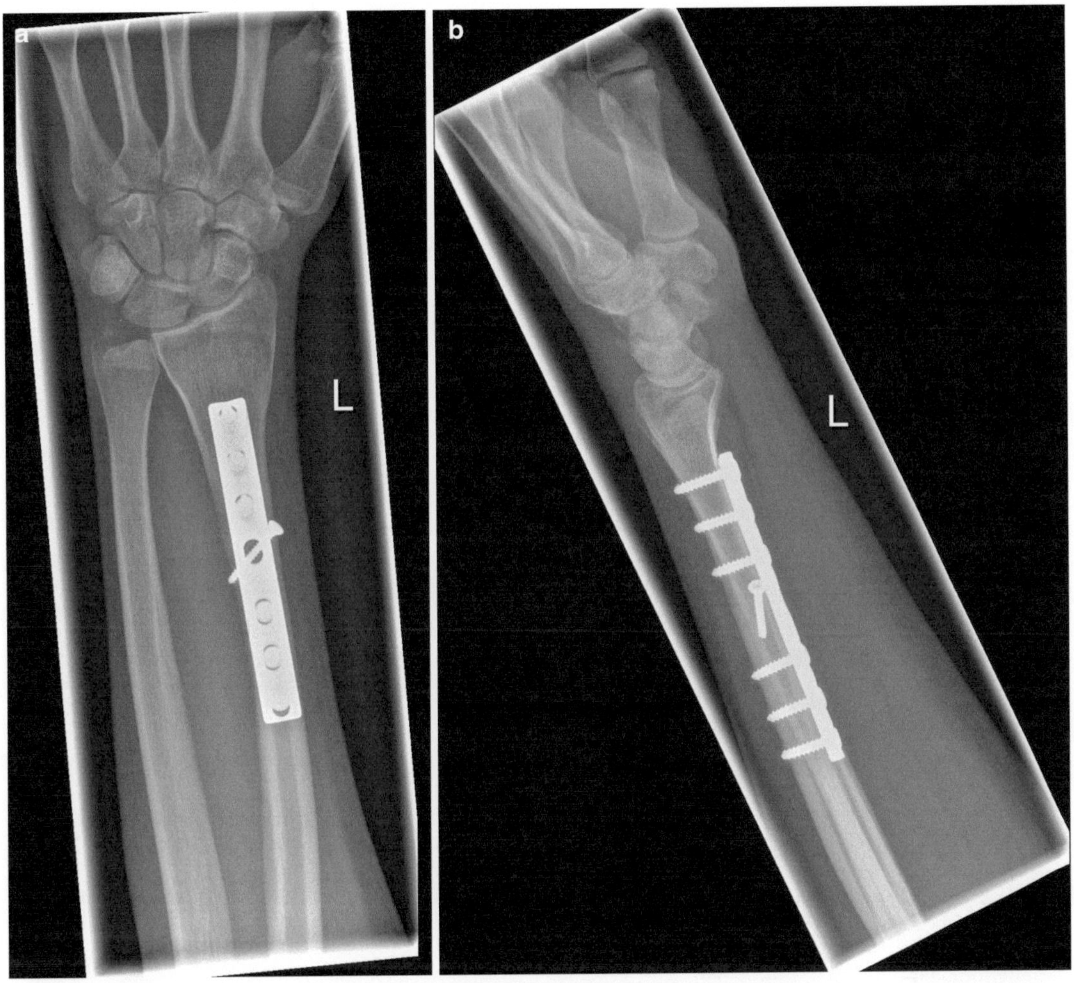

Fig. 22.16 Postoperative radiographs showing the fixation of a Galeazzi fracture with a lag screw and neutralisation plate (**a**, **b**) and a DCP applied in a compression mode (**c**, **d**)

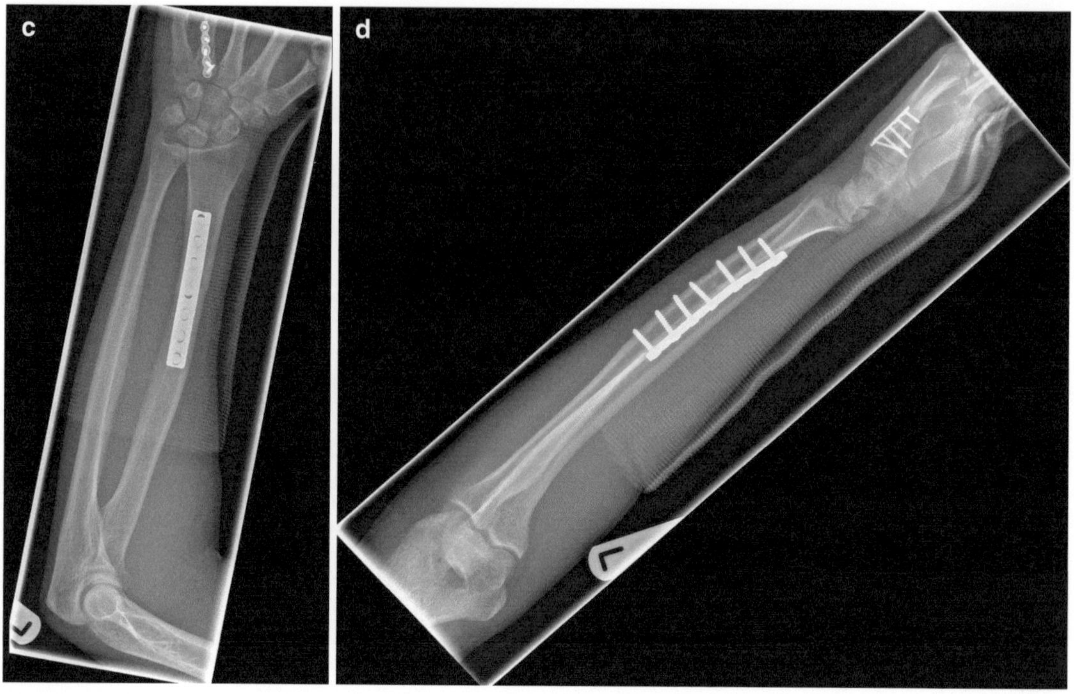

Fig. 22.16 (continued)

References

1. Mikic ZD. Galeazzi fracture-dislocations. J Bone Joint Surg Am. 1975;57:1071–80.
2. Rose-Innes AP. Anterior dislocation of the ulna at the inferior radio-ulnar joint. Case report, with a discussion of the anatomy of rotation of the forearm. J Bone Joint Surg Br. 1960;42-B:515–21.
3. Shiboi R, Kobayashi M, Watanabe Y, et al. Elbow dislocation combined with ipsilateral Galeazzi fracture. J Orthop Sci. 2005;10:540–2.
4. Tsai PC, Paksima N. The distal radioulnar joint. Bull NYU Hosp Jt Dis. 2009;67:90–6.
5. Atesok KI, Jupiter JB, Weiss AP. Galeazzi fracture. J Am Acad Orthop Surg. 2011;19:623–33.

23 Distal Radius Fracture

Georg Gradl

Anatomical Fracture Location

Fractures of the distal forearm have an incidence of 37 out of 10,000 females and 9 out of 100,000 males and are among the most frequent fractures of the adult population above the age of 35 years [1]. Above the age of 85 years, the incidence further increases in females to 120 out of 10,000 citizens [1, 2]. The age has an influence on the accident pattern; in younger adults below the age of 39 years, high-energy trauma is more frequent, leading to a higher percentage of additional carpal ligamentous injuries. This has an impact on both operative strategy and implant selection [3].

Fracture Classification and Analysis

Extra-articular fractures of the distal radius about 2 cm proximal to the joint surface and dorsal displacement are called Colles fractures according to the historical description of Abraham Colles or according to Pouteau who detailed this fracture type as early as 1783. Fractures with palmar displacement are called reversed Colles fractures or Smith fractures (1847). Intra-articular fractures with displacement of the radiocarpal joint were detailed by Barton as early as 1838 with a dorsal articular fragment (Barton fracture) or a palmar articular fragment (reversed Barton). One widespread fracture classification is the AO/ASIF classification according to Maurice E. Müller et al. [4]. The principle of the AO classification is the discrimination between extra- and intra-articular fracture extensions (Fig. 23.1a, b). A meticulous analysis of these fracture patterns on plain X-rays and CT scans is a prerequisite for proper preoperative planning and selection for implants as well as surgical approach. The following treatment algorithm will be based on this classification. Further classification systems are the Frykman classification, which additionally includes fractures of the styloid process (Fig. 23.1c), the Melone classification with four main fragments (shaft, radius styloid, dorsal medial joint fragment, palmar medial joint fragment) and the very detailed Fernandez classification which takes into account the patient's age, type of accident, stability, displacement and nature of fragment.

Extra-articular fractures are the most frequent fracture pattern (43–46%), dominated by simple fractures with a lack of dorsal comminution (A2, 27%), followed by unstable fractures with multiple dorsal metaphyseal fragments (A3, 16%). Partial articular involvement renders one part of

G. Gradl, M.D.
Clinic for Trauma, Orthopedic Surgery, Hand- and Reconstructive Surgery, Spine Surgery, Munich Municipal Hospital Group, Clinic Harlaching, Munich, Germany
e-mail: Georg.Gradl@klinikum-muenchen.de

P.V. Giannoudis (ed.), *Fracture Reduction and Fixation Techniques*,
https://doi.org/10.1007/978-3-319-68628-8_23

Fig. 23.1 (**a**, **b**, **c**) The AO classification discriminates between extra- and intra-articular fracture extension

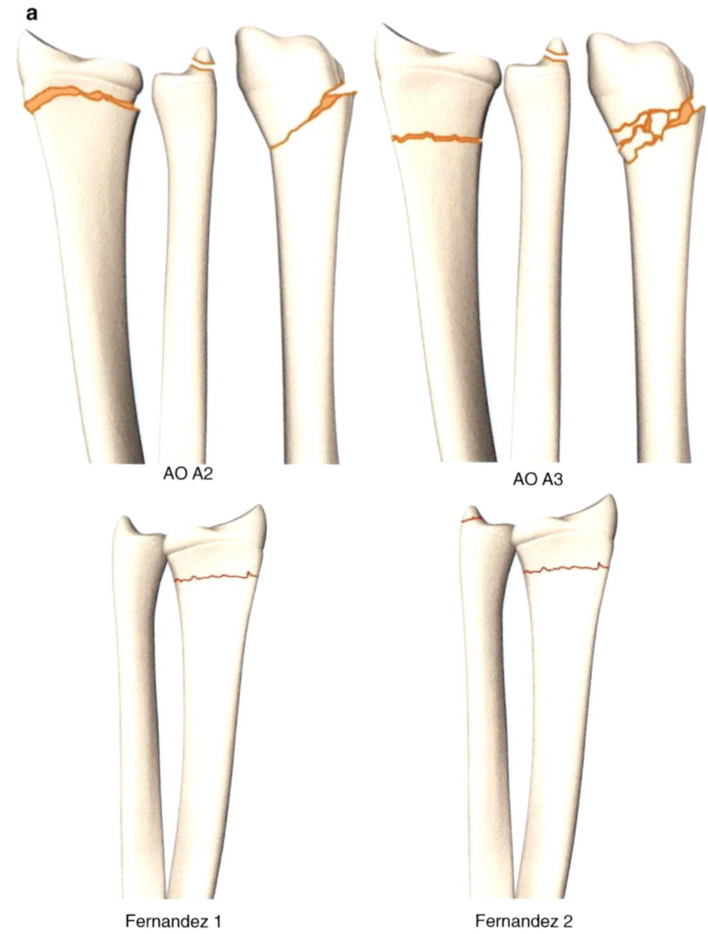

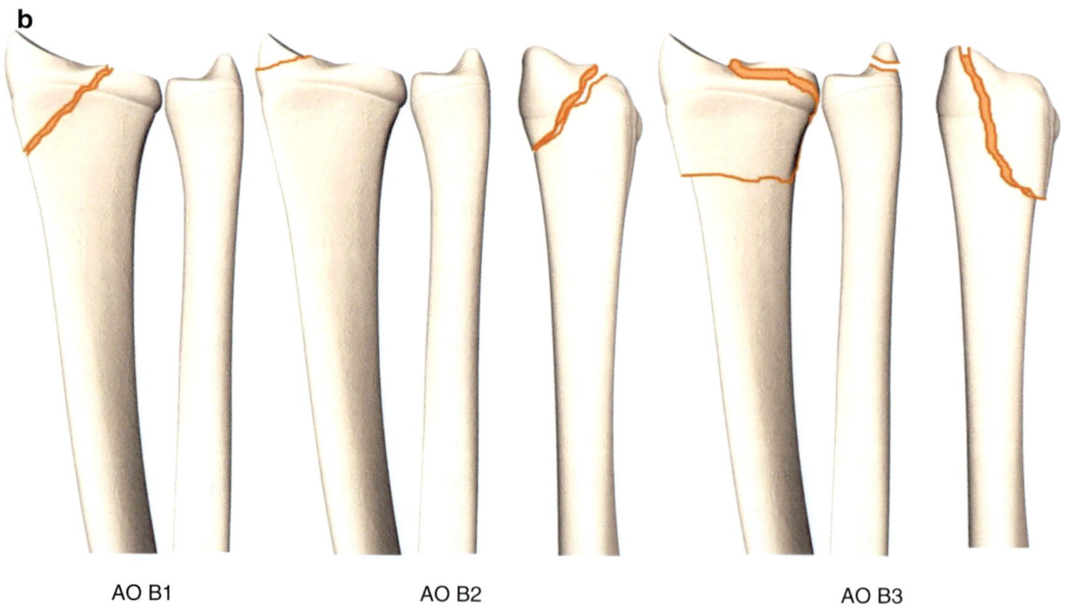

Fig. 23.1 (continued)

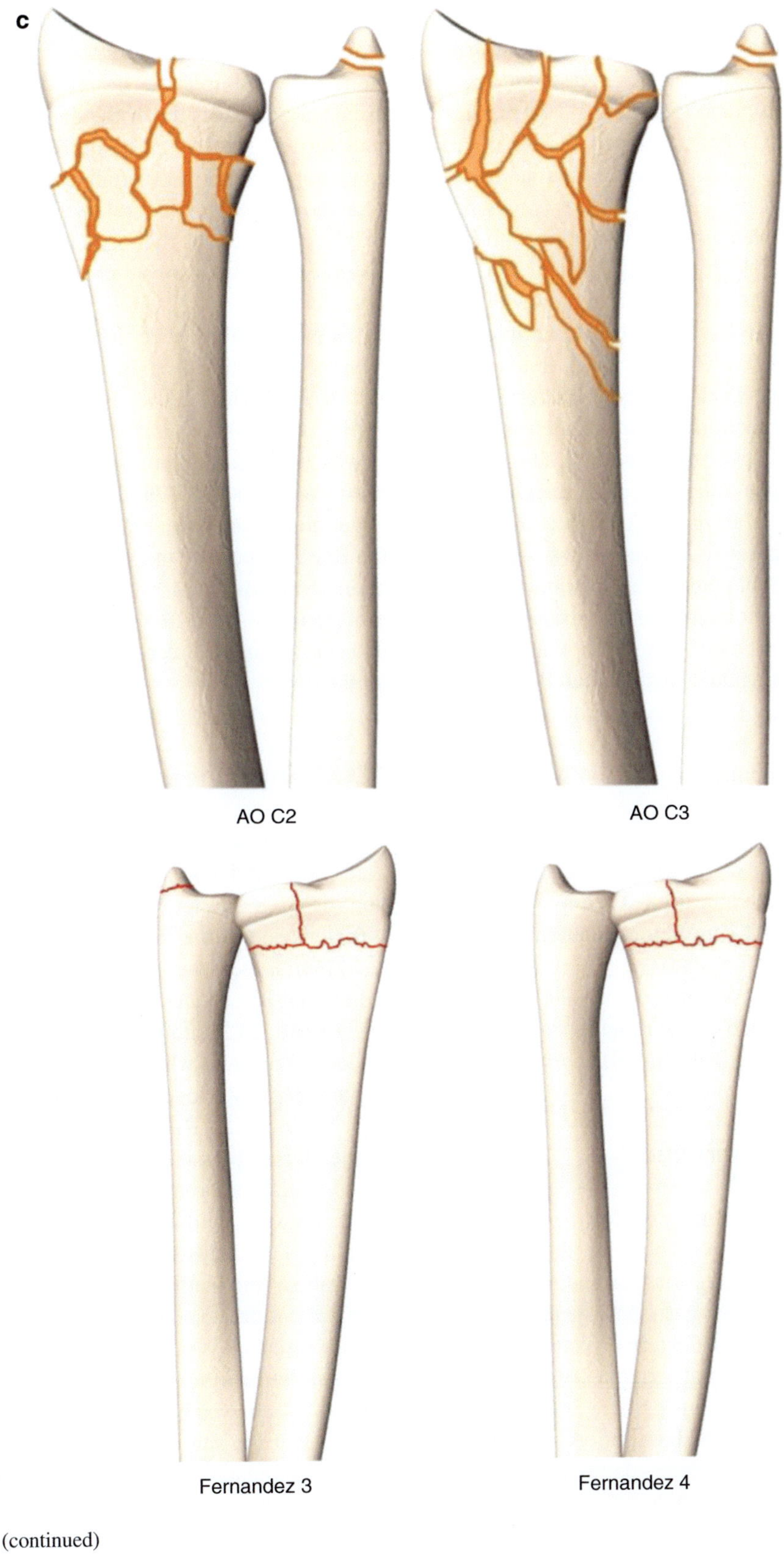

Fig. 23.1 (continued)

the articular surface stable connected to the shaft fragment and is classified as B in the AO/ASIF classification system. B1 fractures are fractures in the sagittal plane (5%) and B2 in the frontal plane (palmar aspect, reversed Barton, 5%; B3, Barton, 6%). Complete intra-articular fractures account for 41–54% of fractures, whereas simple articular involvement in combination with simple metaphyseal fracture is less frequent (C1, 13%) than simple intra-articular fractures with dorsal comminution (C2, 22%) and multiple intra-articular fractures (C3, 7%) [3, 5]. Reduced bone quality promotes extra-articular fractures and has a major influence on fracture incidence, fracture geometry and treatment strategy. On the other hand, multiple intra-articular fractures more often develop after high-velocity trauma [6].

The perioperative accurate analysis of fracture geometry and joint angles is of paramount importance for the choice of therapy strategy, surgical approach and choice of implants. Plain X-rays of the wrist in two planes recommend the lower arm lifted 25° from the horizontal line in the lateral view [7, 8]. CT scans help in terms of evaluation of articular fragments and step-offs. Certain anatomical landmarks need to be defined. Ulnar variance is ideally measured in the middle of the palmar and dorsal radial joint surface [9] and shows a mean value of −0.9 mm with a wide range (−4.2 to 2.3 mm), thus rendering comparison to the uninjured arm necessary in uncertain cases [7]. Palmar inclination or volar tilt presents with a mean value of 10° ranging from 5° to 12°, slowly decreasing with age [9].

Operative Techniques

Among the broad variety of treatment options for distal radius fractures, there are three most frequent treatment categories: closed reduction and immobilisation in a cast, percutaneous fixation with Kirschner wires/external fixation and open reduction and internal fixation. While each has merits and disadvantages, there is no consensus regarding which is the best option.

The distal radius demands for certain prerequisites in implant technology in order to achieve proper reduction and maintenance of reduction. This means easy operation technique and reduction aids; rigid implants, designed to match with the anatomic curvature of the distal radius; interlocking and stable fixation options for fractures involving the joint; and certain fracture fragments like the dorso-ulnar fragment. Accessibility to displaced fragments that need to be reduced and fixed remains an unsolved problem of closed fixation techniques.

Angular stable plate fixation from a volar approach has gained significant attention over the last years. The flexor carpi radialis (FCR) approach allows for limited soft tissue dissection; however, it remains an open technique which in most cases leads to dissection of the pronator quadratus muscle [10]. Fragment displacement to the dorsal aspect of the wrist does not simplify open reduction from palmar which formed the ground for many different reduction techniques that mostly use indirect efforts to restore palmar inclination.

AO A2 and C1 Fractures

These fractures lack a dorsal fracture fragmentation. Closed reduction and maintenance of reduction using a plaster cast may be completely sufficient due to the fact that fracture edges are not comminuted and may be firmly adjusted. Additional Kirschner wire fixation may be helpful. Figure 23.2 shows the typical distraction device of the wrist, where local anaesthesia in the fracture gap helps to lower pain during the reduction manoeuvre. Reduction is performed by gentle dorsal pressure. Figure 23.3a shows an intraoperative approach where the surgeon distracts the wrist with ulnar abduction and palmar bending. This helps to restore the radial length and palmar inclination and thus serves as one standard reduction procedure. Percutaneous K-wire insertion is performed over the tip of the radial styloid (Figs. 23.3b and 23.4). Rotational stability is achieved by using two pins that should not cross at the site of the fracture because this would significantly reduce anti-rotation fixation stability. In case of an undisplaced articular

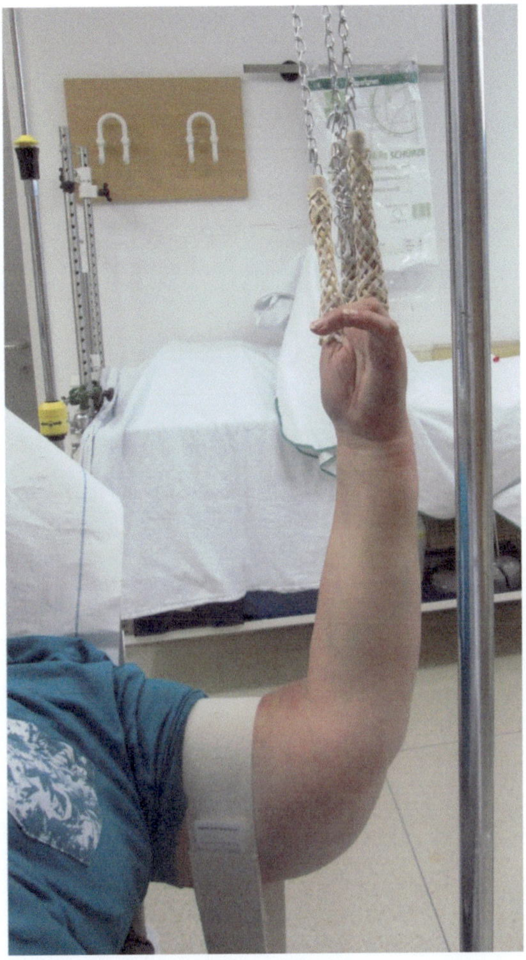

Fig. 23.2 Typical distraction device of the wrist is demonstrated

fracture line, additional pins may be placed parallel to the joint surface. In some cases, however, reduction in a closed manner may not be achieved even in simple fractures, mainly if the palmar cortical edge of the distal fragment fails to fit to the shaft fragment. In these cases, or other cases of difficult restoration of the palmar inclination, a Kapandji wire, inserted from the dorsal aspect of the wrist, through the fracture gap may be helpful (Figs. 23.5 and 23.6).

The Kapandji technique employs a K-wire not smaller than 1.8 mm which is inserted percutaneously from a dorsal approach into the fracture gap and forwarded until the palmar cortex. This is done while bending the K-wire in direction to the dorsum of the hand (Fig. 23.5). Thus, the distal fragment is pushed into the anatomical palmar inclination. Gentle hammer hits may secure the pin in the palmar cortical bone. Alternatively, the K-wire may be forwarded through the palmar cortex machine driven. Special care must be taken in order not to injure the cutaneous branch of the radial nerve, which is at risk during percutaneous pinning through the radial styloid. One pin is, mostly, safe; however, in case of multiple pinning, a limited open approach and careful dissection of the nerve may help to circumvent nerve lesion (Fig. 23.5).

Wrist immobilisation in a palmar splint with 20° of dorsal wrist angulation is recommended, in cases of nonoperative treatment as well as K-wire pinning. A dorsally placed plaster cast

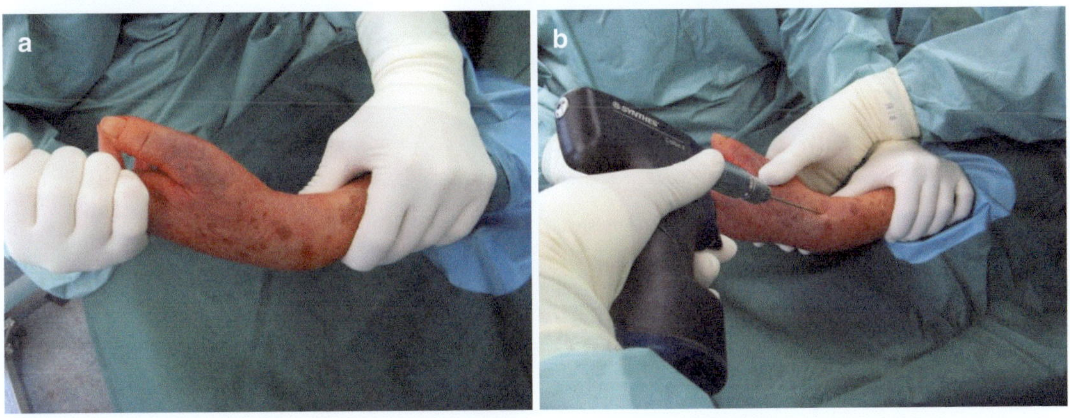

Fig. 23.3 (**a**) Shows an intraoperative approach where the surgeon distracts the wrist with ulnar abduction and palmar bending. (**b**) Percutaneous K-wire insertion is performed over the tip of the radial styloid

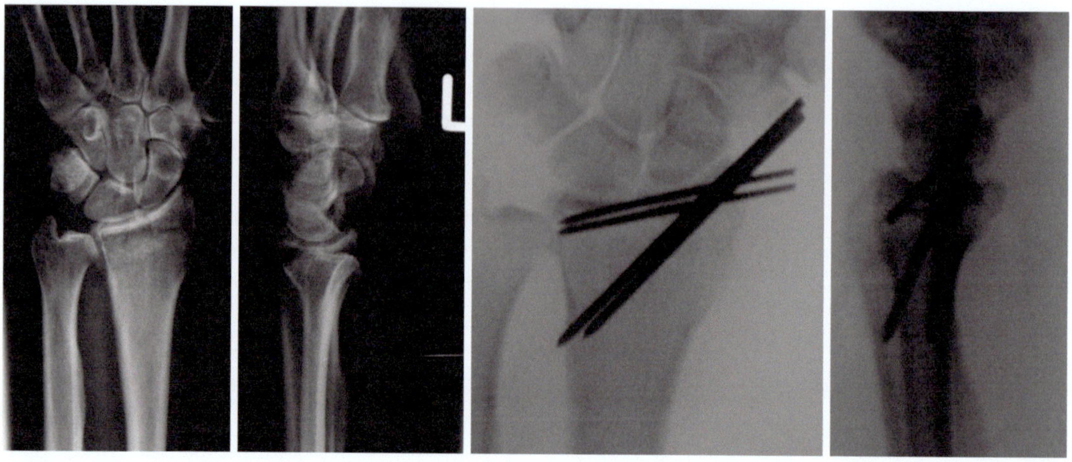

Fig. 23.4 Preoperatively and postoperatively AP and lateral left wrist radiographs showing stabilisation of the fracture with K-wiring

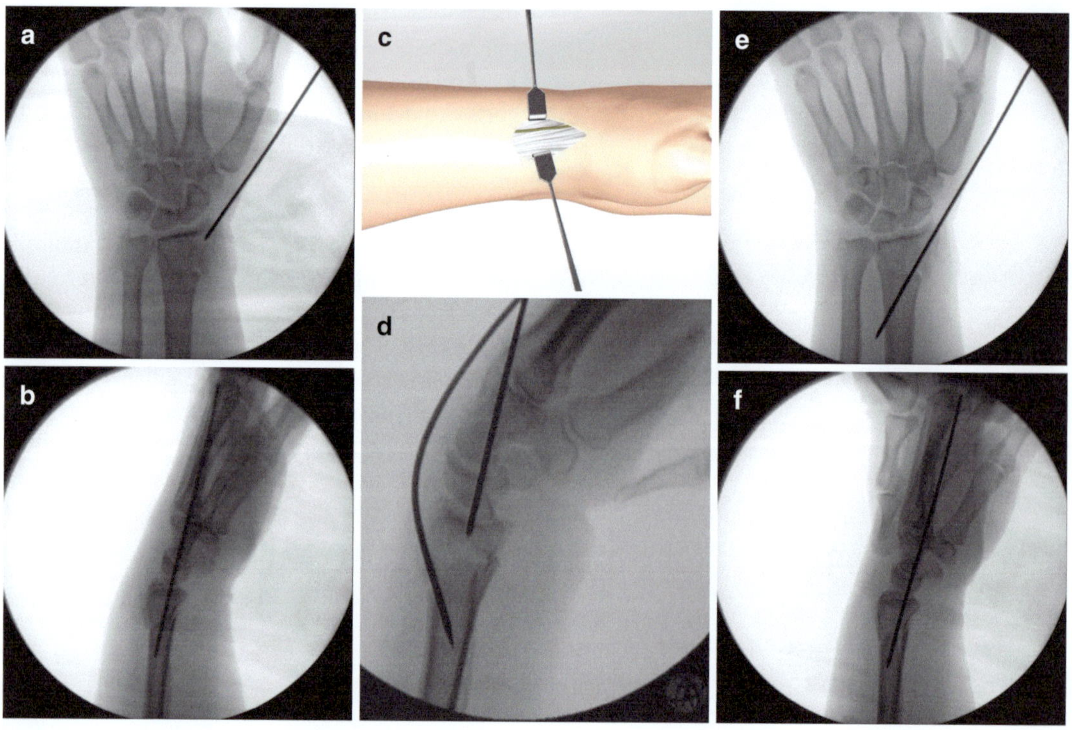

Fig. 23.5 (**a**) Fluoroscopic AP image of right distal radius fracture demonstrating insertion of K-wire through the tip of the radial styloid. (**b**) Fluoroscopic lateral image of right distal radius fracture demonstrating insertion of K-wire through the tip of the radial styloid. (**c**) Demonstration of dorsal incision for access for Kapandji wire insertion. (**d**) Fluoroscopic lateral image of right distal radius fracture demonstrating insertion of Kapandji wire. (**e**) Fluoroscopic AP image of right distal radius fracture demonstrating insertion of K-wire through the tip of the radial styloid across to the opposite cortex. (**f**) Fluoroscopic lateral image of right distal radius fracture demonstrating insertion of K-wire through the tip of the radial styloid with restoration of volar inclination

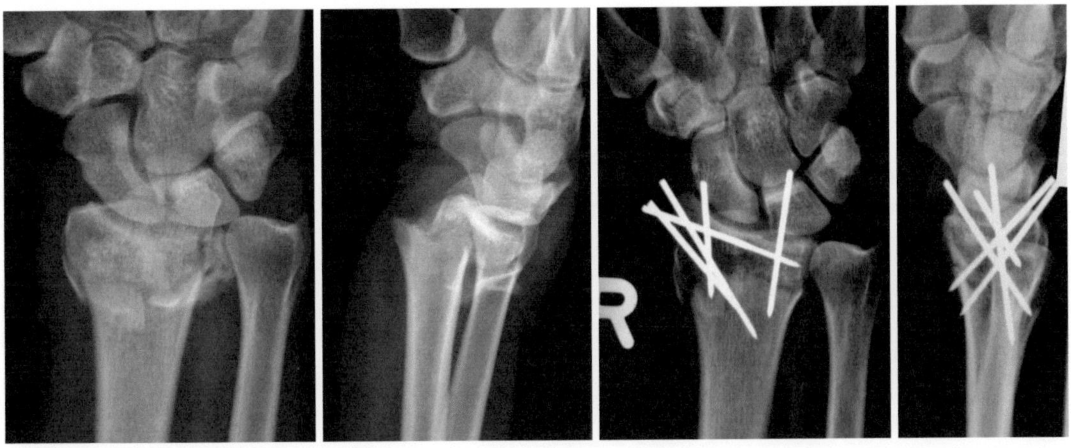

Fig. 23.6 Preoperatively and postoperatively AP and lateral right wrist radiographs showing stabilisation of the intra-articular fracture with K-wiring

with slight dorsal angulation may help to maintain reduction.

Even after multiple K-wire pinning in rare cases of unstable fractures (Fig. 23.6), an additional dorsal or palmar splint is recommended. Implant removal of K-wires takes place 6 weeks after surgery with local anaesthesia if required.

Extra-articular AO A3 Fractures

Extra-articular fractures with dorsal comminution may not qualify for nonoperative treatment due to the fact that they tend to lose initial reduction within the first 2 weeks before initiation of consolidation. However, this may be tolerated in geriatric patients. In this chapter open and semiopen techniques will be described in order to restore anatomy in comminuted extra-articular fractures. Both palmar locking plate fixation and intramedullary nailing are techniques that provide sufficient stability in order to allow for functional after treatment.

Although intramedullary (IM) nailing has not become widely spread, biomechanical studies revealed superiority over plates in terms of fixation stability [11]. Furthermore, there is a large amount of clinical evidence that extra-articular fractures with dorsal displacement are safely treated with IM nailing [12, 13]. Smith fractures, however, may not qualify since they need palmar buttressing [14]. Restoration of anatomy seems to be more demanding in IM nailing, and some studies demonstrate less palmar inclination than in plating procedures [12].

Figure 23.7 demonstrates a technique that helps palmar restoration in IM nailing. Most radial nails are inserted through an approach between the first and second tendon sheet, rendering direct fragment reduction difficult. Thus, joystick techniques are used or more favourable than the Kapandji technique, where the dorsal K-wire is inserted in the fracture gab close to the lunate fossa. A more radial K-wire interferes with the nail. Straight nails without curvature in the anterior-posterior plane tend to direct the distal fragment in a neutral position without the anatomical palmar inclination of 10°. A temporal Kapandji wire may help to circumvent this problem, until the nail is inserted and locked.

There are multiple possibilities to facilitate reduction in palmar plating procedures. One major drawback of palmar plating is that most fractures (Colles) present with dorsal displacement. A palmar approach may thus not be able to reduce the distal fragment directly like a buttressing procedure that works from a dorsal approach in these cases. Having this in mind, all indirect reduction manoeuvres may be used intraoperatively during the palmar approach. I recommend the flexor carpi radialis (FCR) approach radial of the FCR tendon (Fig. 23.8). After closed reduction

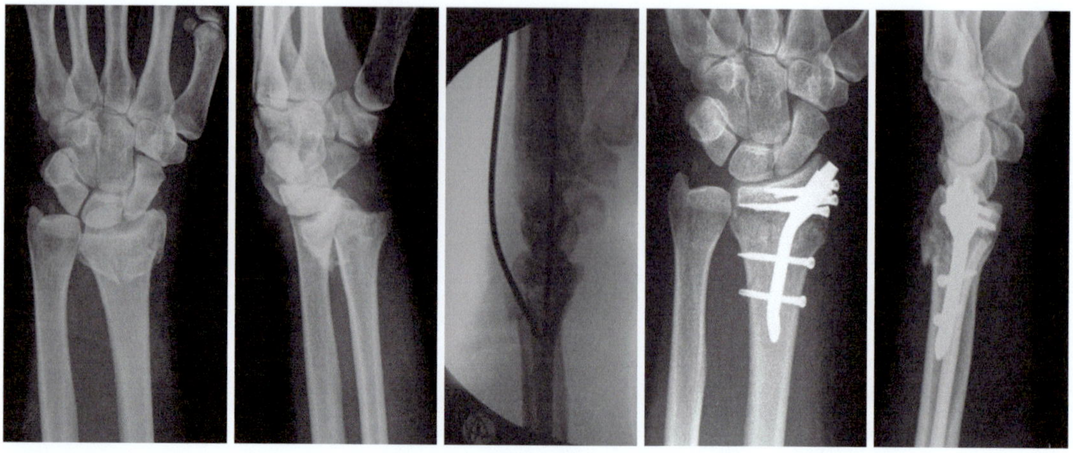

Fig. 23.7 Demonstration of technique facilitating palmar restoration during IM nailing in a right distal radius extra-articular fracture

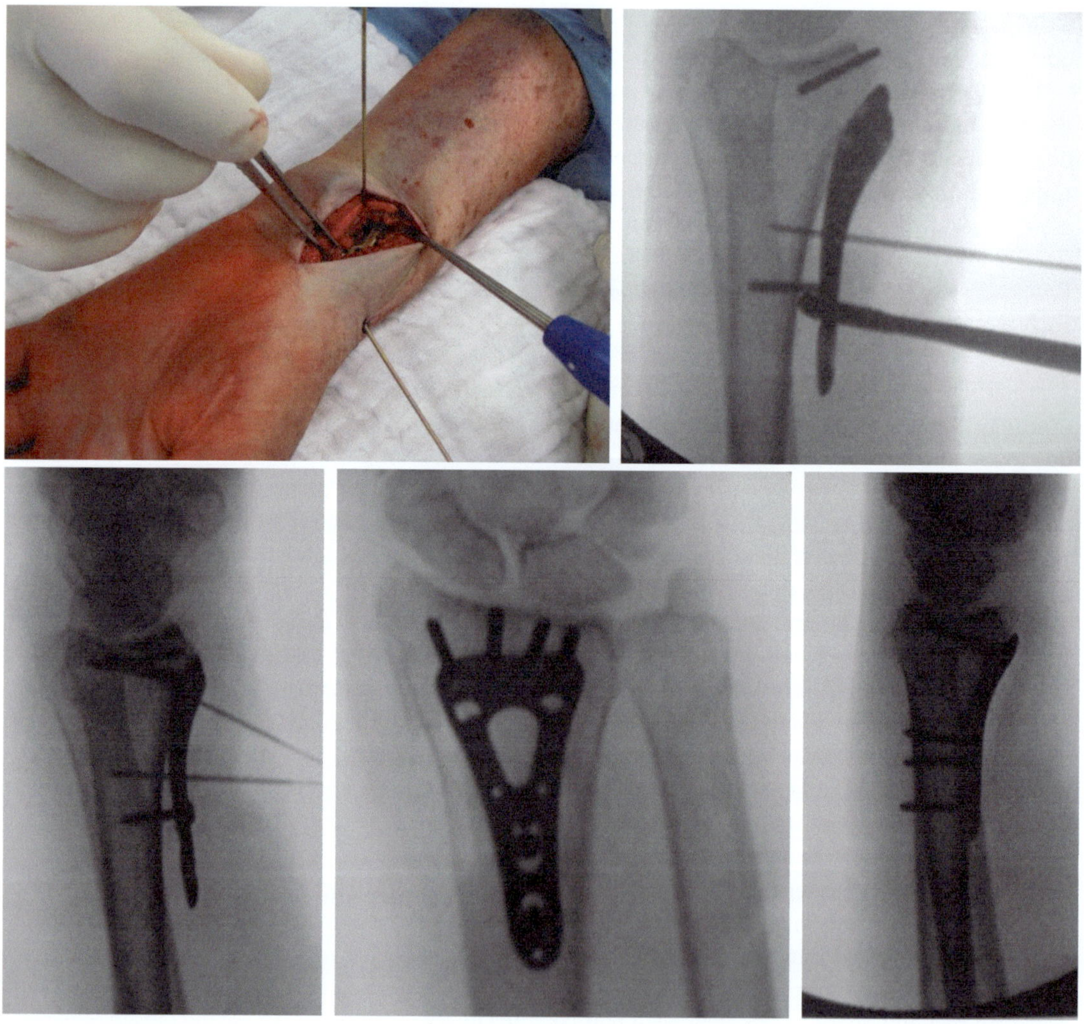

Fig. 23.8 Having used the FCR approach to get access to the distal radius fracture, different intraoperative reduction techniques are demonstrated

a K-wire is placed percutaneously through the radial styloid in order to maintain the reduced fragment in position. Fracture reduction may be facilitated by placing a joystick into the distal fragment or using the Kapandji method. In case of a not ideal reduction, mainly failed restoration of the palmar inclination, the anatomically precurved plate itself may help to achieve better anatomy.

Figures 23.8, 23.9 and 23.10 demonstrate two different reduction techniques. One simple technique of reduction through the precurved

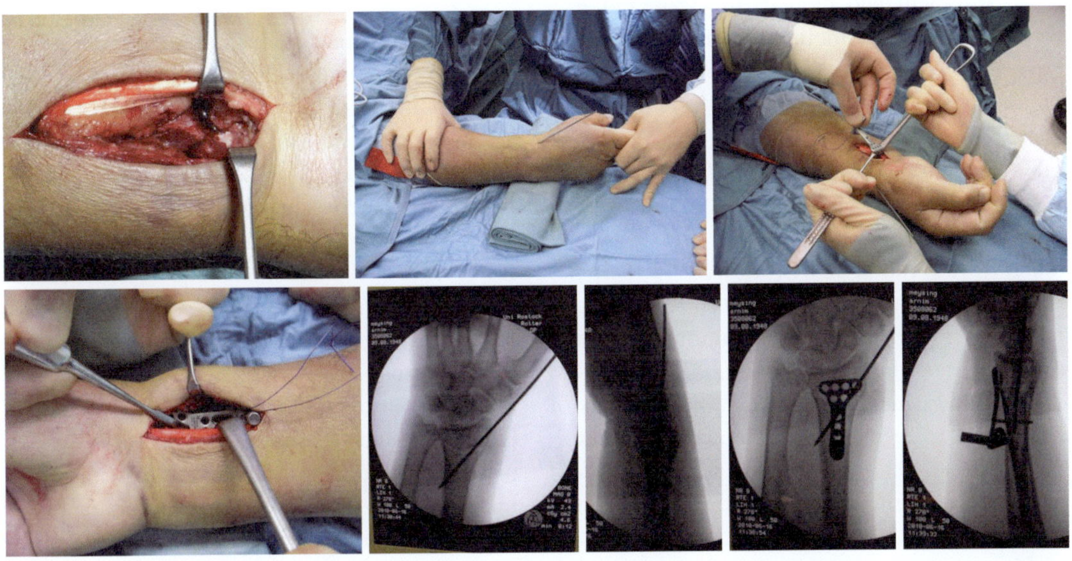

Fig. 23.9 Having used the FCR approach to get access to the distal radius fracture, different intraoperative reduction techniques are demonstrated

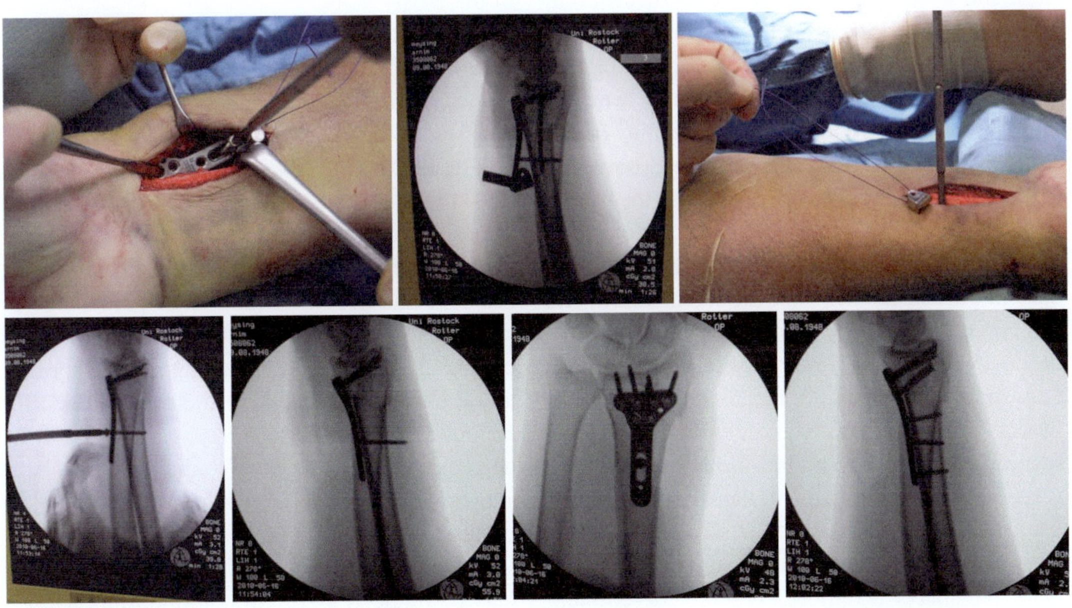

Fig. 23.10 Having used the FCR approach to get access to the distal radius fracture, different intraoperative reduction techniques are demonstrated

plate is the placement of any type of surgical instrument underneath the long aspect of the plate in order to lift it up, prior to insertion of the distal screws. The distal screws (alternatively only K-wires—see Fig. 23.8) are firmly anchored in both the plate (stiff angle) and the fragment. In this manner the plate carries the distal fragment and reduces the fragment in a pronounced radial inclination as soon as the long aspect of the plate is approximated to the radial shaft (Fig. 23.8). There are, however, some obstacles. Since the long aspect of the plate is lifted upwards from the radial shaft, the surgeon loses control of the exact plate positioning. The distal fixation of the plate may not match to the radial shaft followed by malpositioning of the plate. Furthermore, the surgeon has only limited control of the amount of reduction. The more he lifts the plate, the more radial inclination he gets. There is an imminent risk of overaction followed by exaggerated radial inclination angles. This needs to be avoided, since it goes along with severe restriction of wrist motion during dorsal extension.

However, there is another technique that follows the same rules but circumvents the aforementioned shortcomings. Figures 23.9 and 23.10 show the technique, where a spacer of different sizes is mounted underneath the plate. The first step is the FCR approach to the distal radius. After indirect reduction and K-wire placement through the radial styloid, the surgeon may detect a less favourable palmar inclination, however, sufficient reconstruction of radial length. In this case, the surgeon may place the plate prior to the distal fragment fixation—like the standard procedure in palmar plating—on the radial shaft. The surgeon chooses the size of the spacer in dependence upon the previously achieved reduction. Less palmar inclination means bigger spacer. Direct control of plate fixation to the radial shaft securely circumvents malpositioning. The plate is securely anchored to the radial shaft with a longer screw, since the spacer lifts the plate up. After insertion of the distal screws in the T-shaped plate, the spacer is removed and the curved plate further reduces the distal fragment. Figure 23.10 demonstrates how highly effective the spacer technique restores the palmar inclination, although the primary attempt of closed reduction was less successful.

Intra-articular AO B1–3 Fractures and C2–3 Fractures

The abovementioned techniques that help reduction and maintenance of reduction are well suitable for intra-articular fractures, given that the articular fragment is attached to the joint capsule and not separated. This serves as a prerequisite for indirect reduction applying distraction and flexion or using precurved plates. In general, the full arsenal of reduction techniques, a meticulous analysis of fracture geometry and available implants are necessary to manage these fractures. Palmar or dorsal shearing fractures (Barton and reversed Barton fractures) have no IM nailing indication since the nail could well further displace the fracture on its way through the small intramedullary canal [14]. These fractures need exact preoperative planning; CT scan can be helpful and is highly recommended. Thus, the surgeon is capable to choose the adequate operative approach either from dorsal or palmar aspect of the wrist.

Figure 23.11 demonstrates a dorsal shearing injury, involving the dorso-ulnar fragment. Open reduction and maintenance of reduction were achieved by employing a dorsal buttress plate.

Figure 23.12a shows a palmar shearing fracture (reversed Barton) with luxation of the wrist joint. These fractures most often follow a high-energy trauma like in this case of a road traffic accident and present with a high percentage of soft tissue injuries. Palmar shearing fractures may well be reduced through a palmar approach and a buttress plate, where there is no need for angular stability. The ulnar styloid which may be neglected in most cases of radius fractures was addressed using a suture anchor due to complete rupture of the TFC complex (Fig. 23.12b).

Articular step-offs and separated fragments may be reduced by direct manipulation, using a rasp or other instruments, or indirectly with the aid of K-wire joysticks (Fig. 23.13). A separated

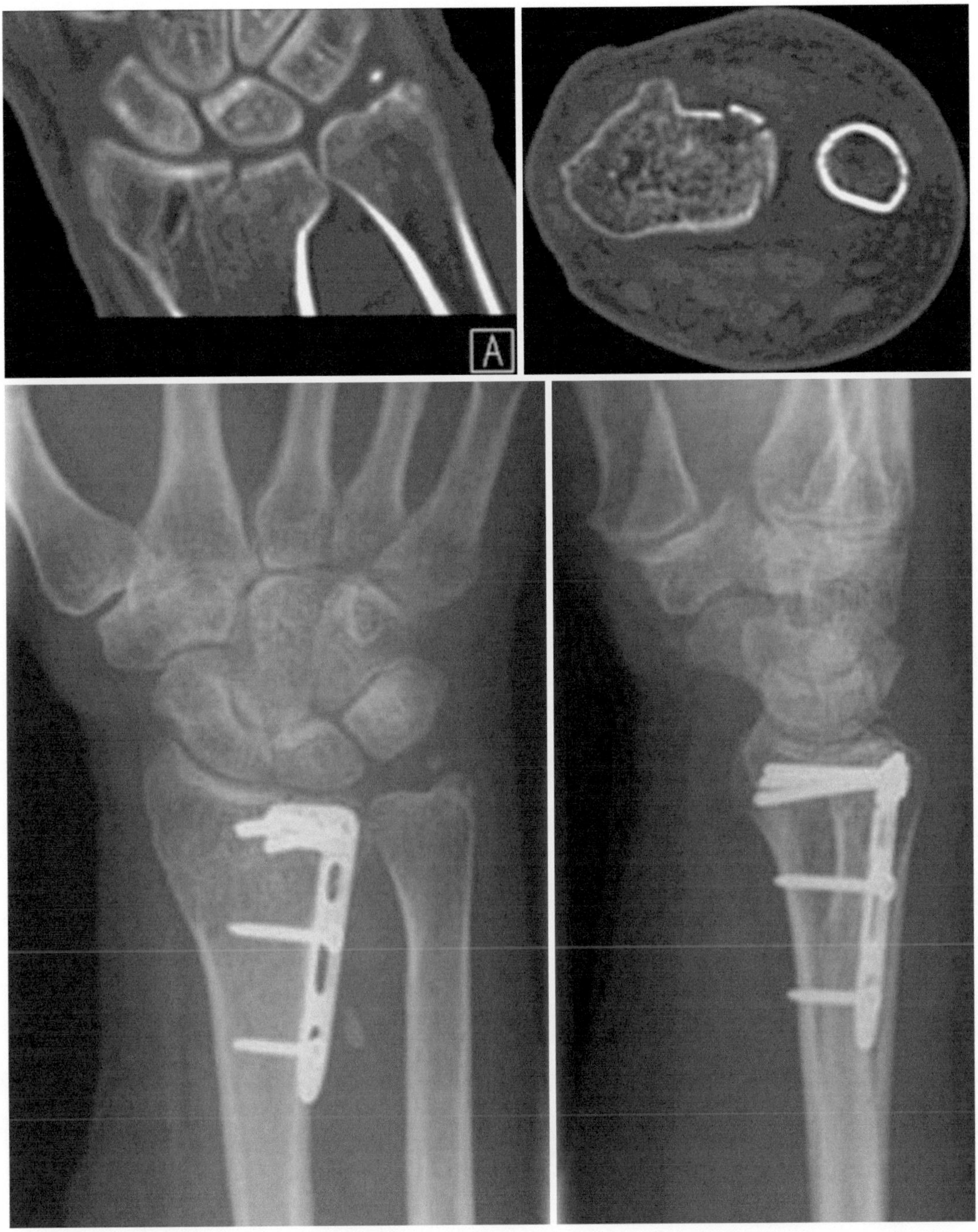

Fig. 23.11 Demonstration of a dorsal shearing injury, involving the dorso-ulnar fragment. Open reduction and maintenance of reduction were achieved by employing a dorsal buttress plate

radial styloid may be partly detached from the brachioradialis muscle in order to facilitate reduction. If a K-wire is used, the diameter should not be less than 1.6 mm and inserted in a steep angle in order to facilitate manipulation of the styloid fragment. The angle may be lowered during the insertion, and the K-wire may securely be anchored in the ulnar fragment or

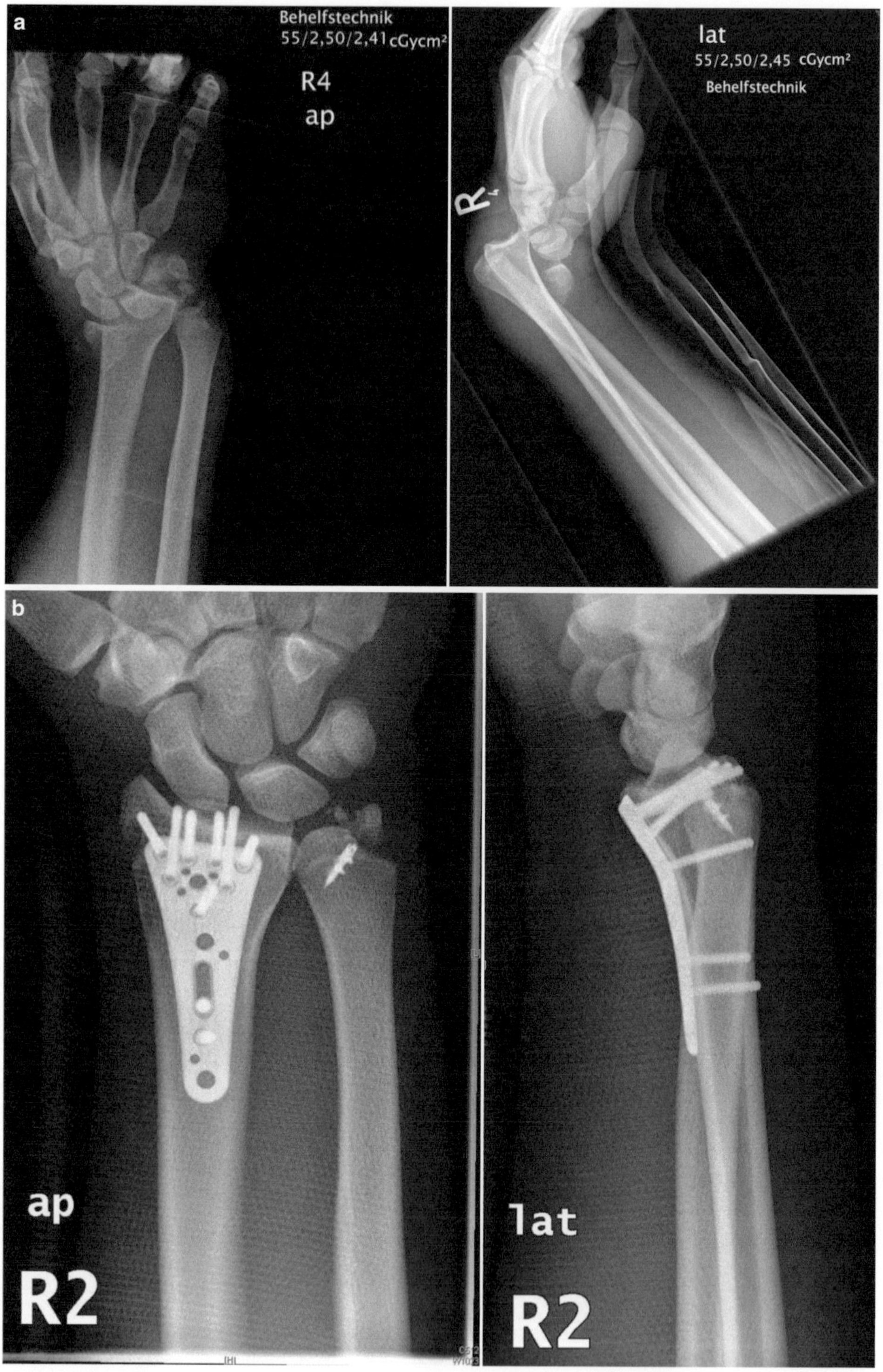

Fig. 23.12 (**a**) Demonstrates a palmar shearing fracture (reversed Barton) with dislocation of the wrist joint. (**b**) Fracture was approached via a palmar approach. A buttress plate was used for stabilisation. The ulnar styloid fracture was addressed using a suture anchor due to complete rupture of the TFC complex

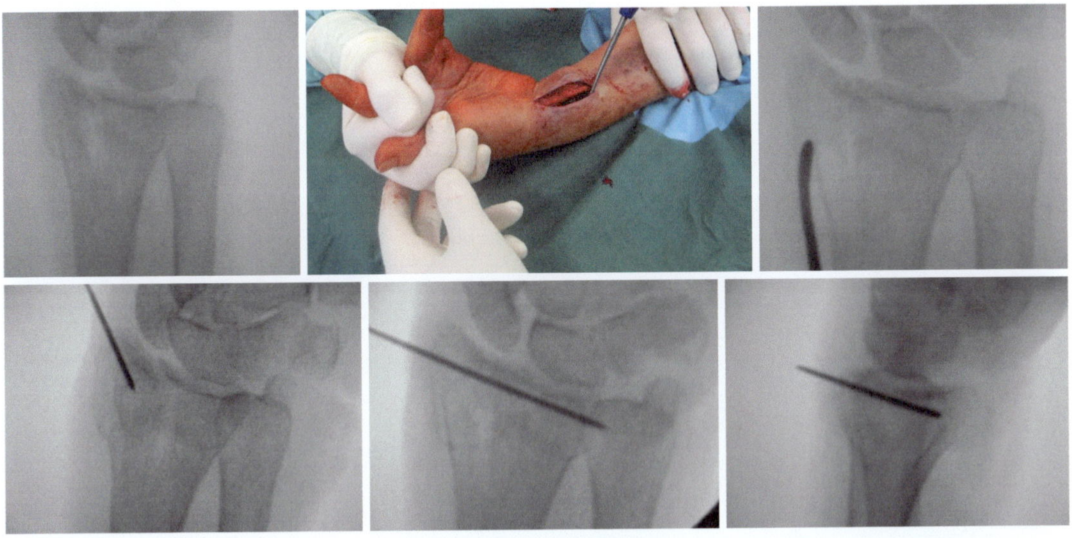

Fig. 23.13 Intraoperative picture and fluoroscopic images demonstrating a case with articular step-off. The separated fragment was reduced by direct manipulation, using a rasp and a K-wire as a joystick, which was then advanced to maintain reduction

even in the ulnar head, when used temporarily [13]. The creation of a stable articular block is highly recommended.

Figure 23.14 gives an example of a fracture with multiple articular involvement and a separated radial styloid. In this case the palmar approach was chosen even though a dorsal approach might have given the chance of direct fragment manipulation. Three different reduction tools are used in this case simultaneously. Through a small dorsal extra incision, a rasp passed guided through the metaphyseal fracture line in order to lift the dorsal articular surface (Fig. 23.14a). A K-wire joystick helped to reduce and fix the separated styloid fragment. No special care was taken for reconstruction of the palmar inclination. A malreduction of 0° was initially tolerated, which helped to restore the joint surface (Fig. 23.14b). The palmar plate was then inserted carrying a spacer. The spacer removal and reduction of the palmar inclination by the curved plate finalised the reduction manoeuvre (Fig. 23.14c).

Radius fractures with dorsal comminution in combination with articular fragments of the dorsal rim, however, qualify nicely for open reduction buttress plating. K-wires that fix the articular block need not be removed (Fig. 23.15). Double plating without separation or removal of the Lister tubercle and the use of an extensor retinaculum flap help to avoid extensor tendon dysfunction/injuries.

In case of severe joint depression and metaphyseal comminution (AO C3 fractures), especially in reversed Barton fractures with additional dorsal wedge, the combination of palmar and dorsal plating is one standard procedure. However, this is highly invasive and may go along with soft tissue problems and prolonged healing time.

One possible technique, especially in the elderly, is the combination of external fixation and palmar plating. Distraction and slight ulnar as well as palmar deviation help to reduce the articular surface without direct manipulation of small fragments. Figure 23.16 shows a case of a C3 fracture (Fig. 23.16a), where the external fixation alone gains radial length; however, it fails to reduce the frontal articular line (Fig. 23.16b). Additional palmar plating serves (a) as a buttress function of the palmar fragment and (b) helps to create a firm block with the dorsal articular part using both angular stable and compression screws (Fig. 23.16c).

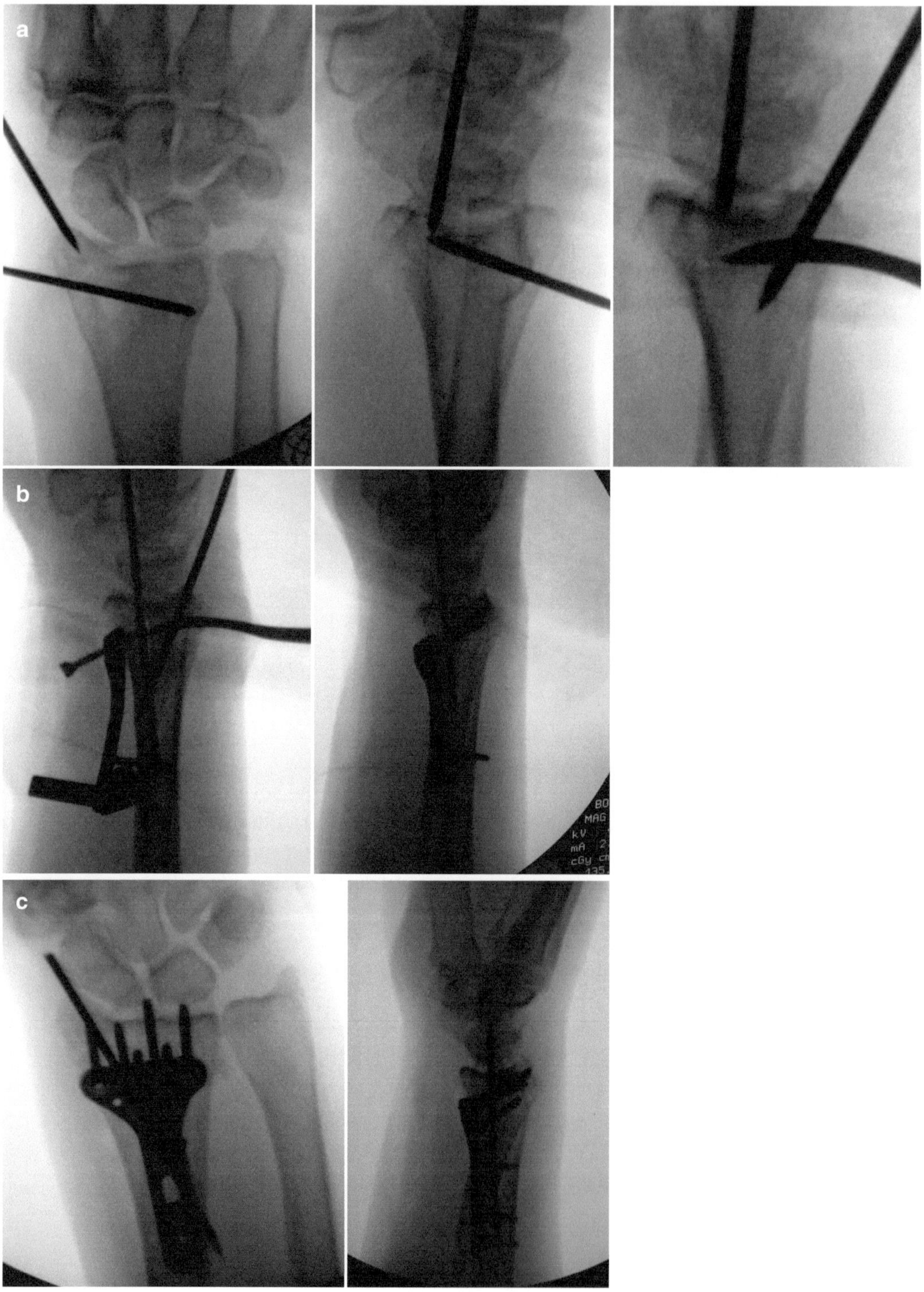

Fig. 23.14 (**a**, **b**, **c**) Images demonstrate a distal radius fracture with multiple articular involvements and a separated radial styloid fragment. The palmar approach was chosen. Through a small dorsal extra incision, a rasp passed through the metaphyseal fracture line in order to lift the dorsal articular surface. A K-wire joystick helped to reduce and fix the separated styloid fragment. The palmar plate was then inserted carrying a spacer. The spacer removal and reduction of the palmar inclination by the curved plate finalised the reduction manoeuvre

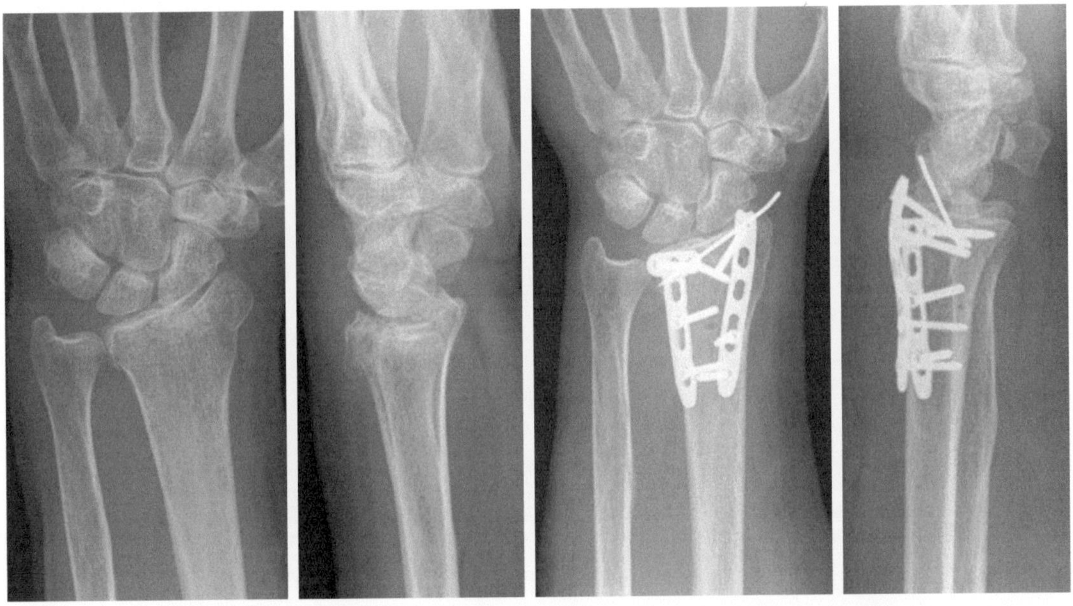

Fig. 23.15 Distal radius fracture with dorsal comminution in combination with articular fragmentation of the dorsal rim. Open reduction and stabilisation with buttress plating were carried out. The K-wires used for reduction do not need to be removed. Double plating without separation or removal of the Lister tubercle and the use of an extensor retinaculum flap help to avoid extensor tendon dysfunction/injuries

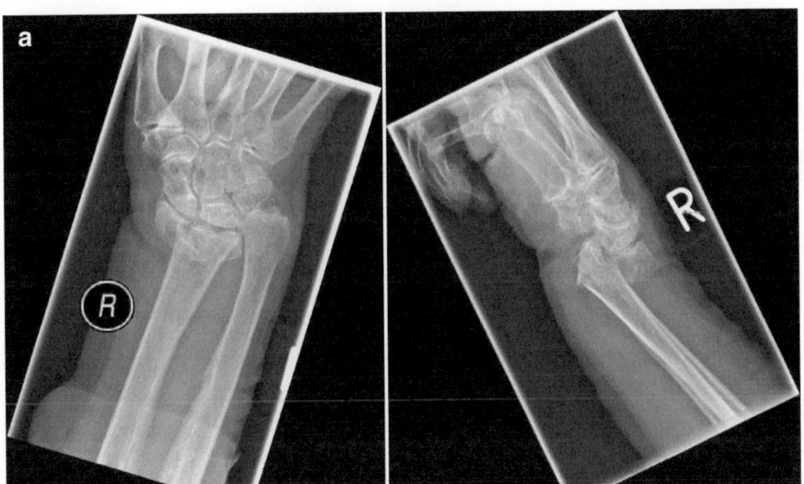

Fig. 23.16 (**a**, **b**, **c**) In this case (type C3 fracture), a combination of external fixation and palmar plating is demonstrated. External fixation alone gains radial length; however, it fails to reduce the frontal articular line. Additional palmar plating serves as a buttress function of the palmar fragment and also helps to create a firm block with the dorsal articular part using both angular stable and compression screws

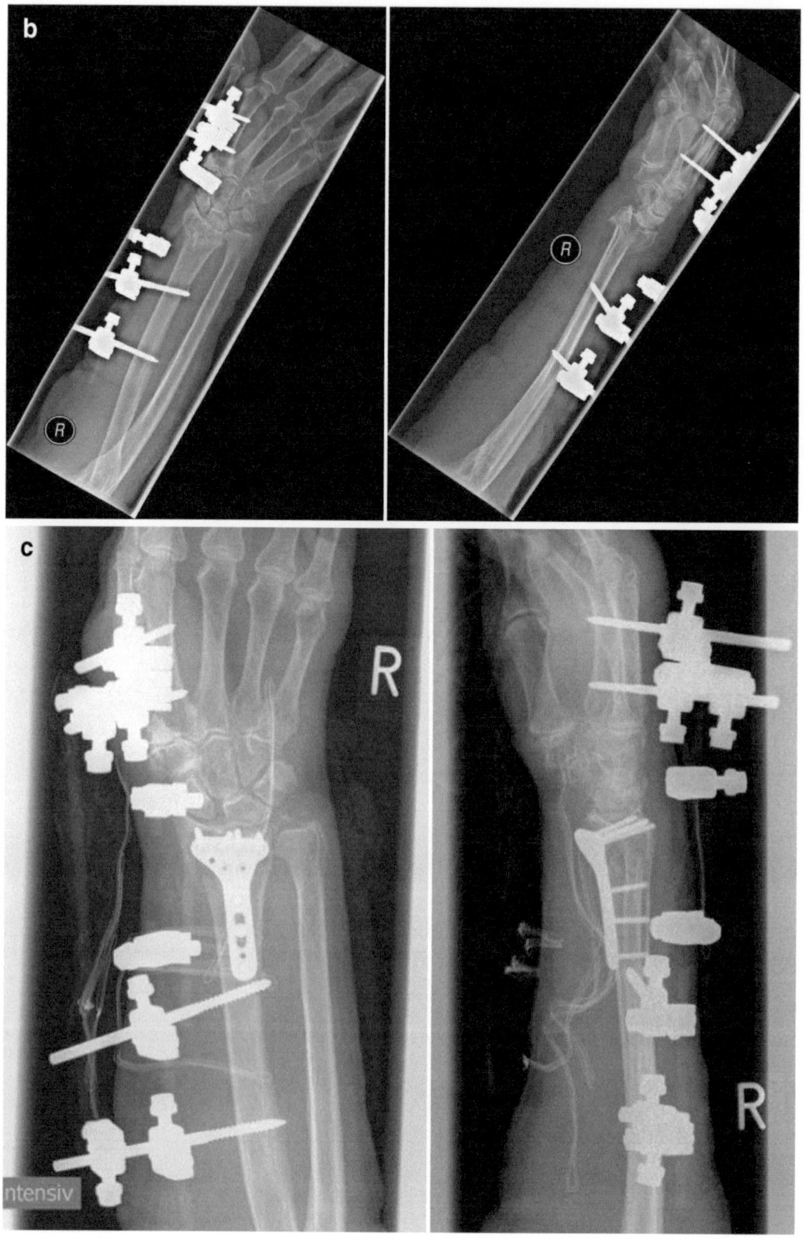

Fig. 23.16 (continued)

External Fixation for A3 and C1–3 Fractures

External fixation has lost clinical relevance; however, it may be highly effective for indirect reduction and maintenance of reduction in both extra-articular and intra-articular fractures.

One major obstacle is the problem of wrist overdistraction and long-term immobilisation.

There are in principal two possibilities to mount an external fixation. One is wrist spanning and the other one non-spanning. The so-called radio-radial external fixator is motion preserving and suitable for both extra- and intra-articular fractures [15–18].

Figure 23.17a–c demonstrate the technique of first wrist spanning assembly, fracture reduction employing distraction, ligamentotaxis and K-wire fixation of the distal fragment.

The examples of Fig. 23.18a, b show (a) the assembly using a standard small fixator and (b) a precurved bar compatible with a Ilizarov hybrid technique that accommodates several pins/K-wires that are forwarded in the distal fragment. The pins range in diameter from 1.6 to 2.0 mm. Up to six threaded or unthreaded pins may be placed in the distal fragment from different angles and may cross the fracture line. Figure 23.19a presents highly comminuted fractures, extending into the joint which was treated by a wrist non-spanning external fixator. The pins were first securely anchored in the distal fragment and then connected to the external fixator bars in order to achieve reduction employing direct fragment movement. Additional pins were inserted without connection to the external fixator as shown in Fig. 23.19b, c. Implant removal may be prolonged until 98 weeks post-surgery in order to safely ensure fracture consolidation (Fig. 23.19d).

Tips, Tricks and Pitfalls

- Palmar locking plating has indeed advanced to one standard technique in the treatment of distal radius fractures. However, there remain certain obstacles and pitfalls.
- Restoration of palmar inclination and maintenance of reduction during the healing period remain an issue [10]. Angular stable screws tend to cut through comminuted fragments of the dorsal rim and thus promote secondary loss of reduction. Length measurement failures with concomitant screw overlength may lead to extensor tendon affection. Another disadvantage of palmar plating remains the placement of a plate on top of the bone. Even though current plate designs address somehow ideally the distal radius bony geometry, still it appears that plates and prominent screws lead to discomfort in the wrist region. Different plate designs either refer to the watershed line or the palmar rim. The later are located more distally. It is of paramount

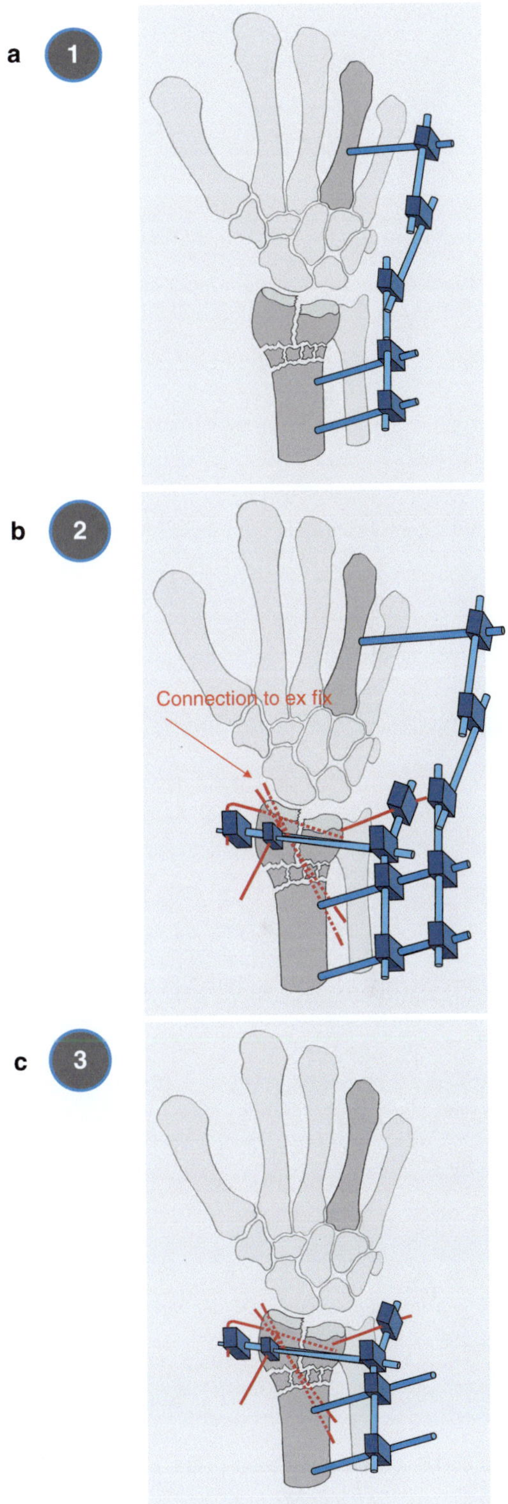

Fig. 23.17 (**a**, **b**, **c**) Figures demonstrate the technique of wrist spanning assembly, fracture reduction employing distraction, ligamentotaxis and K-wire fixation of the distal fragment

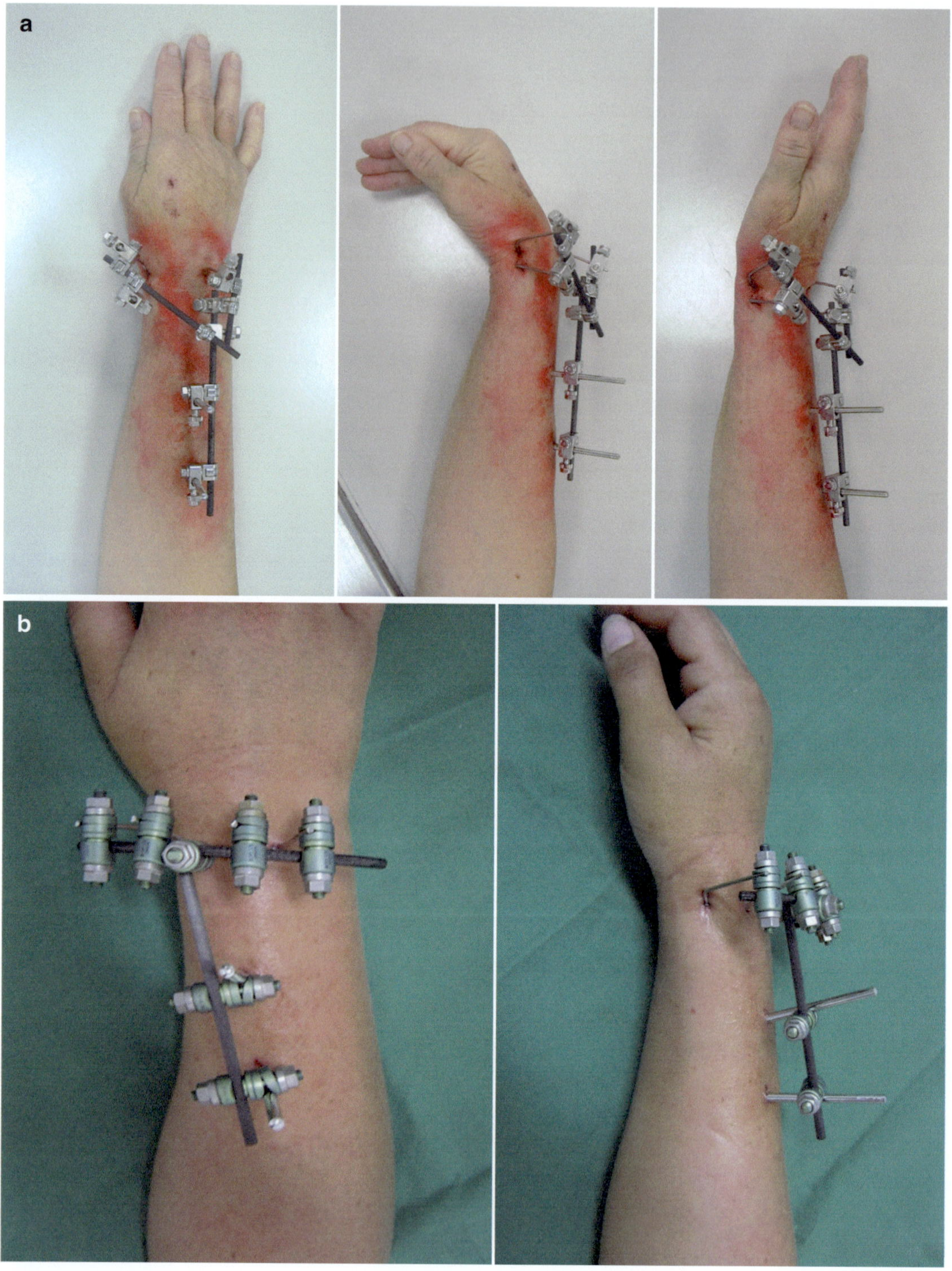

Fig. 23.18 (**a**) Demonstration of the assembly using a standard small fixator. (**b**) A precurved bar compatible with an Ilizarov hybrid technique that accommodates several pins/K-wires that are forwarded in the distal fragment. Up to six threaded or unthreaded pins may be placed in the distal fragment from different angles and may cross the fracture line

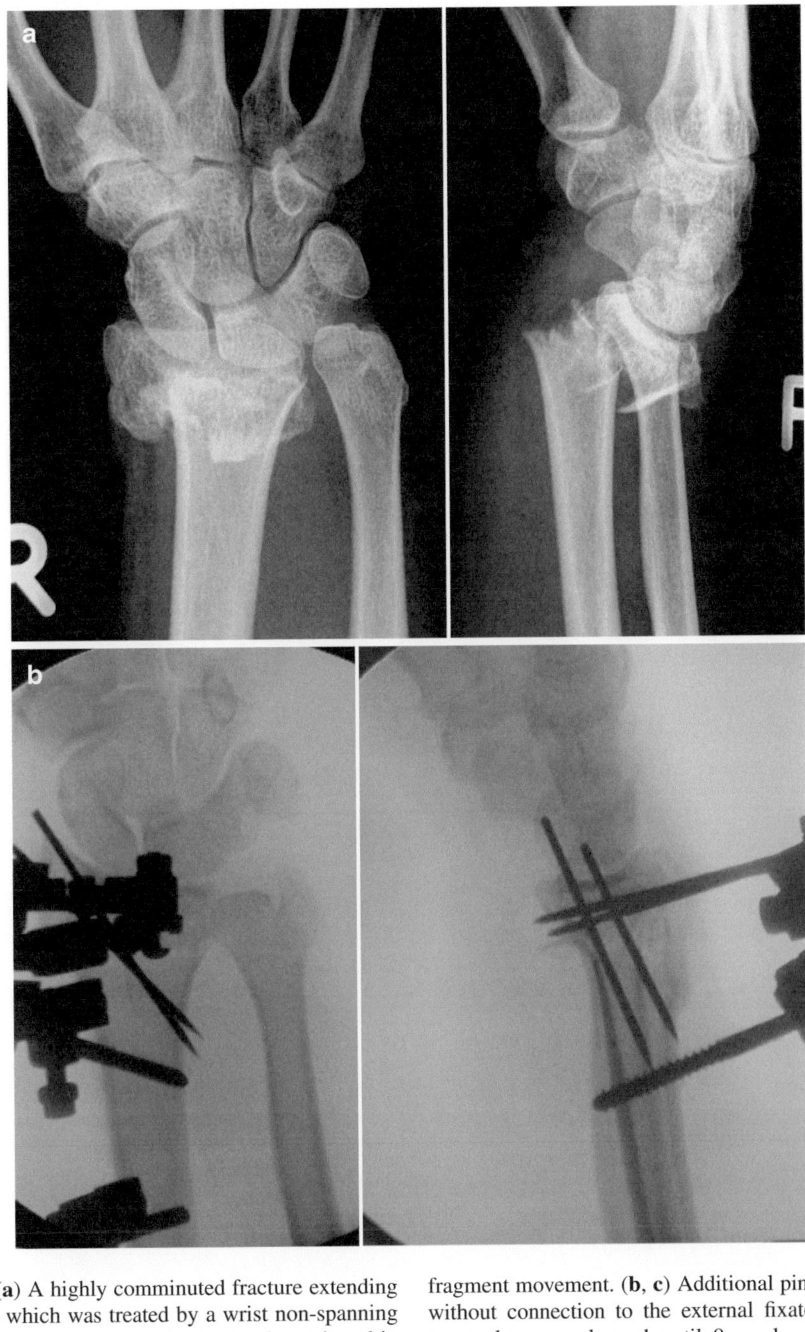

Fig. 23.19 (**a**) A highly comminuted fracture extending into the joint which was treated by a wrist non-spanning external fixator. The pins were first securely anchored in the distal fragment and then connected to the external fixator bars in order to achieve reduction employing direct fragment movement. (**b**, **c**) Additional pins were inserted without connection to the external fixator. (**d**) Implant removal was prolonged until 9 weeks post-surgery in order to safely ensure fracture consolidation

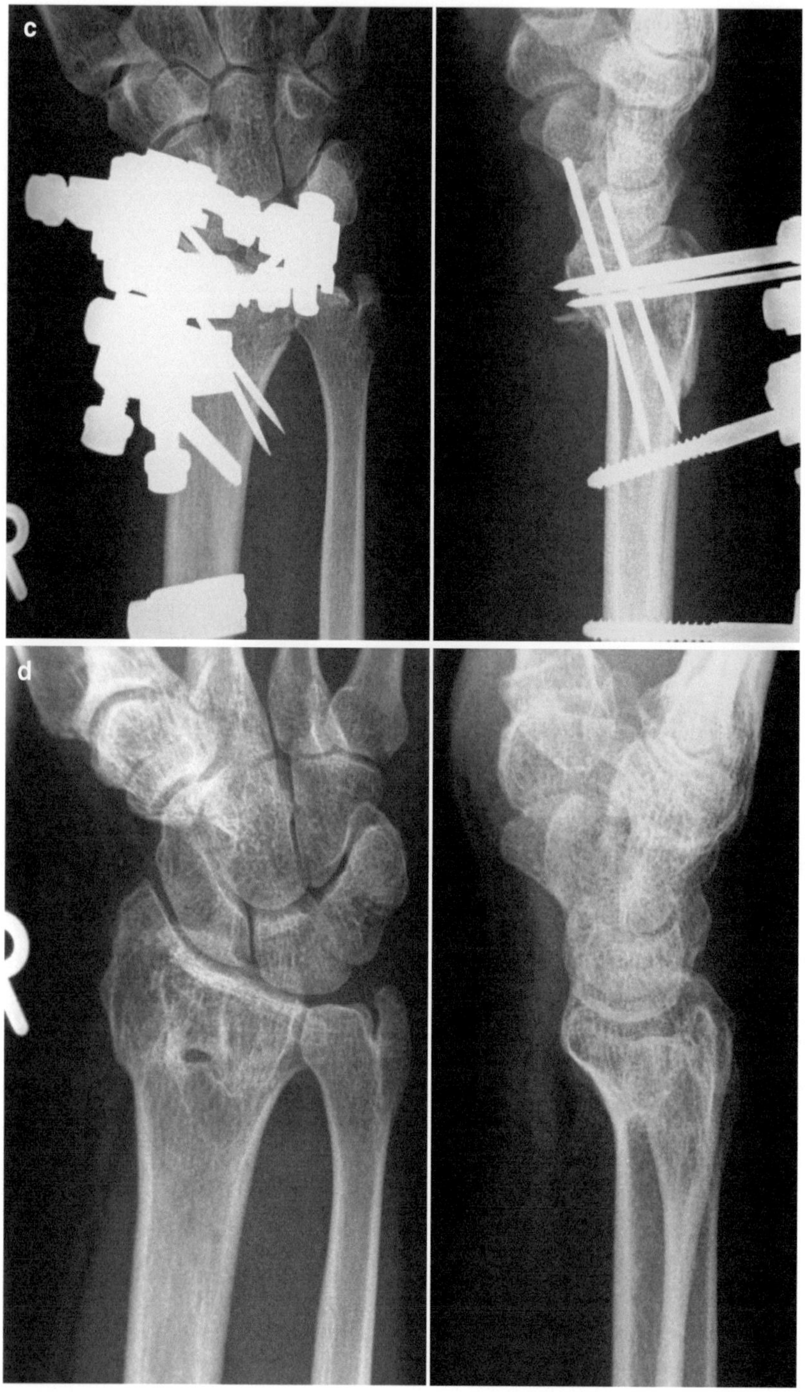

Fig. 23.19 (continued)

importance to place these plates in the right position. Plates may not be located ideally and stiff angle screws may thus penetrate the joint. Furthermore, preoperative and intraoperative analysis of soft tissue injuries, mainly ruptures of the scapholunate ligaments, needs to be performed, no matter which fixation technique is used.

- Figure 23.20 demonstrates a typical case of palmar plate fixation of an extra-articular comminuted fracture with concomitant weak bone stock. During the healing period, the angular stable screws were not able to preserve palmar inclination and cut through. Until now it is not clear as to whether a second "line of defence" using the second row of screws may help to address the problem of secondary loss of palmar inclination of dorsally displaced comminuted fractures. Dorsal buttress plate fixation is an additional way to securely provide fixation stability in cases of weak bone stock and imminent dorsal re-displacement.
- The problem of correct plate and screw position is shown in Fig. 23.21a. The plate is placed too far proximal, and angular stable screws were placed through the joint surface. Plates with a multidirectional angular stable screw design may help to circumvent this problem as well as intraoperative X-ray control of correct plate position. However, a multidirectional screw provides the risk of surgeon-based mistakes. Figure 23.21b demonstrates an angular stable screw that diverges extremely in order to fix the radioulnar fragment. Post-surgery CT scan revealed malposition of the screw into the radioulnar joint. If there is any doubt on post-surgery X-rays, CT scans are recommended to securely rule out any intra-articular screw placement.
- One further surgeon-based mistake is false measurement of the screw length. This is of importance both in the distal and the proximal fragment. Screw overlength may cause severe tendon affections as well as tendon ruptures. Figure 23.22 demonstrates screw overlength after palmar plate fixation. During implant removal, contrast material was injected in the bony canal and exposes the tendon sheet as a sign of tendon irritation.

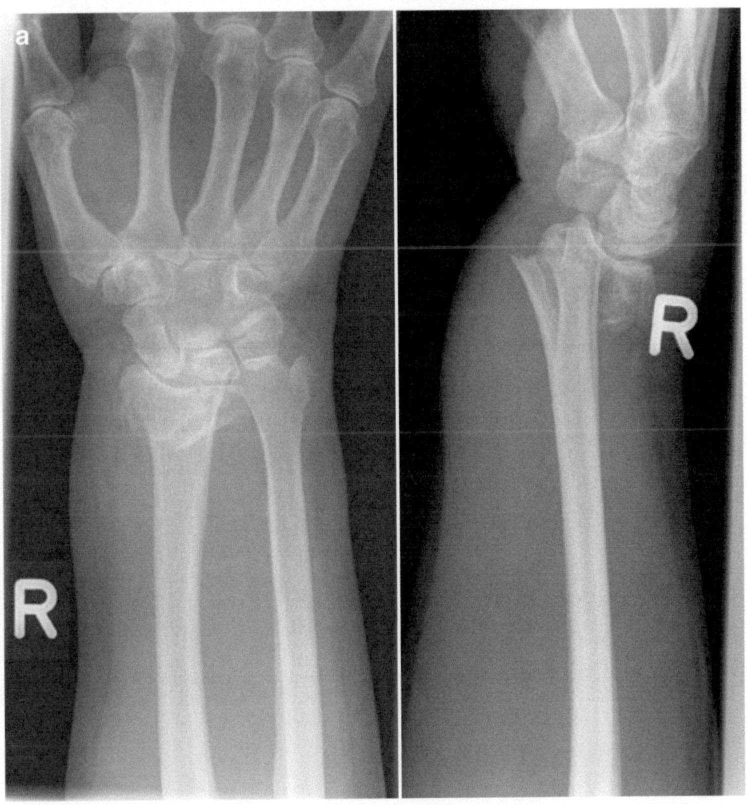

Fig. 23.20 (a, b, c) Preoperative and postoperative radiographs demonstrating a typical case of palmar plate fixation of an extra-articular comminuted fracture with concomitant weak bone stock. During the healing period, the angular stable screws were not able to preserve palmar inclination and cut through

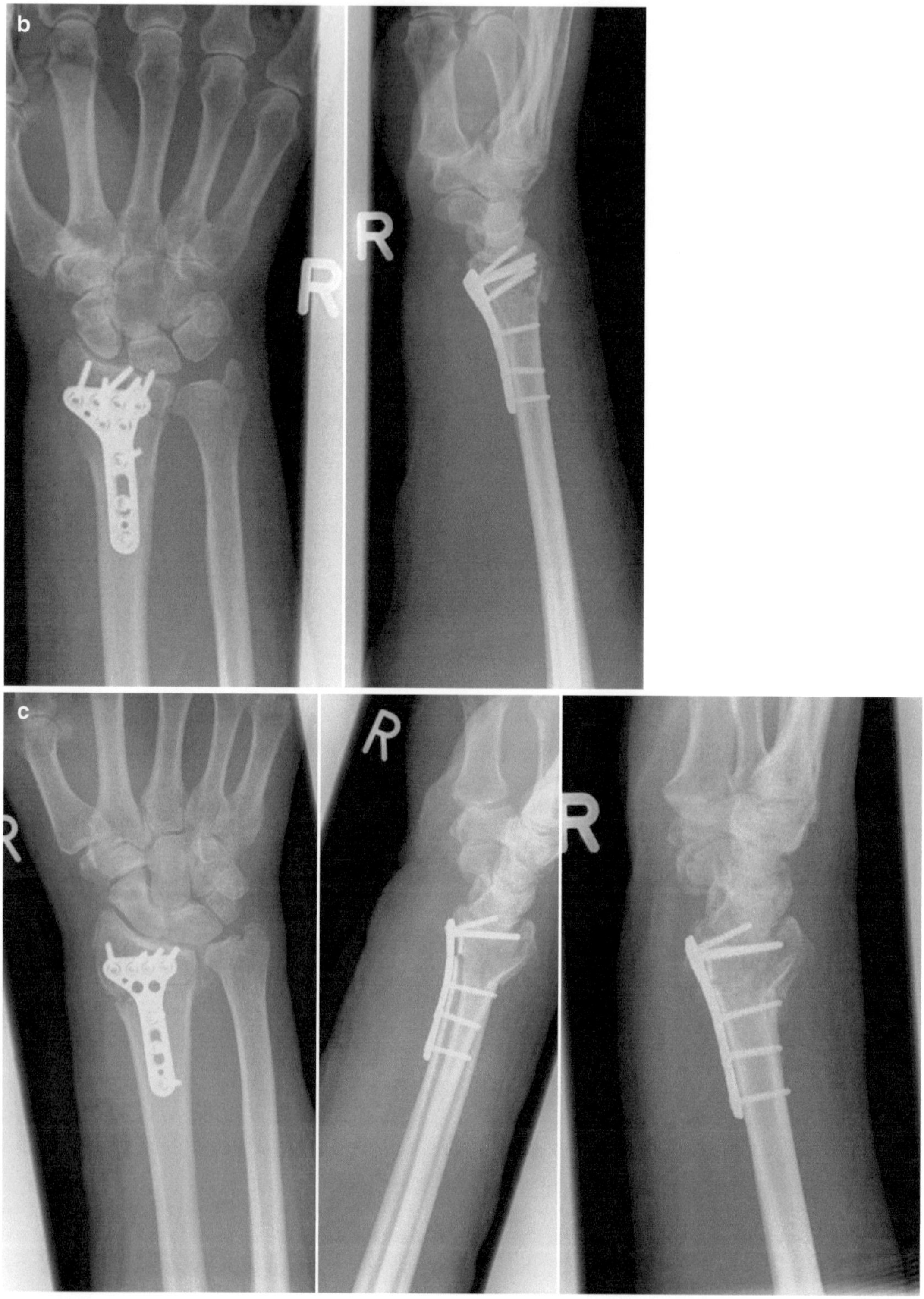

Fig. 23.20 (continued)

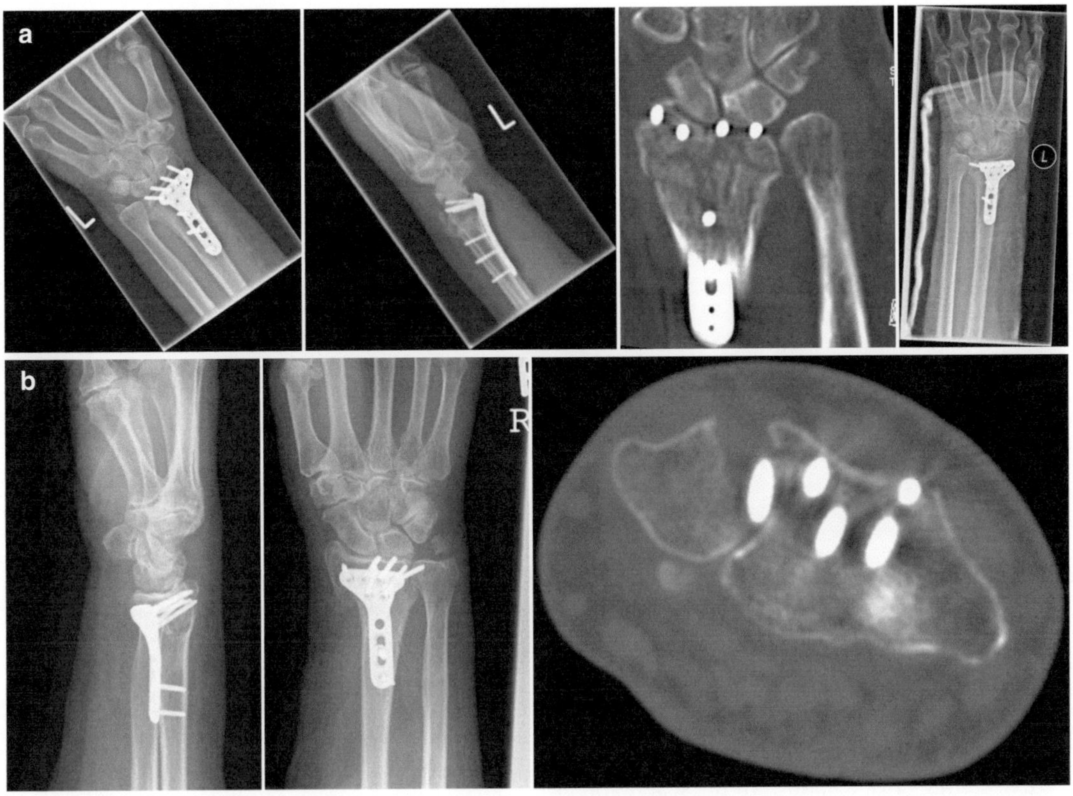

Fig. 23.21 (**a**) This case demonstrates that the plate is placed too far proximal and angular stable screws were placed through the joint surface. (**b**) In this case an angular stable screw diverging extremely in order to fix the radioulnar fragment is demonstrated. Post-surgery CT scan revealed malposition of the screw into the radioulnar joint

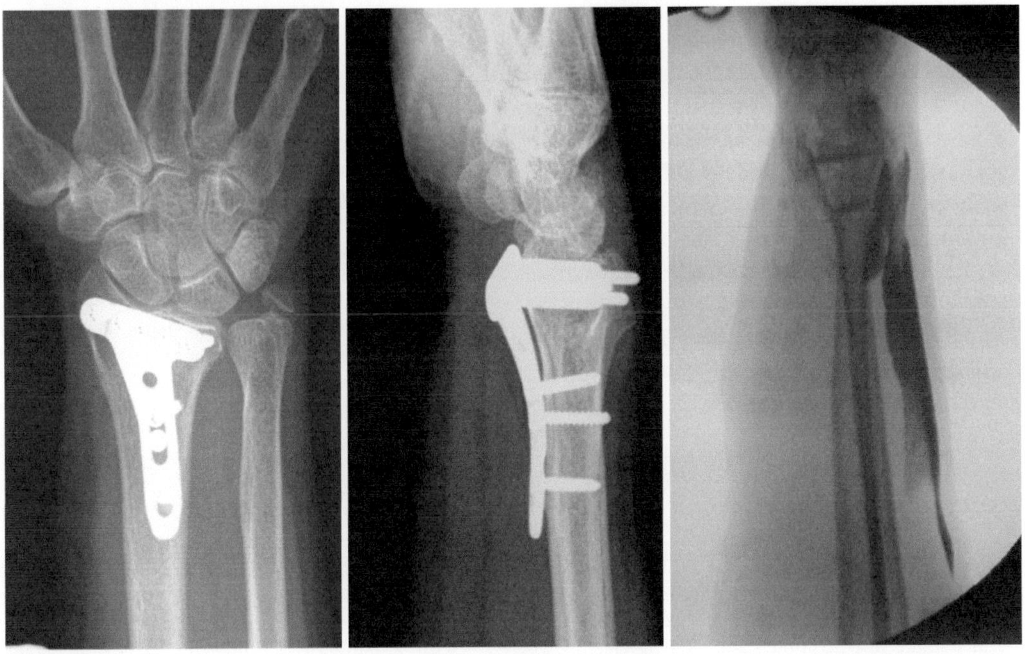

Fig. 23.22 Demonstration of screw overlength after palmar plate fixation. During implant removal, contrast material was injected in the bony canal and exposes the tendon sheet as a sign of tendon irritation

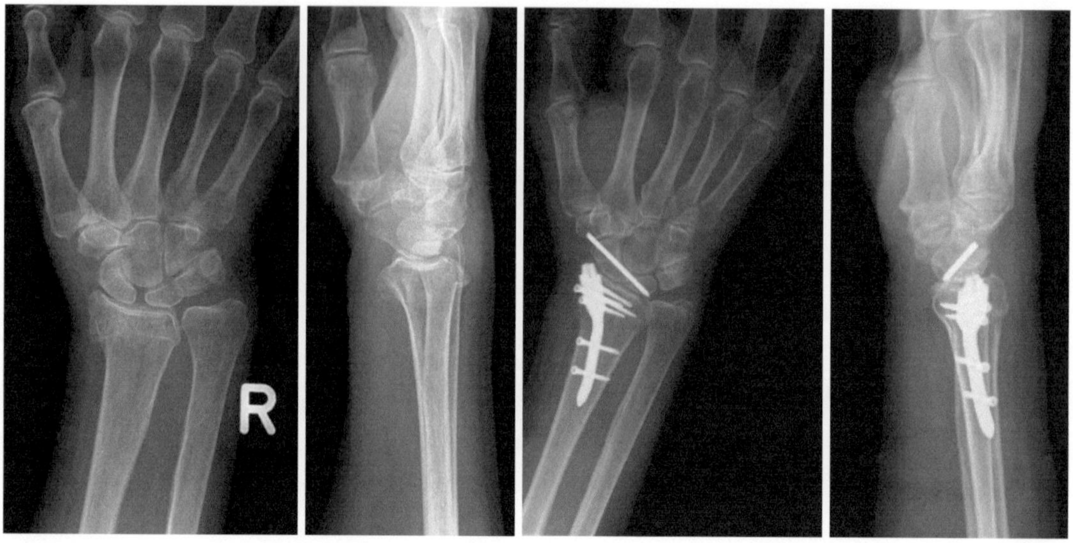

Fig. 23.23 Demonstration of a case associated with scapholunate interosseous ligament (SLD) damage which was fixed surgically with open ligament repair and temporary K-wire fixation together with an IM nailing procedure

- Soft tissue injuries are frequent mainly in intra-articular distal radius fractures and need to be meticulously analysed in the perioperative setting [19]. Ruptures of the scapholunate interosseous ligament (SLD) are most frequent and go along with severe degenerative changes of the wrist if neglected. However, plane radiographs are moderately reliable and are better at ruling out than ruling in SLD. In patients at risk with suspicious results on plain X-rays, further evaluation using CT scans or at least dynamic C-arm evaluation during surgery is necessary [17]. In case of acute injury, primary fixation is recommended. Immediate treatment is capable to restore hand function in the same way as if there was no carpal injury [20]. Figure 23.23 presents a SLD which was fixed surgically with open ligament repair and temporary K-wire fixation together with an IM nailing procedure.

References

1. O'Neill TW, Cooper C, Finn JD, Lunt M, Purdie D, Reid DM, Rowe R, Woolf AD, Wallace WA, Colles UK. Fracture Study Group. Incidence of distal forearm fracture in British men and women. Osteoporos Int. 2001;12:555–8.
2. Thompson PW, Taylor J, Dawson A. The annual incidence and seasonal variation of fractures of the distal radius in men and women over 25 years in Dorset, UK. Injury. 2004;35:462–6.
3. Pechlaner S, Gabl M, Lutz M, Krappinger D, Leixnering M, Krulis B, Ulmer H, Rudisch A, Arbeitsgruppe A. Distal radius fractures—aetiology, treatment and outcome. Handchir Mikrochir Plast Chir. 2007;39:19–28.
4. Müller ME, Nazarian S, Koch P, Schatzker J. The comprehensive classification of fractures of long bones. New York: Springer; 1990. p. 106–15.
5. Cuenca J, Martínez AA, Herrera A, Domingo J. The incidence of distal forearm fractures in Zaragoza (Spain). Chir Main. 2003;22:211–5.
6. Vogt MT, Cauley JA, Tomaino MM, Stone K, Williams JR, Herndon JH. Distal radius fractures in older women: a 10-years follow-up study of descriptive characteristics and risk factors. The study of osteoporotic fractures. J Am Geriatr Soc. 2002;50:97–103.
7. Hollevoet N, Van Maele G, Van Seymortier P, Verdonk R. Comparison of palmar tilt, radial inclination and ulnar variance in left and right wrists. J Hand Surg Br. 2000;25:431–3.
8. Lundy DW, Quisling SG, Lourie GM, Feiner CM, Lins RE. Tilted lateral radiographs in the evaluation of intra-articular distal radius fractures. J Hand Surg [Am]. 1999;24:249–56.
9. Medoff RJ. Essential radiographic evaluation for distal radius fractures. Hand Clin. 2005;21:279–88.
10. Arora R, Lutz M, Hennerbichler A, Krappinger D, Espen D, Gabl M. Complications following internal fixation of unstable distal radius fracture with a palmar locking-plate. J Orthop Trauma. 2007;21:316–22.

11. Burkhart KJ, Nowak TE, Gradl G, Klitscher D, Mehling I, Mehler D, Mueller LP, Rommens PM. Intramedullary nailing vs. palmar locked plating for unstable dorsally comminuted distal radius fractures: a biomechanical study. Clin Biomech (Bristol, Avon). 2010;25(8):771–5. https://doi.org/10.1016/j.clinbiomech.2010.06.004. Epub 7 Jul 2010
12. Gradl G, Falk S, Mittlmeier T, Wendt M, Mielsch N, Gradl G. Fixation of intra-articular fractures of the distal radius using intramedullary nailing: a randomized trial versus palmar locking plates. Injury. 2016;47(Suppl 7):S25–30. https://doi.org/10.1016/S0020-1383(16)30850-6.
13. Falk SS, Mittlmeier T, Gradl G. Results of geriatric distal radius fractures treated by intramedullary fixation. Injury. 2016;47(Suppl 7):S31–5. https://doi.org/10.1016/S0020-1383(16)30851-8.
14. Gradl G. Distal radius fractures. Z Orthop Unfall. 2009;147(5):621–35. https://doi.org/10.1055/s-0029-1186133. quiz 636-7. Epub 5 Oct 2009. German. No abstract available
15. Windolf M, Schwieger K, Ockert B, Jupiter JB, Gradl G. A novel non-bridging external fixator construct versus volar angular stable plating for the fixation of intra-articular fractures of the distal radius—a biomechanical study. Injury. 2010;41(2):204–9. https://doi.org/10.1016/j.injury.2009.09.025. Epub 9 Oct 2009
16. Gradl G, Jupiter JB, Gierer P, Mittlmeier T. Fractures of the distal radius treated with a nonbridging external fixation technique using multiplanar k-wires. J Hand Surg [Am]. 2005;30(5):960–8.
17. Gradl G, Gradl G, Wendt M, Mittlmeier T, Kundt G, Jupiter JB. Non-bridging external fixation employing multiplanar K-wires versus volar locked plating for dorsally displaced fractures of the distal radius. Arch Orthop Trauma Surg. 2013;133(5):595–602. https://doi.org/10.1007/s00402-013-1698-5 . Epub 2013 Feb 19.
18. Gradl G, Mielsch N, Wendt M, Falk S, Mittlmeier T, Gierer P, Gradl G. Intramedullary nail versus volar plate fixation of extra-articular distal radius fractures. Two year results of a prospective randomized trial. Injury. 2014;45(Suppl 1):S3–8. https://doi.org/10.1016/j.injury.2013.10.045. Epub 4 Nov 2013
19. Gradl G, Neuhaus V, Fuchsberger T, Guitton TG, Prommersberger KJ, Ring D. Science of Variation Group. Radiographic diagnosis of scapholunate dissociation among intra-articular fractures of the distal radius: interobserver reliability. J Hand Surg [Am]. 2013;38(9):1685–90. https://doi.org/10.1016/j.jhsa.2013.05.039. Epub 30 Jul 2013
20. Gradl G, Pillukat T, Fuchsberger T, Knobe M, Ring D, Prommersberger KJ. The functional outcome of acute scapholunate ligament repair in patients with intraarticular distal radius fractures treated by internal fixation. Arch Orthop Trauma Surg. 2013;133(9):1281–7. https://doi.org/10.1007/s00402-013-1797-3. Epub 23 Jun 2013

24 Distal Ulna Fractures

Tristan E. McMillan and Alan J. Johnstone

Introduction and Fracture Patterns

Isolated fractures of the distal ulna are relatively rare and usually result from a direct force or crush injury. However, ulna fractures do occur more commonly in association with fractures of the distal radius, with up to 65% of fractures of the distal radius having associated distal ulna fractures [1]. Fractures of the distal ulna can be overlooked; however, due to the distal ulna's direct interaction with the bony anatomy of the distal radius and complex soft tissue attachments of the interosseous membrane (IOM), distal radioulnar joint (DRUJ) itself, ulnocarpal ligaments and the triangular fibrocartilage complex (TFCC), a mistreated injury can have significant long-term consequences on wrist function through persistent symptoms or reduced function.

We have defined fractures of the distal ulna as those that occur distal to the IOM. The most distal fibres of the IOM, named the distal oblique bundle (DOB), originate from the distal one sixth of the ulna shaft coinciding with the proximal border of the pronator quadratus (PQ) muscle [2]. Fractures proximal to the insertion of the DOB should be considered as ulnar shaft fractures.

T.E. McMillan, M.B.Ch.B., M.R.C.S.
Trauma and Orthopaedics, Aberdeen Royal Infirmary, Aberdeen, Scotland, UK

A.J. Johnstone, F.R.C.S. (✉)
Trauma and Orthopedic Surgery, Aberdeen Royal Infirmary, Aberdeen, Scotland, UK
e-mail: alanjjohnstone@me.com

Thereafter, we have classified distal ulna fractures anatomically into styloid tip, styloid base, ulnar head and ulnar metaphysis (neck)/distal diaphysis, as shown in Fig. 24.1. This has similarities to the *Comprehensive Classification of Fractures*, where distal ulna fractures associated with distal radius fractures have been classified using a Q modifier; Q1 designates a fracture of the ulnar styloid, whilst Q2 and Q3 are fractures of the ulnar neck, Q4 and Q5 are fractures involving the ulnar head and Q6 is a fracture of the distal ulnar shaft [3]. Our reasoning for this sub-classification is the distinct significance of each of these anatomical regions and their influence on fracture patterns and their subsequent management:

- Styloid tip, avulsion through its attachment to the ulnar collateral ligament
- Styloid base, avulsion or involvement of the TFCC
- Ulnar head, intra-articular nature and associated disruption to the DRUJ
- Metaphysis/distal diaphysis, classical radial displacement of the proximal fragment due to the action of PQ and IOM, as shown in Fig. 24.2

P.V. Giannoudis (ed.), *Fracture Reduction and Fixation Techniques*,
https://doi.org/10.1007/978-3-319-68628-8_24

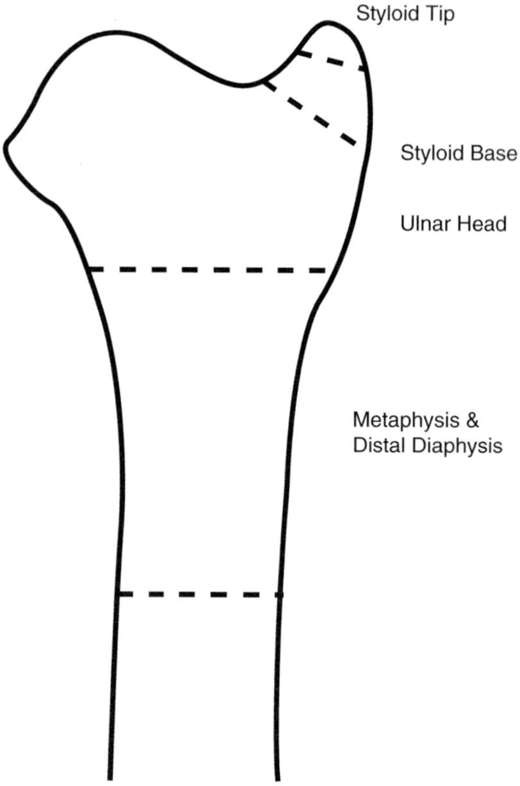

Fig. 24.1 Diagram illustrating the anatomical classification of fractures of the distal ulna

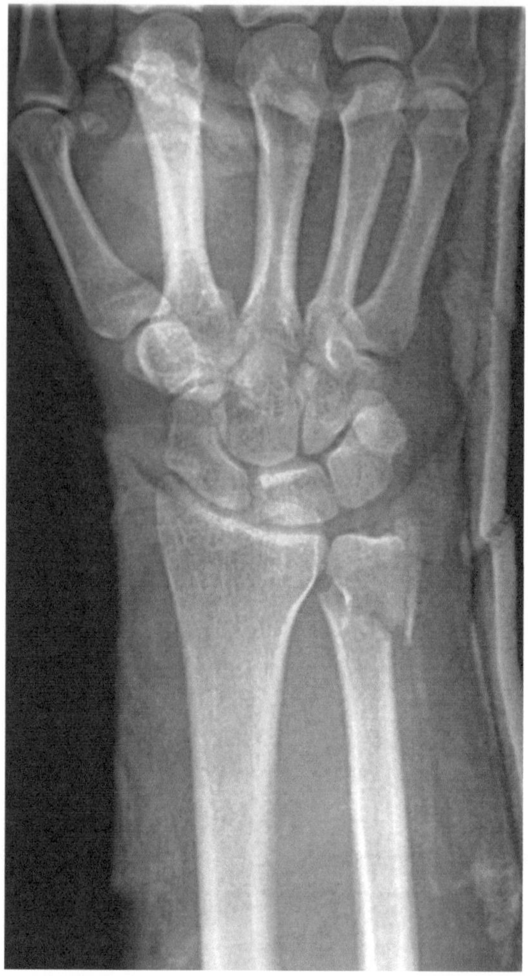

Fig. 24.2 Radiograph showing a neck fracture of the distal ulna, with classic medial displacement of the proximal fragment due to the action of the pronator quadratus and interosseous membrane

Decision to Treat and Preoperative Planning

Frequently the most difficult decision that is associated with distal ulna fractures is whether to treat operatively or nonoperatively.

Absolute indications for surgical management include:

- Open fractures
- Neurovascular compromise usually affecting the ulnar nerve

Relative indications for surgical management include:

- Displaced metaphysis/distal diaphysis, particularly those with significant shortening
- Displaced head fractures with intra-articular extension
- Any distal ulna fracture with associated DRUJ instability
- Unstable fractures of the ulna in association with unstable fractures of the distal radius, whereby reduction and stabilisation of the ulna facilitate the treatment of the distal radius fracture

As a minimum, good-quality anteroposterior and lateral preoperative radiographs of the distal radius and DRUJ are required to evaluate the wrist for co-existing injury keeping in mind that Essex-Lopresti-type injuries may need more

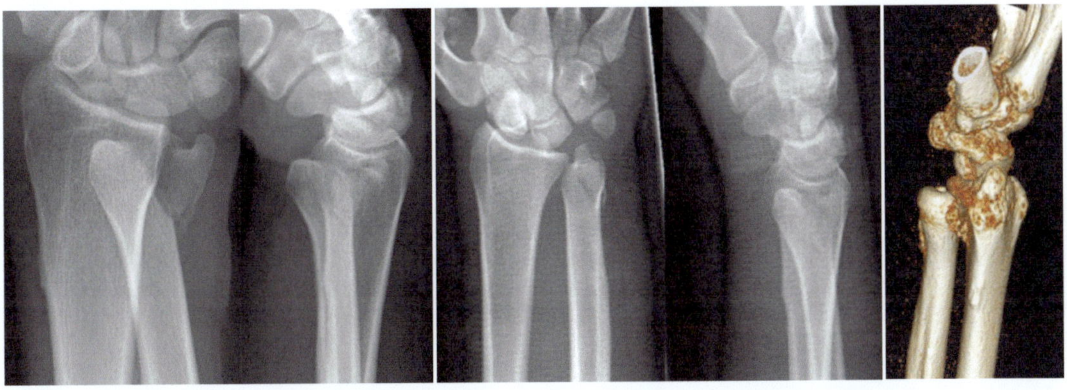

Fig. 24.3 Case of a young gentleman with a large base of styloid fracture and DRUJ dislocation, treated out with our unit with prolonged cast immobilisation. He represented 3 months later with wrist pain and loss of pronation and supination, at which point a CT confirmed DRUJ dislocation and fracture non-union

detailed radiographs to assess the whole of the forearm including the wrist and elbow. A widened distal radioulnar space on the anteroposterior radiographs should raise suspicion of a DRUJ injury, and a true lateral of the wrist should be obtained to assess for dislocation or subluxation of the DRUJ. We advocate that cases with DRUJ instability, especially those that can be visualised on true lateral radiographs of the wrist, should be treated operatively in most cases to prevent chronic instability or dislocation. This is highlighted in Fig. 24.3.

In those patients where the extent of the associated DRUJ bony injury or soft tissue injury is unclear, computed tomography (CT) or magnetic resonance imaging (MRI) can aid clinical decision making and surgical planning.

Although a large percentage of ulnar styloid fractures will go on to non-union, surgical fixation of these injuries remains controversial with some studies demonstrating no effect upon clinical outcome, providing any associated distal radius fracture is suitably reduced and stabilised [4, 5]. On the other hand, Dar et al. advocate that a more vigorous approach to treating these injuries is adopted to reduce weakness and ulnar-sided wrist pain [6]. Due to the potential disruption to the stabilising ligaments of the distal ulna and TFCC, and subsequent effect upon the stability of the DRUJ, we advocate fixation of large base fractures with >2 mm of displacement, using a percutaneous Kirschner wire (K-wire) or a tension band construct. We have also managed to treat these fractures successfully with single mini-fragment screws, so as to avoid the need for removal of hardware, but have found this technique to be labour intensive and of no long-term clinical advantage to the patient.

Overall we advocate that the majority of styloid tip fractures should be treated conservatively, although patients should be educated about the incidence of ulnar-sided wrist pain and the potential for a slower recovery of grip strength and wrist flexion, although these should improve within 12 months of injury [7].

Patient Set-Up in Theatre

Patient set-up is similar to that used for fixation of the distal radius. The patient is supine, and the arm is draped free so that the forearm can be supinated or pronated on a radiolucent arm table, or, through flexing the elbow, the arm can be held in mid-pronation whilst the hand is held vertically. Following positioning, the operating table is then rotated by 90 degrees, as seen in Fig. 24.4, to provide more room for the operating surgeon and to facilitate easier positioning and use of the image intensifier intraoperatively.

Although not always required, if the surgeon envisages the need for a bloodless operative field, a tourniquet is applied to the upper arm and the patient is prepped and draped to a suitable level, proximal to the elbow. We are increasingly seeing the use of extremity drapes with an incorporated elastic aperture, and whilst we appreciate their benefit in ease of use and effective isolation, there is a concern with regard to the potential venous tourniquet effect of the elastic aperture. We therefore choose to use two large adhesive drapes as shown in Fig. 24.5.

The surgeon positions themselves at the caudal aspect of the hand table for the management of any associated distal radius fracture, then moving to the cranial aspect with the forearm pronated to address the distal ulna fracture. The reverse is true depending upon the arm being operated upon and of course the hand dominance of the surgeon.

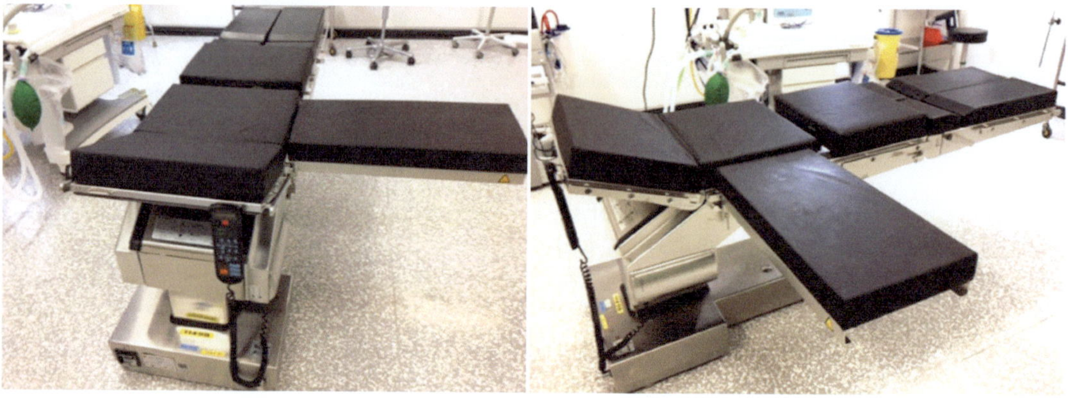

Fig. 24.4 Operative table set-up with radiolucent arm table attached and table rotated 90° to ease the placement and use of intraoperative fluoroscopy

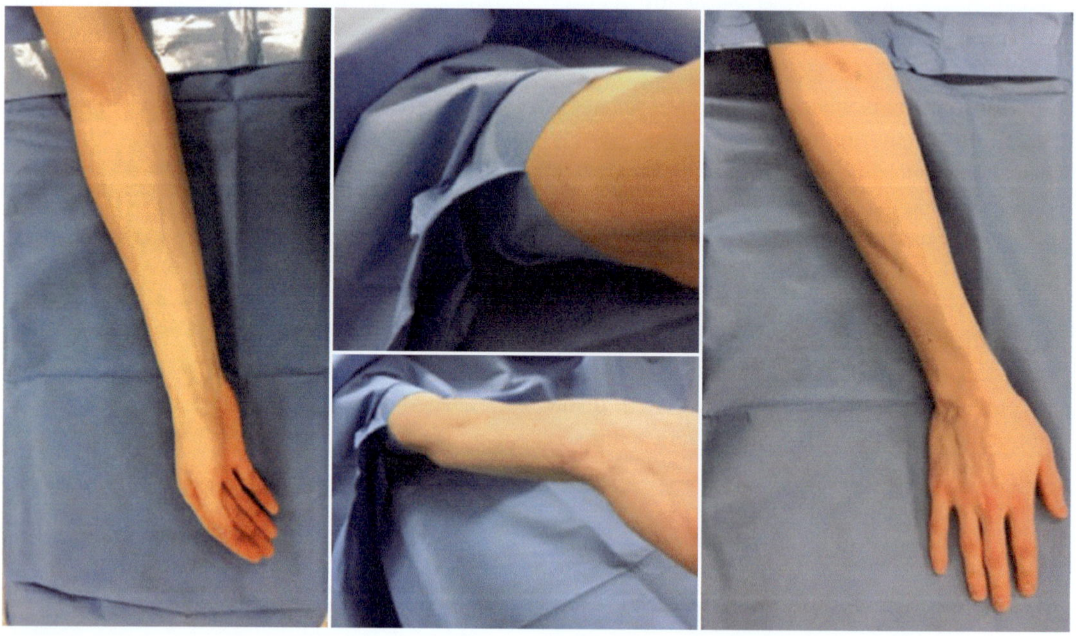

Fig. 24.5 Draping technique, utilising two large adhesive drapes to isolate and drape the limb, whilst still allowing free movement of the limb and, importantly, avoiding the potential tourniquet effect of elasticated extremity drapes

Closed Reduction Manoeuvres

Due to the relatively subcutaneous nature of the distal ulna, reduction can sometimes be achieved with closed manipulation. Importantly, restoration of alignment is significantly aided by first restoring the length and alignment of any associated distal radius fracture. The radius fracture must therefore be addressed first, with assessment of the alignment and stability of the ulna fracture once this has been achieved.

Closed reduction of an ulnar styloid fracture is technically difficult due to its small size and to the deforming forces through the attachment of the ulnar collateral ligament, dorsal carpal ligament and TFCC. Therefore, where it is considered necessary to achieve accurate reduction of these fractures, they usually require an open or 'mini-open' approach.

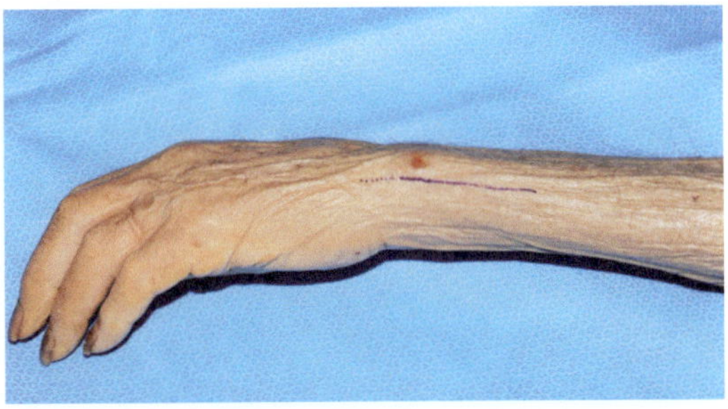

Fig. 24.6 The longitudinal incision along the subcutaneous border of the ulna, volar to the dorsal prominence

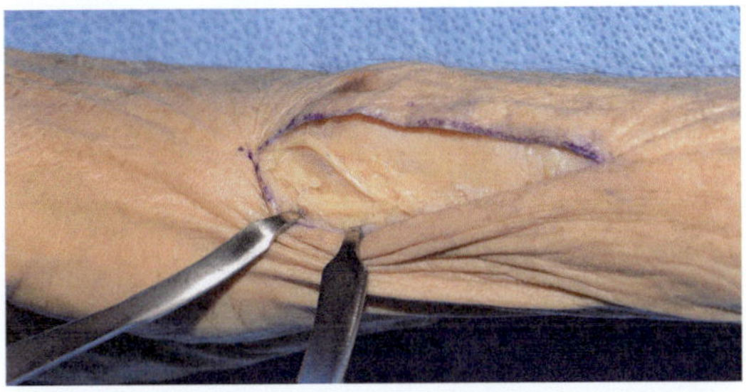

Fig. 24.7 Cadaveric dissection showing the dorsal branch of the ulnar nerve crossing the subcutaneous border of the distal ulna, from palmar to dorsal

Surgical Approach

For most distal ulna fractures, a longitudinal incision is made along the subcutaneous border of the ulna (Fig. 24.6). The intended inter-nervous plane lies between the extensor carpi ulnaris (posterior interosseous nerve) and flexor carpi ulnaris (ulnar nerve). Careful superficial dissection to allow identification and protection of the dorsal branch of the ulnar nerve as it passes from volar to dorsal is essential. Cadaveric research on the course of the dorsal branch of the ulnar nerve has shown that the nerve passes dorsal to the flexor carpi ulnaris and pierces the deep fascia where it becomes subcutaneous on the ulnar aspect of the forearm approximately 5 cm proximal to the pisiform [8]. It crosses from palmar to volar at that distal aspect of the ulna as shown in Fig. 24.7. There is variation in the exact point at which it crosses the subcutaneous border of the ulna making it vulnerable to iatrogenic injury. Although Puna and Poon demonstrated that the dorsal branch of the ulnar nerve crosses on average 0.2 cm proximal to the tip of the ulnar styloid [9], this range varied from 2.5 cm proximal to 2.5 cm distal to the tip of the styloid.

To achieve suitable exposure of the distal ulna, after defining and establishing the plane between the tendons of extensor and flexor carpi ulnaris using sharp dissection, both tendons are retracted dorsally and volarly, respectively, using a self-retainer or two small Hohmann retractors. Subperiosteal dissection, shown in Fig. 24.8, provides suitable exposure to facilitate fixation of fractures of the ulna neck/distal diaphysis and simple fractures of the ulnar head. If, however, the ulnar head fracture is comminuted, direct visualisation of the articular surface may be required. Although limited, this can occasionally be achieved through the same incision, by developing the plane between the fifth and sixth extensor compartments. Subsequent radial retraction of extensor digiti minimi then allows direct visualisation of the dorsal aspect of the ulnar head and the articular surface.

Whilst this allows some degree of exposure to the DRUJ, if a more extensive exposure is needed, a separate volar or dorsal approach is indicated. The authors favour a dorsal approach particularly when there is an ulnar head fracture with significant intra-articular comminution, or if DRUJ

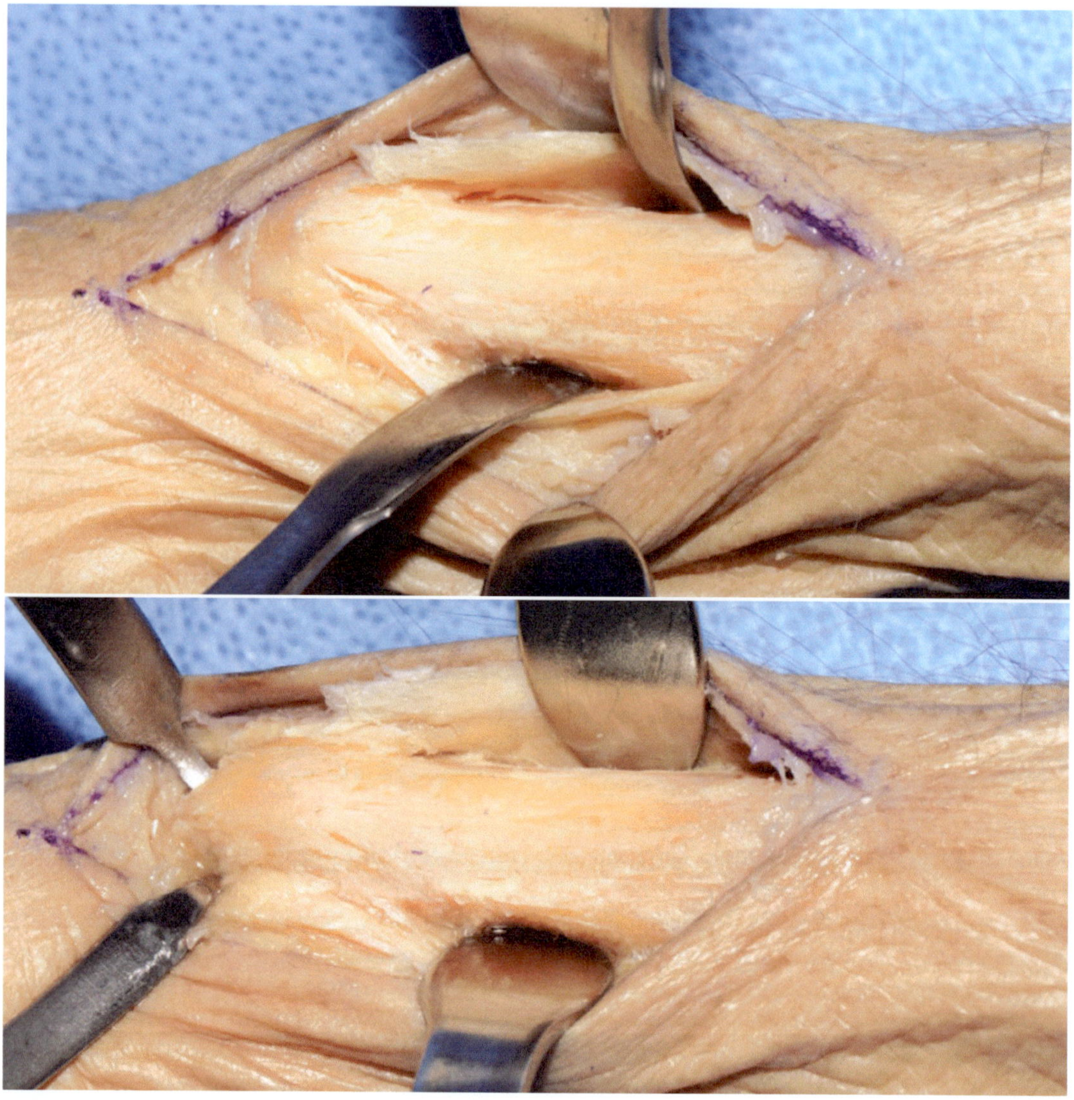

Fig. 24.8 Cadaveric subperiosteal dissection to expose the ulna. The incision and dissection can be extended distally to expose the styloid

reconstruction is indicated since the dorsal ligaments usually require to be repaired. This is performed through a longitudinal incision in line with the fifth extensor compartment. After extensor digiti minimi is retracted radially, the joint is approached through the floor of the fifth compartment. Bain et al. describe incising the retinaculum and capsule as one, creating an ulnar-based thick capsular-retinacular flap that allows suitable exposure of the joint and a stable repair at the end [10].

Open Reduction Manoeuvres

The main aim is to restore length, rotation and natural bone alignment. With open reduction, head, neck and distal diaphyseal fractures can be reduced using a combination of gentle traction and direct manipulation using bone reduction forceps.

Fractures of the styloid can be reduced using pointy reduction forceps. An alternative, and arguably more effective, method for these fragments is the placement of a K-wire into the distal styloid fragment whilst using a drill sleeve to control the fragment and to protect the adjacent soft tissues. The wire is then used to 'joystick' the fragment back to its anatomical position, before finally securing it by advancing the wire.

As previously mentioned, fractures of the distal metaphysis/diaphysis tend to result in radial displacement of the proximal fragment, thereby requiring reduction by applying an ulnar force to the shaft to correct alignment. We recommend that this is achieved by placing a toothed reduction clamp on the proximal fragment before applying a force ulnarwards, perpendicular to the shaft, as shown in Fig. 24.9. By applying only the tips of the forceps to the shaft, it is usually possible to slide a suitable plate through the gap between the jaws in the forceps, to lie in an optimal position on the distal ulna.

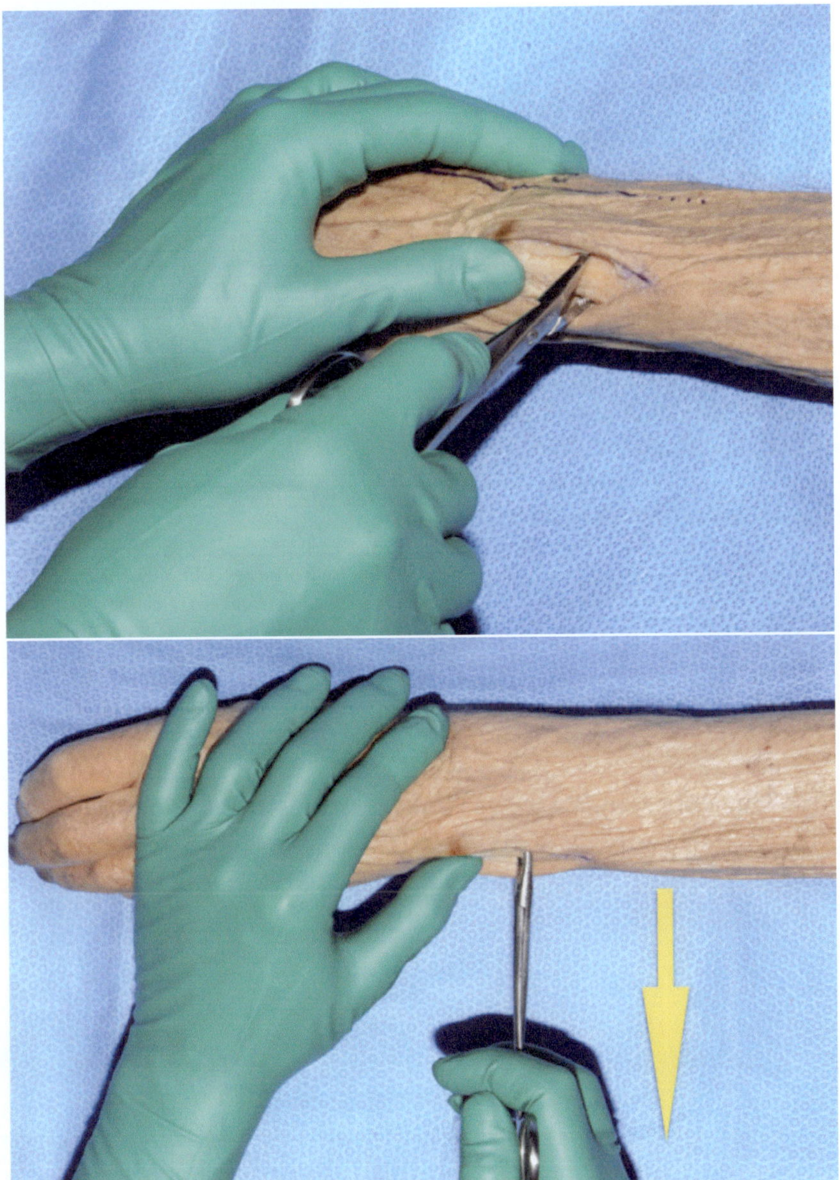

Fig. 24.9 A toothed reduction clamp is applied to the proximal fragment with force applied in the direction shown (ulnarwards). This is opposed by direct pressure with the surgeon's thumb over the ulna head, thereby enabling reduction

Implant Insertion

When deciding whether to fix an associated styloid base fracture, it is essential to assess the stability of the DRUJ clinically and radiologically intraoperatively. Clinically this can be achieved with flexion of the elbow to 90°, placing the forearm in neutral rotation whilst the surgeon attempts to translate the distal ulna in dorsal, volar and ulnar directions. If there is any doubt about the clinical findings, the same process should be repeated using fluoroscopy to 'visualise' the stability of the DRUJ.

Whilst K-wires have a role in styloid fractures, their role in fractures of the ulna head or neck should be limited to simple, non-comminuted fractures. Where possible they should be avoided in those with osteoporotic bone due to the poor hold and increased risk of loosening and/or loss of reduction. An example of this is seen in Fig. 24.10.

Open reduction and internal fixation on the other hand have the potential benefit of secure fixation and early mobilisation. Due the thin soft tissue envelope and the shape of the distal ulna, traditional standard plates were not well suited for fixation of fractures of the distal ulna. Through their bulk and prominence under the skin (Fig. 24.11), many required to be removed after fracture union. Moreover, with their limited screw options, it was difficult to achieve more than one or two screw fixation within the distal fragment resulting in poor fracture stability that was prone to mechanical failure. This has led to the evolution and increased use of low-profile (Fig. 24.12), anatomical locking

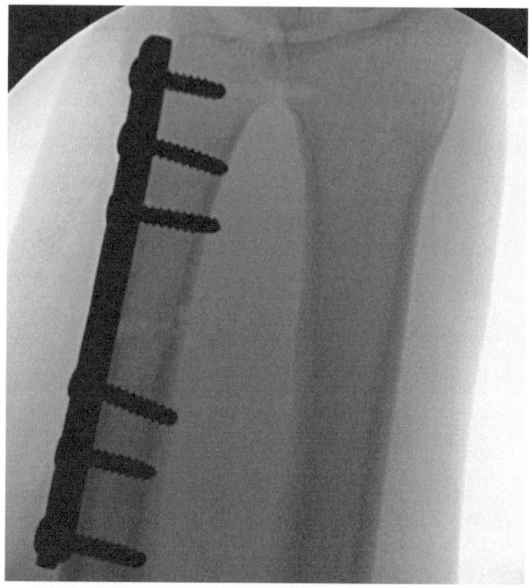

Fig. 24.11 Intraoperative image highlighting the bulky nature of the more traditional non-locking plates used for the fixation of distal ulna fractures. This was acceptable in this case due to the proximity of the fracture and a greater than normal soft tissue envelope

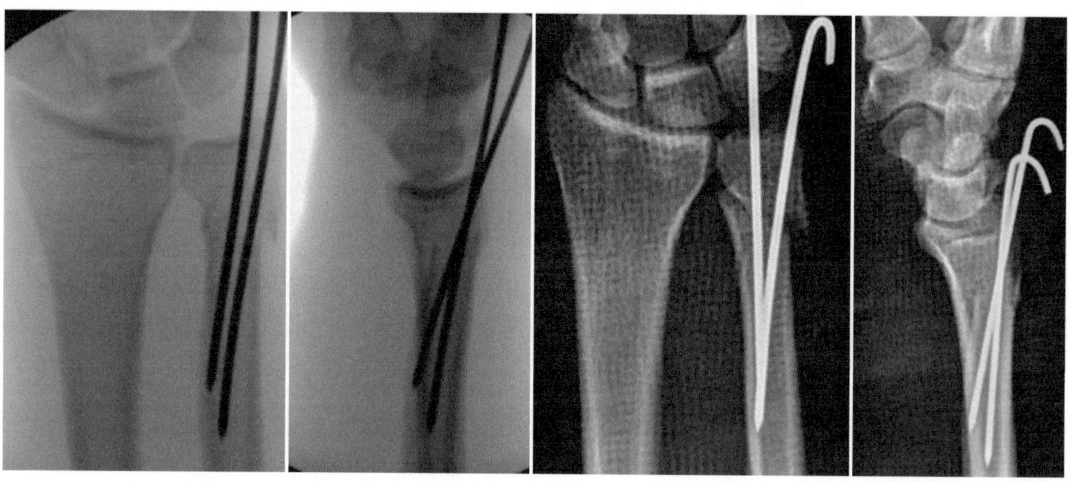

Fig. 24.10 Radiographs of a distal diaphysis/metaphyseal fracture reduced closed and fixed with two percutaneous K-wires and subsequent loss of reduction

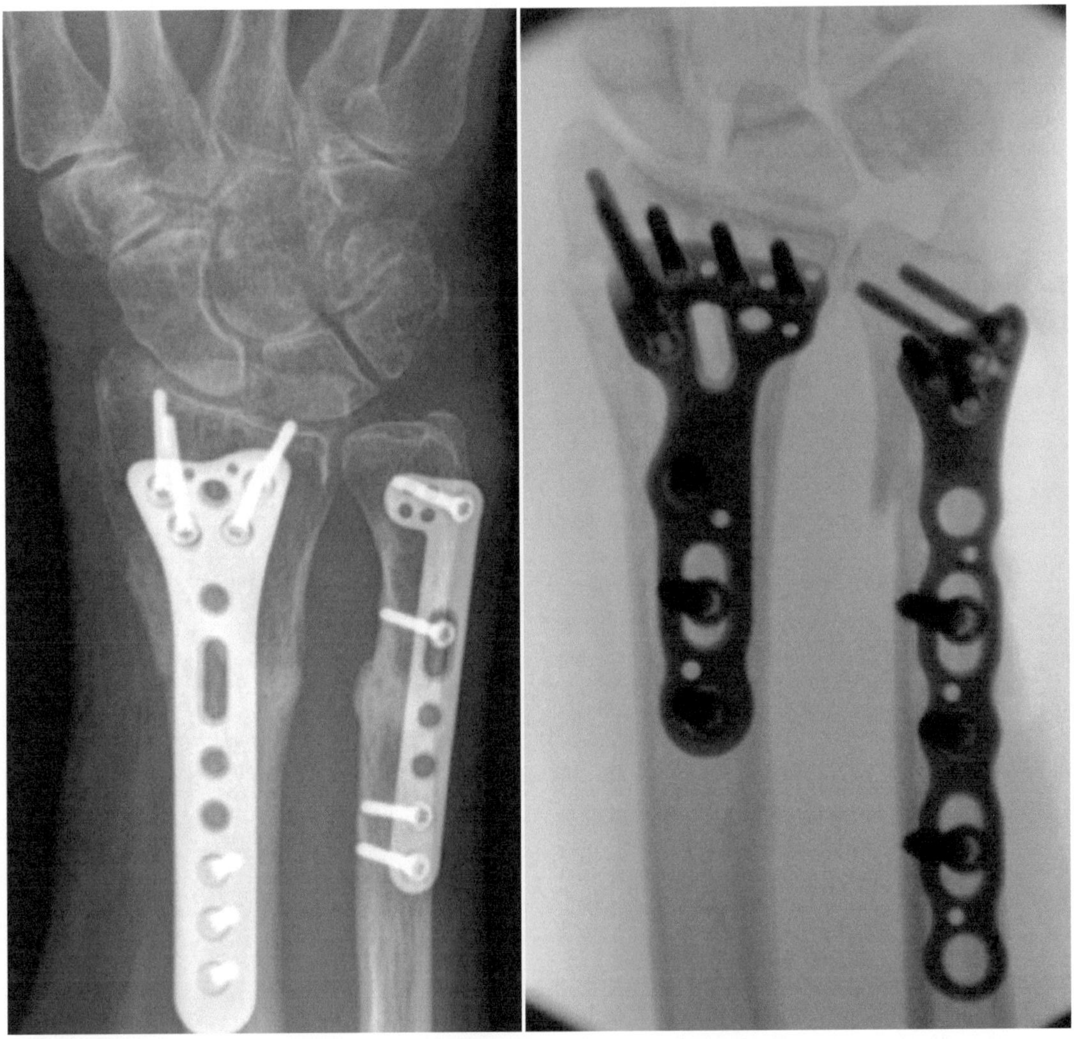

Fig. 24.12 Postoperative and intraoperative radiographs of two different low-profile plates used to treat fractures of the distal ulna. These particular images have been selected to highlight the importance of careful anatomical placement of the plates to reduce their prominence

plates. These plates lend themselves much better to fixation of fractures of the ulna head, neck and distal diaphysis. Even with extremely distal fractures, the modern anatomical plates permit the insertion of several tightly packed angled screws through the distal part of the plate improving overall fragment hold. Also, through the introduction of locking screw technology, fixed-angle stability has enhanced the pull-out strength of the screws, especially where the screws inserted into each fracture fragment are inserted in different planes.

Summary of Tips, Tricks and Pitfalls

The key to treating ulnar fractures is to assess their importance to overall wrist alignment, fracture stability and long-term function. Although it may not be immediately apparent, understanding the associated soft tissue disruption that accompanies these fractures is paramount to treating and obtaining an optimal result. Overall, surgical exposure of the distal ulna is not challenging provided the dorsal branch of the ulnar nerve is identified and carefully protected throughout the procedure. However, there is little doubt that the small size of the distal ulnar fragment, especially since fracture comminution is common, provides the real challenge to obtaining stable fracture fixation and correct fracture alignment. Modern low-profile locking plate technology has revolutionised the treatment of these fractures when compared to traditional plate designs, except for ulnar styloid tip and ulnar styloid base fractures, where K-wire fixation remains a good method for treating these injuries.

Acknowledgements We would like to thank the Department of Anatomy and the Department of Medical Illustrations at the University of Aberdeen for their assistance and expertise in the preparation of this chapter.

References

1. Sammer DM, Shah HM, Shauver MJ, Chung KC. The effect of ulnar styloid fractures on patient-rated outcomes after volar locking plating of distal radius fractures. J Hand Surg [Am]. 2009;34(9):1595–602.
2. Noda K, Goto A, Murase T, Sugamoto K, Yoshikawa H, Moritomo H. Interosseous membrane of the forearm: an anatomical study of ligament attachment locations. J Hand Surg [Am]. 2009;34(3):415–22.
3. Müller ME, Koch P, Nazarian S, Schatzker J. The comprehensive classification of fractures of long bones. Berlin, Heidelberg: Springer; 1990.
4. Kim JK, Koh Y-D, Do N-H. Should an ulnar styloid fracture be fixed following volar plate fixation of a distal radial fracture? J Bone Jt Surg Am. 2010;92(1):1–6.
5. Sawada H, Shinohara T, Natsume T, Hirata H. Clinical effects of internal fixation for ulnar styloid fractures associated with distal radius fractures: a matched case-control study. J Orthop Sci. 2016;21(6):745–8.
6. Dar I, Wani I, Mumtaz U, Jan M. Effect of ulnar styloid fracture on functional outcome of Colle's fractures: a comparative analysis of two groups. Int Surg J. 2015;2(4):556–9.
7. Daneshvar P, Chan R, Macdermid J, Grewal R. The effects of ulnar styloid fractures on patients sustaining distal radius fractures. J Hand Surg [Am]. 2014;39(10):1915–20.
8. Botte MJ, Cohen MS, Lavernia CJ, von Schroeder HP, Gellman H, Zinberg EM. The dorsal branch of the ulnar nerve: an anatomic study. J Hand Surg [Am]. 1990;15(4):603–7.
9. Puna R, Poon P. The anatomy of the dorsal cutaneous branch of the ulnar nerve. J Hand Surg Eur Vol. 2010;35(7):583–5.
10. Bain GI, Pourgiezis N, Roth JH. Surgical approaches to the distal radioulnar joint. Tech Hand Up Extrem Surg. 2007;11(1):51–6.

25 Scaphoid Fracture

Anica Herlyn and Alice Wichelhaus

Anatomical Fracture Location

The scaphoid bone connects both carpal rows, synchronizes the motions of the carpal bones, and serves as an intercalated anchor. The scaphoid is situated at a 45° plane to the horizontal and longitudinal axes of the carpus that leads to specific fracture patterns with typical trauma mechanisms such as a fall on the dorsiflexed wrist. Consequently, the scaphoid proximal pole remains fixated between the distal radius and radioscaphocapitate ligament. The mobile distal pole has a less protected position, with an increasing degree of dorsiflexion and a dorsally directed acting force vector [1]. During impact, when radial adduction is combined with dorsiflexion, distal scaphoid fractures are caused by palmar positioning of the scaphoid. A combination of ulnar adduction and dorsiflexion with dorsal scaphoid inclination leads to distal scaphoid fractures [2]. Proximal pole fractures result from initial subluxation of the scaphoid prior to forced supination.

A. Herlyn (✉) • A. Wichelhaus
Dept. of Trauma, Hand and Reconstructive Surgery, University of Rostock, Medical Center, Rostock, Germany
e-mail: anica.herlyn@med.uni-rostock.de

The precarious blood supply to the scaphoid is largely retrograde through the dorsal and volar branches of the radial artery. Seventy to eighty percent of the proximal scaphoid is supplied via the dorsal ridge, whilst the volar branch supplies the remaining 20–30% via the scaphoid tubercle [3, 4]. Unfortunately, 60% of scaphoid fractures affect the modestly supplied scaphoid waist; 15% involve the scarcely supplied proximal and densely supplied distal third; and 10% involve the tuberculum ossis scaphoidei. Scaphoid fractures are at risk of delayed union and nonunion because of its peculiar blood supply and the fact that more than two-thirds is covered by articular cartilage [5].

To identify fractures that are appropriate for operative treatment, the Herbert and Fisher classification [6] is most commonly used in British and American literature. Type A fractures involving non-dislocated fractures of the tuberosity (A1) or scaphoid waist (A2) are stable and associated with superior union rates. Type B fractures including the oblique distal one-third (B1), proximal fractures (B3), waist fractures with displacement (B2) or fracture dislocations (B4), and comminuted fractures (B5) are defined as potentially unstable and most likely require operative treatment (Fig. 25.1). Type C and D fractures correspond to delayed union and nonunion [7].

P.V. Giannoudis (ed.), *Fracture Reduction and Fixation Techniques*,
https://doi.org/10.1007/978-3-319-68628-8_25

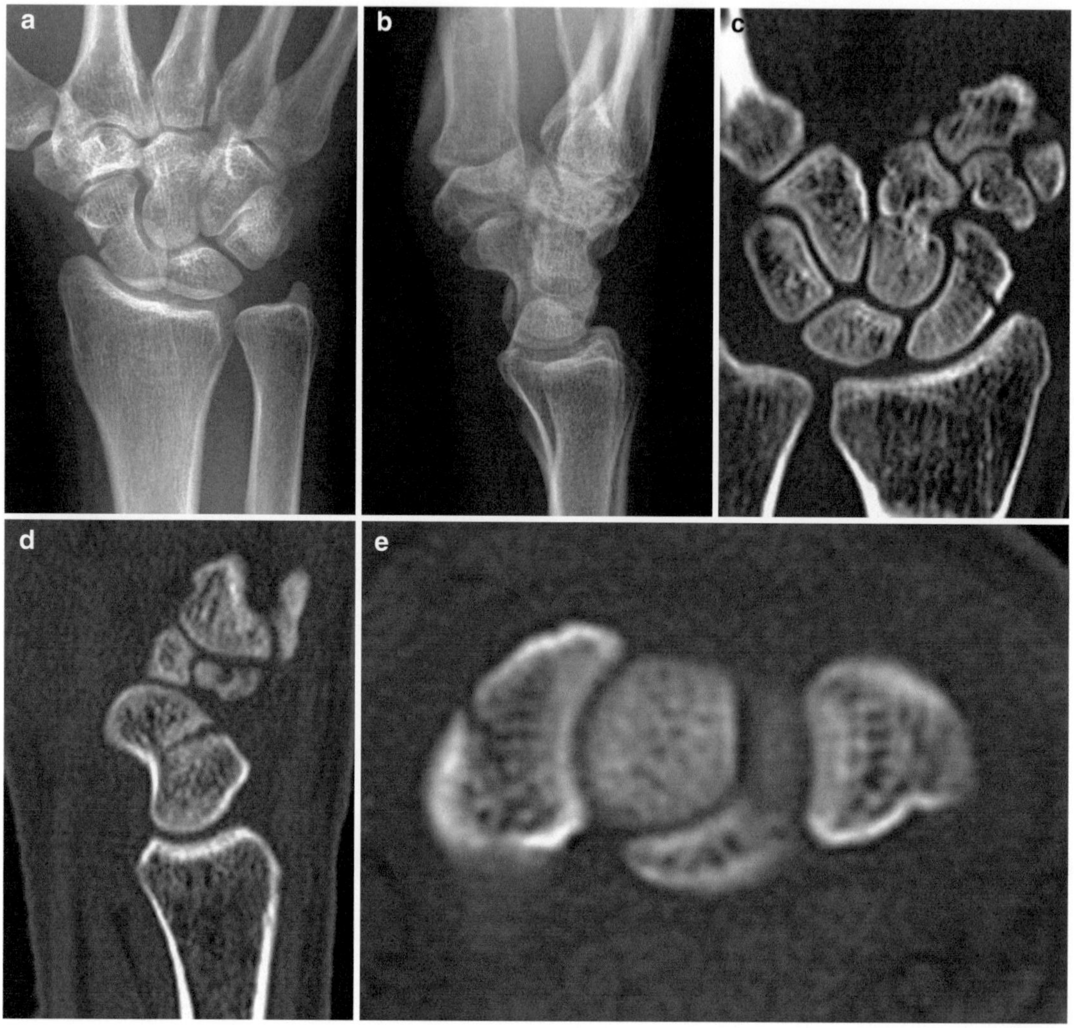

Fig. 25.1 (a–e) Radiographs in anteroposterior (**a**), lateral (**b**) views and CT scans (**c**, **d**, **e**) of a type B scaphoid fracture pattern according to Herbert and Fisher [6]

Brief Preoperative Planning

For scaphoid fractures with any pathologic angulation, displacement (type B), or carpal malalignment, arthroscopic-assisted or open reduction and fixation are recommended if any concerns exist regarding fracture stability. Some authors recommend minimally invasive arthroscopic-assisted reduction and percutaneous fixation; however, current literature has not demonstrated the mid- or long-term benefits, as compared with open reduction and internal fixation, which we believe is the current standard treatment and facilitates reduction considerably.

The commonly used implants are cannulated titan double-threaded (tip and head) compression screws, self-tapping, and self-drilling.

The implant is characterized by two threaded screw parts that are both broader than the unthreaded screw shank. To allow compression of the fracture gap, the thread pitch of the screw head is smaller than the tip, allowing for an axial force vector. With both threads anchored in the bone, compression is applied to the fracture gap to help further tighten the screw.

A broad variety of cannulated screws can be purchased in different threads, pitches, and sizes. Moreover, larger screws have demonstrated lower rates of implant failure [8–10]. However, no study has demonstrated significant differences in outcomes with different screw characteristics, except for commonly used cannulated screws that allow for improved central screw positioning, as compared with the original Herbert screw [11].

Patient Set-Up in Theatre

A radiolucent 'hand' table is commonly used. Few authors have described the positioning directly at the image intensifier collector [12].

Patients are placed in a supine position with their shoulder abducted and their forearm supinated for a volar approach or pronated for a dorsal approach. The wrist is extended dorsally for a volar approach or flexed for a dorsal approach using a roll of cotton cloth.

Figure 25.2 shows patient positioning with the main surgeon sitting on the radial side, a surgical assistant on the opposite side, and a surgical nurse and an image intensifier in extension of the patient's arm. The image intensifier is placed so it maintains a dorsal and volar course with respect to the beam projection during the whole operation.

For arthroscopic techniques, the wrist may be placed in a traction tower to facilitate arthroscopy. As described by Slade and Jaskwhich [13], a mini C-arm may be placed laterally. Duckworth and Ring [12] placed the image intensifier in a vertical position and fixed the wrist in extension with the carpus vertical to the beam using towels.

Closed Reduction Manoeuvres

Only a few fractures can be reduced solely using extension and radial deviation. A roll of cotton cloth may help gain reduction; however, a surgical assistant has to ensure maximum extension throughout the whole procedure (Fig. 25.3). The complex scaphoid shape and carpal anatomy make intraoperative image intensification extremely challenging. Arthroscopic visualization may aid reduction for experienced surgeons.

Reduction Instruments

No specific reduction instruments are required; all necessary instruments are within a standard hand operation set:

- K wire(s) (1.2–1.5 mm) used as a joystick for reduction
- K wire (0.8–0.9 mm) used as a guidewire for screw insertion
- Elevator

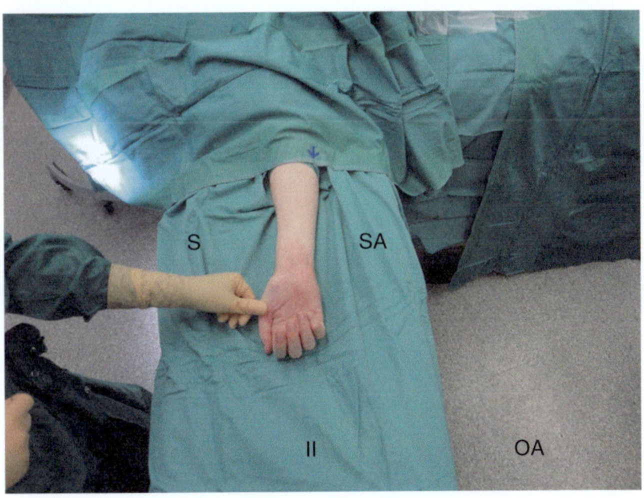

Fig. 25.2 Intraoperative positioning of a patient on a hand table for a volar approach with the surgeon sitting at the patient's radial site (S), the surgical assistance sitting at the ulnar site (SA). The operating assistant (OA) and image intensifier (II) are positioned in extension of the patients arm

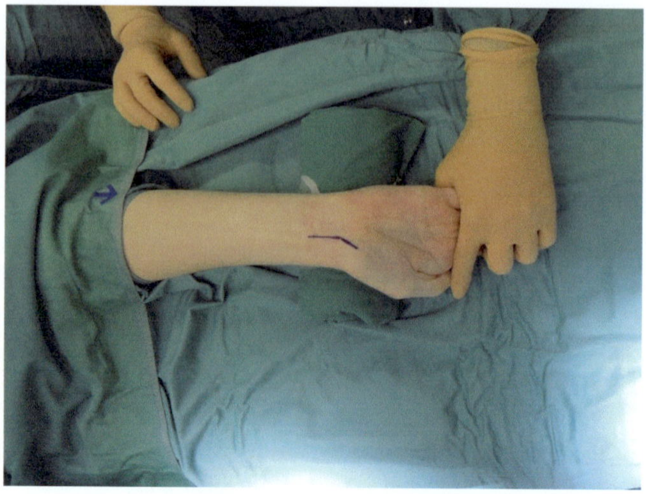

Fig. 25.3 A closed reduction manoeuvre with maximum extension and radial deviation using a towel roll. Incision for an open volar approach is marked

Surgical Approach

Open Dorsal Approach for Proximal Pole Scaphoid Fractures

Proximal pole scaphoid fractures are believed to be unstable because of rotational forces from the scapholunate ligament. This issue coupled with a high risk of nonunion and the peculiar blood supply leads to a common approach involving a small, open dorsal incision that offers the surgeon the advantage of being able to visually check fracture alignment. An open approach enables optimal implant positioning and application of two K wires that function as joysticks and can be applied to each fragment to facilitate reduction.

For the open dorsal approach, a 3- to 4-cm radiocarpal incision is created that is centred oblique relative to and above the extensor pollicis longus tendon. The third compartment is opened, and the extensor pollicis longus tendon is retracted radially. The second compartment and dorsal wrist joint capsule that is close to the dorsal radiotriquetral ligament is incised, and the proximal pole is exposed. Maximum dorsiflexion of the wrist is important for optimal viewing of the fracture site.

Care should be exercised during incision because of the dorsal ridge vessels.

Open Volar Approach for Scaphoid Waist Fractures

Waist fractures and dislocated or unstable (oblique) distal third scaphoid fractures are commonly treated using a volar open or minimally invasive approach. An advantage of the palmar approach is a lower risk of injury to the vascular supply [14].

A 4- to 5-cm slightly bowed incision is performed starting distal to the distal scaphoid pole that crosses the transverse wrist wrinkle along the flexor carpi radialis tendon. The tendons sheath is opened, and the flexor carpi radialis tendon is retracted in an ulnar direction (Fig. 25.4a). Care should be taken if the superficial radial artery is a hindrance and necessitates distal retraction or ligation. After visualization of the wrist joint capsule, an incision is created longitudinal to the scaphoid to visualize the fracture line (Fig. 25.4b). Fracture hematomas usually dissipate after incision of the capsule. To spare as much of the crossing radioscaphocapitate ligament as possible, the incision should be started at the distal pole and proceed proximally until the fracture is adequately visualized.

Potential disadvantages are higher rates of scaphotrapezial osteoarthrosis over the years that anyhow remain mostly asymptomatic [15].

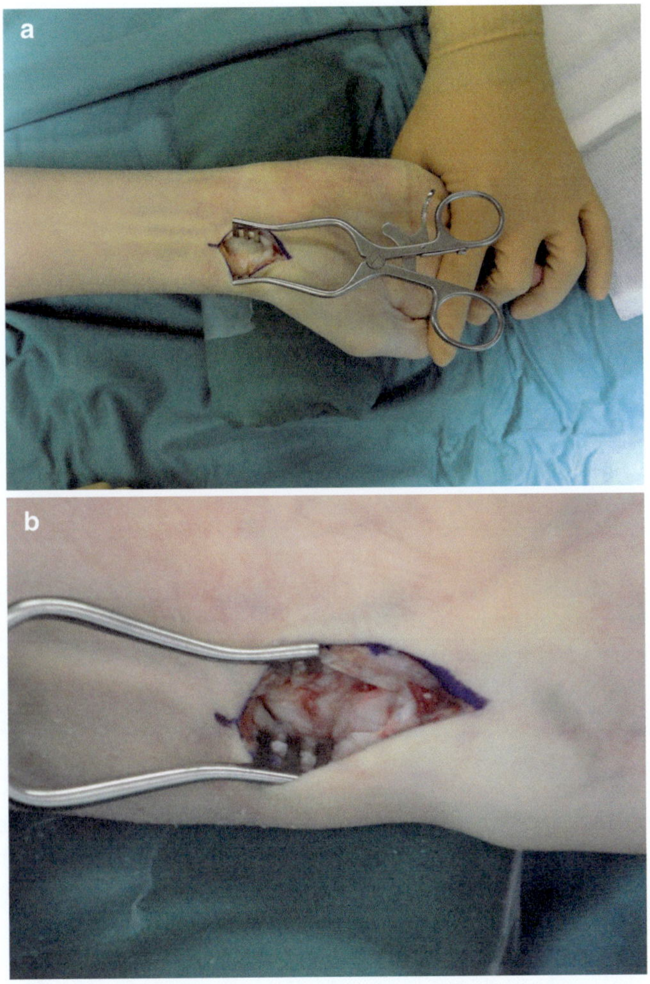

Fig. 25.4 (**a**, **b**) Intraoperative exposure of an open volar approach for a scaphoid waist fracture. The flexor carpi radialis tendon sheath is opened, and the tendon is retracted in an ulnar direction to visualize the wrist joint capsule (**a**). Incision of the wrist joint capsule is created longitudinal to the scaphoid in order to visualize the fracture (**b**)

Percutaneous or Minimally Invasive Arthroscopic-Assisted Approach for (Stable) Scaphoid Waist Fractures

Percutaneous or minimally invasive arthroscopic-assisted techniques have the advantage of sparing the volar carpale capsule and tendons and, therefore, may allow for less postoperative immobilization because of improved stability [16].

Visualization of the scaphotrapezial joint space with fluoroscopy is followed by the creation of a 1-cm-maximum percutaneous stab incision in a volar-radial course above the scaphotrapezial joint and the insertion of a guidewire. If a minimally invasive dorsal approach with a small open incision is used, there is an increased risk of lesions to the posterior interosseous nerve, extensor indicis proprius tendon, or extensor digitorum tendon [17].

For a stark arthroscopic approach, a midcarpal portal (3/4 or 4/5) allows for the best.

Open Reduction Manoeuvres

Most scaphoid fractures require direct reduction manoeuvres that are facilitated by the use of K wires (preferably 1.2–1.5 mm) drilled into each fragment that serve as joysticks:

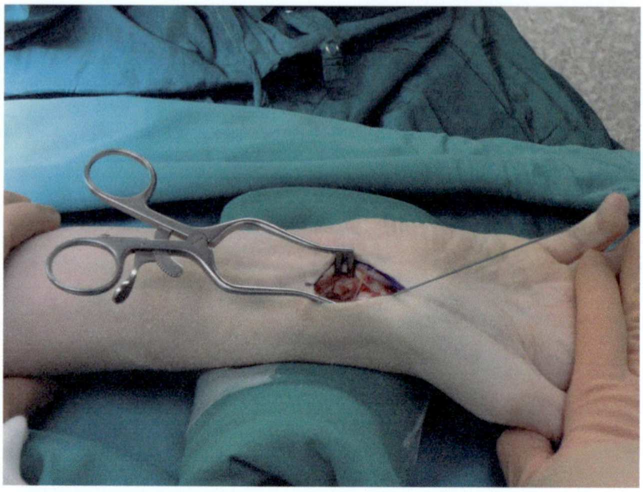

Fig. 25.5 Reduction manoeuvre using a K wire as a joystick

In case of a volar approach, the wrist is positioned in maximum extension to allow for optimal visualization of the fracture. Ulnar deviation may aid the reduction, as well as a dorsally positioned towel roll beneath the wrist. For the joystick technique, a K wire is inserted into each fragment at an angle to the pole, gripping the maximum possible diameter to increase strength. Slight off-centre positioning of the joysticks to the longitudinal axis of the fragments is important to spare the fracture line and to allow correct guidance and positioning of the wire that corresponds with the central axis of the scaphoid. If the approach allows for use of only one K wire, the distal fragment displays the more important one covering the dislocated fragment (Fig. 25.5). To prevent a respective fragment from evading an elevator may be placed below the proximal pole. Using the K wires as a joystick, rotation and positioning of both fragments can be controlled until the guidewire is positioned.

For dorsal and arthroscopic approaches (versus percutaneous), an analogous proceeding may be performed.

For slightly displaced or comminuted fractures, the guidewire itself may be used as a joystick if it is drilled into the first fragment to be retained for reduction manoeuvres and to be advancement crossing past the fracture line.

With unstable fractures, a second guidewire may be used to control rotation if the fragment is unstable during both the drilling and screw insertion phases.

For comminuted fractures, bone grafting has to be considered to facilitate reduction and stimulate union.

For a stark arthroscopic approach, fracture reduction is performed using a manoeuvre of extension and radial deviation, followed by volar percutaneous guidewire stabilization [12, 16].

Implant Insertion

Any of these approaches, along with reduction, is followed by guidewire insertion. Its positioning is of uppermost importance to the success of the operation. It helps to keep in mind that the scaphoid is positioned at a 45° plane to the horizontal and longitudinal axes of the wrist.

For a volar approach, the ideal insertion point for the guidewire is distal through the scaphoid tubercle, allowing for central wire placement in the proximal scaphoid pole, which is often slightly radial to the tuberculum. Under the image intensifier in the anteroposterior, lateral, and oblique supinated/pronated views, the guidewire is drilled longitudinally along the long axis of the scaphoid to the proximal

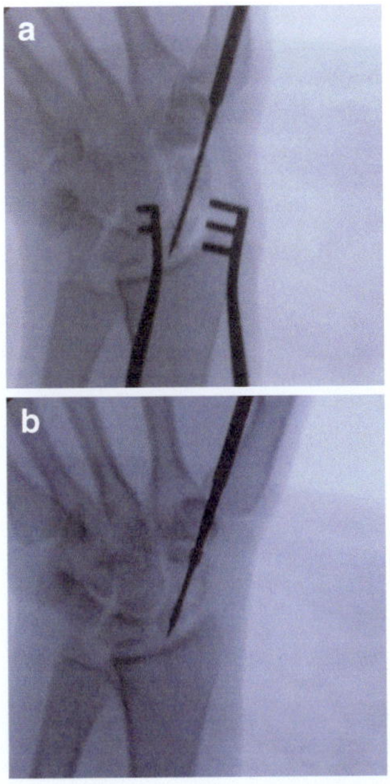

Fig. 25.6 (**a**, **b**) Intraoperative image intensifier views after bicortical guidewire insertion (**a**) and fracture fixation using a cannulated self-drilling double-threaded compression screw (**b**)

pole using a guide sleeve. A virtual line parallel to the adducted thump may serve as an auxiliary line. The K wire should be placed bicortical without injuring the proximal cartilage (Fig. 25.6a). If the positioning is inadequate, a second K wire may be used that is positioned parallel to the first one in a more optimal position. In some cases, the trapezial bone interferes with wire positioning, leading to suboptimal wire positioning that is too volar or horizontal and necessitates repositioning under fluoroscopic control. Therefore, in rare cases, it is necessary to insert the wire through the trapezium that does not seem to increase morbidity [18]. During image intensifier control, it is important to keep the wrist at maximum flexion to prevent wire bending. Therefore, the anteroposterior view is only possible with the forearm in a vertical position.

After correct guidewire positioning and fluoroscopic guidance, control of reduction length measurement is ensued. The screw length is usually 22–26 mm. To prevent screw prominences at any end that would necessitate implant removal at a later time, it is recommended to use a <2-mm screw in case of any doubt. With a percutaneous approach, measurements using a sleeve measure may be difficult because of the surrounding soft tissues; therefore, preoperative estimation of length using CT scans or a second K wire of the same length to approximate the difference is recommended. Some authors have indicated that they drilled the wire further into the trapezoid bone to fix it [18]. This injurs crossing cartilage, so the authors do not recommend this method.

In case no self-drilling screw is available, predrilling can be performed with the guidewire in place. Drilling should be stopped if any resistance is encountered as the guidewire may bend and be at risk of breakage. A bent wire can usually be drilled further until the straight part of the wire is encountered. After drilling, a cannulated screw is carefully inserted under visualization via image intensifier to avoid loss of reduction secondary to rotational forces or fragment distraction. Whilst inserting the screw, palpable compression of the fracture gap and tight anchoring of the implant are noted (Fig. 25.6b).

Following wire extraction and final image intensifier viewing, anteroposterior, lateral, and oblique supinated/pronated views should enable approximation of central screw positioning without joint penetration in either scaphotrapezial or radiocarpal aspects. Non-penetrating subchondral screw positioning should be obtained under direct view if an open approach is performed. Postoperative and follow-up radiographs are shown in Fig. 25.7.

Summary of Tips, Tricks, and Pitfalls

- The use of self-tapping and self-drilling screws reduces the risk of loss of fracture reduction during fixation.
- An open approach facilitates reduction considerably because of direct visualization of the fracture.
- During the whole procedure, secure maximum extension is necessitated for a palmar approach, or maximum flexion is necessitated for a dorsal approach.

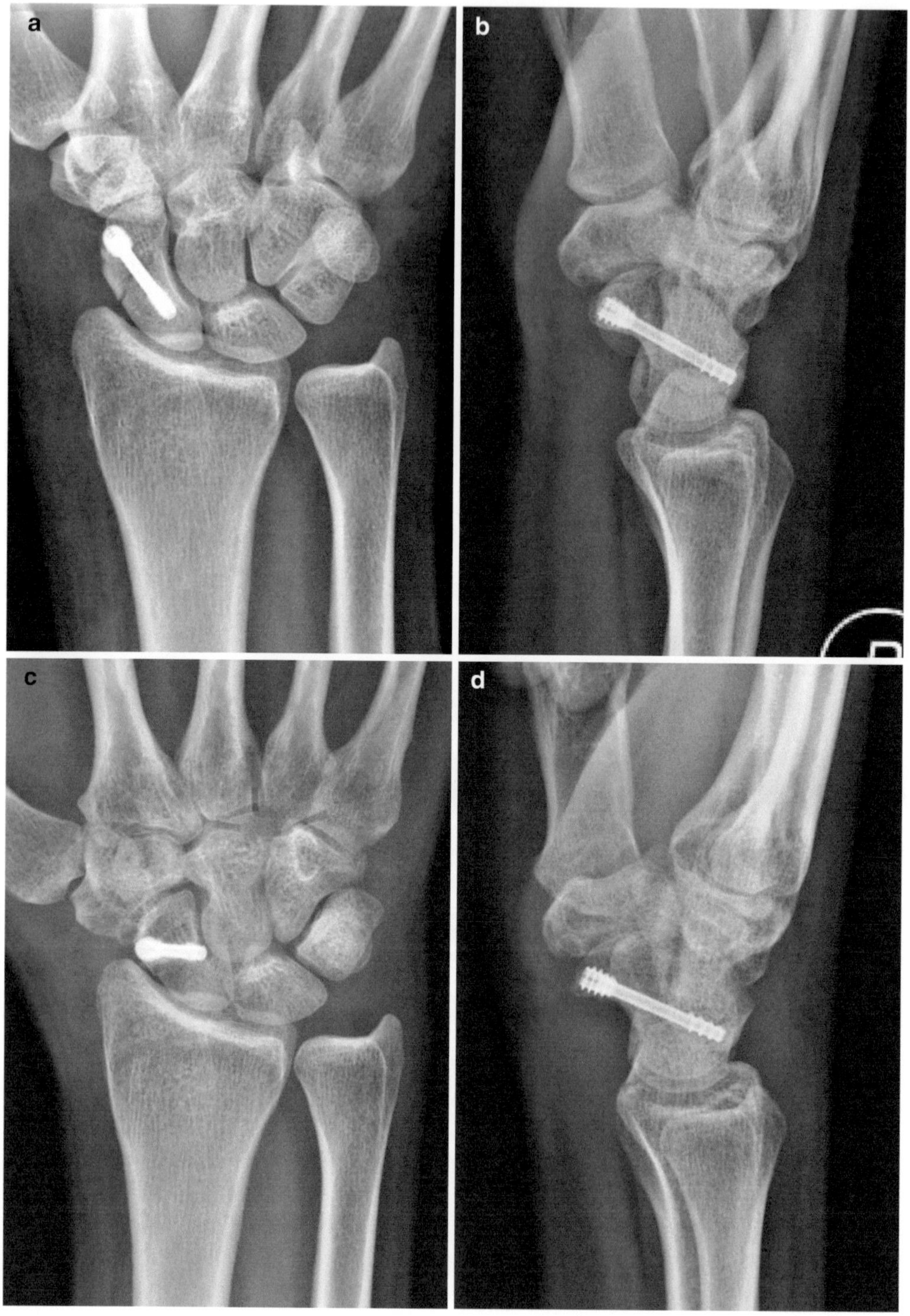

Fig. 25.7 (**a**–**d**) Postoperative (**a**, **b**) and follow-up radiographs 8 weeks after surgery (**c**, **d**) following open reduction and screw fixation using an open volar approach

References

1. Schmitt R, Lanz U. Bildgebende Diagnostik der Hand. Stuttgart, Germany: Thieme; 2013.
2. Taleisnik J. Fractures of the carpal bones. In: Green DP, editor. Operative hand surgery, vol. 2. New York: Churchill Livingstone; 1988. p. 813–40.
3. Reigstad O, Grimsgaard C, Thorkildsen R, et al. Scaphoid non-unions, where do they come from? The epidemiology and initial presentation of 270 scaphoid non-unions. Hand Surg. 2012;17(3):331–5. https://doi.org/10.1142/S0218810412500268.
4. Slutsky DJ, Slade JFIII. The scaphoid. Stuttgart: Thieme; 2010.
5. Duckworth AD, Ring D. Carpus fractures and dislocations. In: Court-Brown CM, Heckmann JD, McQueen MM, et al., editors. Rockwood and Green's fractures in adults, vol. 1. Philadelphia: Wolters Kluwer; 2015. p. 1008–9.
6. Herbert TJ, Fisher WE. Management of the fractured scaphoid using a new bone screw. J Bone Joint Surg Br. 1984;66(1):114–23.
7. Duckworth AD, Ring D. Carpus fractures and dislocations. In: Court-Brown CM, Heckmann JD, McQueen MM, et al., editors. Rockwood and Green's fractures in adults, vol. 1. Philadelphia: Wolters Kluwer; 2015. p. 1010–7.
8. Sugathan HK, Kilpatrick M, Joyce TJ, et al. A biomechanical study on variation of compressive force along the Acutrak 2 screw. Injury. 2012;43(2):205–8. https://doi.org/10.1016/j.injury.2011.07.011.
9. Beadel GP, Ferreira L, Johnson JA, et al. Interfragmentary compression across a simulated scaphoid fracture—analysis of 3 screws. J Hand Surg [Am]. 2004;29(2):273–8.
10. Oduwole KO, Cichy B, Dillon JP, et al. Acutrak versus Herbert screw fixation for scaphoid non-union and delayed union. J Orthop Surg. 2012;20(1):61–5.
11. Trumble TE, Clarke T, Kreder HJ. Non-union of the scaphoid. Treatment with cannulated screws compared with treatment with Herbert screws. J Bone Joint Surg Am. 1996;78(12):1829–37.
12. Duckworth AD, Ring D. Carpus fractures and dislocations. In: Court-Brown CM, Heckmann JD, McQueen MM, et al., editors. Rockwood and Green's fractures in adults, vol. 1. Philadelphia: Wolters Kluwer; 2015. p. 1019–25.
13. Slade JFIII, Jaskwhich D. Percutaneous fixation of scaphoid fractures. Hand Clin. 2001;17(4):553–74.
14. Dias JJ, Singh HP. Displaced fracture of the waist of the scaphoid. J Bone Joint Surg Br. 2011;93(11):1433–9. https://doi.org/10.1302/0301-620X.93B11.26934.
15. Vinnars B, Pietreanu M, Bodestedt A, et al. Nonoperative compared with operative treatment of acute scaphoid fractures. A randomized clinical trial. J Bone Joint Surg Am. 2008;90(6):1176–85. https://doi.org/10.2106/JBJS.G.00673.
16. Sauerbier M, Schaedel-Hoepfner M, Mehling IM. Die Behandlung der frischen Skaphoidfraktur. Handchirurgie Scan. 2013;2(4):313–33. https://doi.org/10.1055/s0033-1359021.
17. Adamany DC, Mikola EA, Fraser BJ. Percutaneous fixation of the scaphoid through a dorsal approach: an anatomic study. J Hand Surg [Am]. 2008;33(3):327–31. https://doi.org/10.1016/j.jhsa.2007.12.006.
18. Geurts G, van Riet R, Meermans G, et al. Incidence of scaphotrapezial arthritis following volar percutaneous fixation of nondisplaced scaphoid waist fractures using a transtrapezial approach. J Hand Surg [Am]. 2011;36(11):1753–8. https://doi.org/10.1016/j.jhsa.2011.08.031.

26 Perilunate Dislocation

Laurent Obert, Francois Loisel, and Daniel Lepage

Anatomical Fracture Location

Perilunate dislocation of the carpus is defined as loss of contact between the capitate and the lunate; it accounts for 5–10% of all carpal injuries. These dislocations follow multiple trauma in 10% of cases and always result from high-energy injuries, when the wrist is more or less locked in hyperextension (motorcycle handlebars) or resulting from falls from a height. The distal row of the carpus is very solidly attached to the metacarpals, and the proximal row is blocked between the radius and the distal row; the lesions therefore occur in the proximal row (Fig. 26.1).

Brief Preoperative Planning

Oedema and thickening of the wrist are different from what is observed in fractures of the distal radius. If the patient is conscious, there is pain on both sides of the wrist, sometimes with paresthesia of the median nerve, but the clinical picture is poor, with slight cracking noises upon examination of the wrist that has only slightly increased in volume. There is nonetheless an important sign: it is difficult to extend the fingers. The diagnosis can be made based on AP X-rays (the lunate has a pyramid-like aspect, the Gilula lines are disturbed) and lateral X-rays (the lunate has lost its normal ratios with the radius and the capitate, it is dislocated forward or backward from the radius) (Fig. 26.2). In one quarter of cases, posterior perilunate dislocation is not detected because of a lack of diagnostic rigor and/or a poorly interpreted or absent lateral X-ray. However, in the context of a patient that needs to be resuscitated, an AP X-ray alone can be misleading and the absence of a lateral image can lead to misjudging the lesions. The capitate is displaced backward from the radius, and the lunate can remain under the radius (stages I and II) (Fig. 26.3) or be dislocated forward (stage III). Two-thirds of the perilunate dislocations are dorsal and associated with scaphoid fractures (Fig. 26.4); in this case, the trauma forces were applied to the scaphoid rather than to the scapholunate ligament. In two-thirds of cases, there is another associated fracture caused by the severity of the injuring forces: lesions in the antebrachial area (distal radioulnar dislocation, Galeazzi fracture) or in the elbow, as well as intracarpal lesions with osteochondral fractures of the top of the capitate, the tip of the styloid, and avulsions of the anterior pole of the triquetrum.

L. Obert, M.D. (✉) • F. Loisel, M.D.
D. Lepage, M.D., Ph.D.
Orthopedic, Traumatology, and Hand Surgery Unit, University Hospital CHRU Besancon, Medical School, University of Bourgogne - Franche Comte, Research Unit: Nano Medicine, Besancon, France
e-mail: laurentobert@yahoo.fr; lobert@chu-besancon.fr

P.V. Giannoudis (ed.), *Fracture Reduction and Fixation Techniques*,
https://doi.org/10.1007/978-3-319-68628-8_26

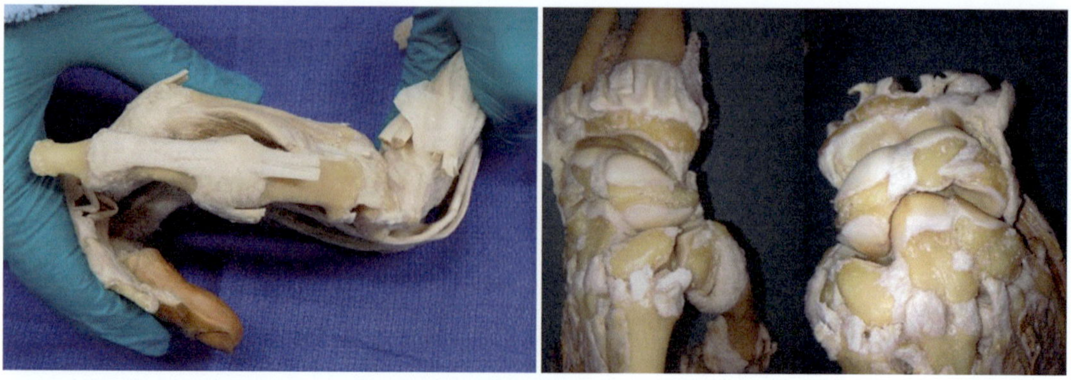

Fig. 26.1 Perilunate dislocation is a spectrum of injuries secondary to high-energy trauma at wrist level, in extension at radiocarpal level but with a flexion at finger level. Palmar capsule is a weak zone

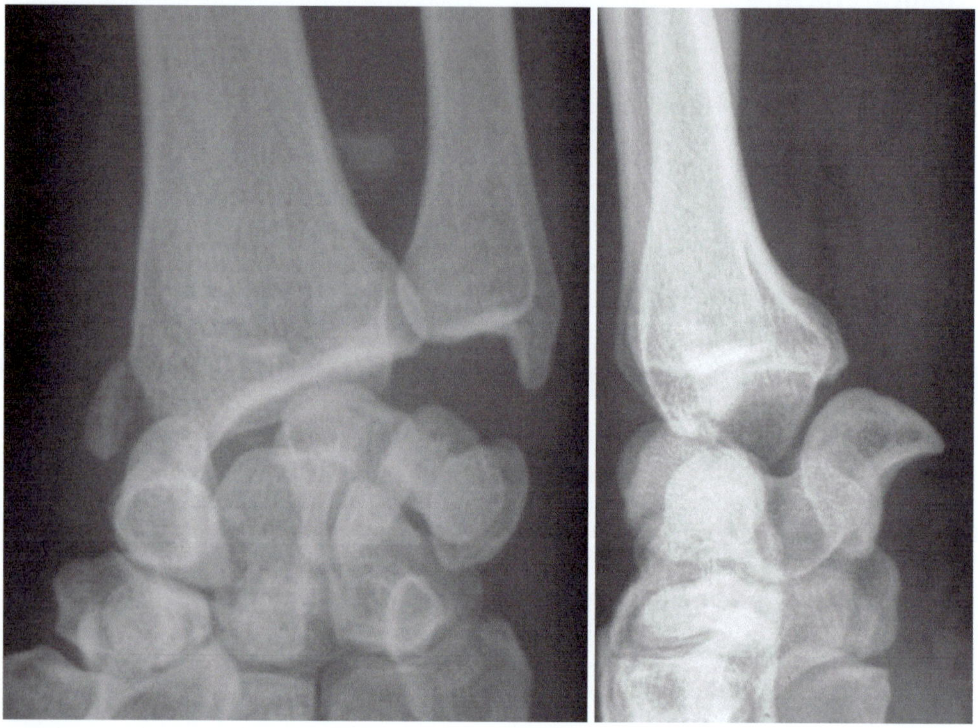

Fig. 26.2 An example of perilunate dislocation with styloid fracture which contains the radio carpal ligaments. In this case the fixation of the styloid and the reinsertion of radio carpal ligaments both allow to stabilize the radiocarpal joint

Patient Set-Up in Theatre

Standard table is used, patient in supine position, surgeon on the side of the patient's head (depending on the dominant hand of the surgeon), and image intensifier coming from lateral side positioning, under tourniquet (250 mmHg) (Fig. 26.5).

Closed Reduction Manoeuvres

The injury must be reduced as soon as possible under general anaesthesia in the operating room, with 5–7 kg of traction, possibly using a digital traction system. With the wrist flexed, the thumb pushes forward on the lunate, whereas the index

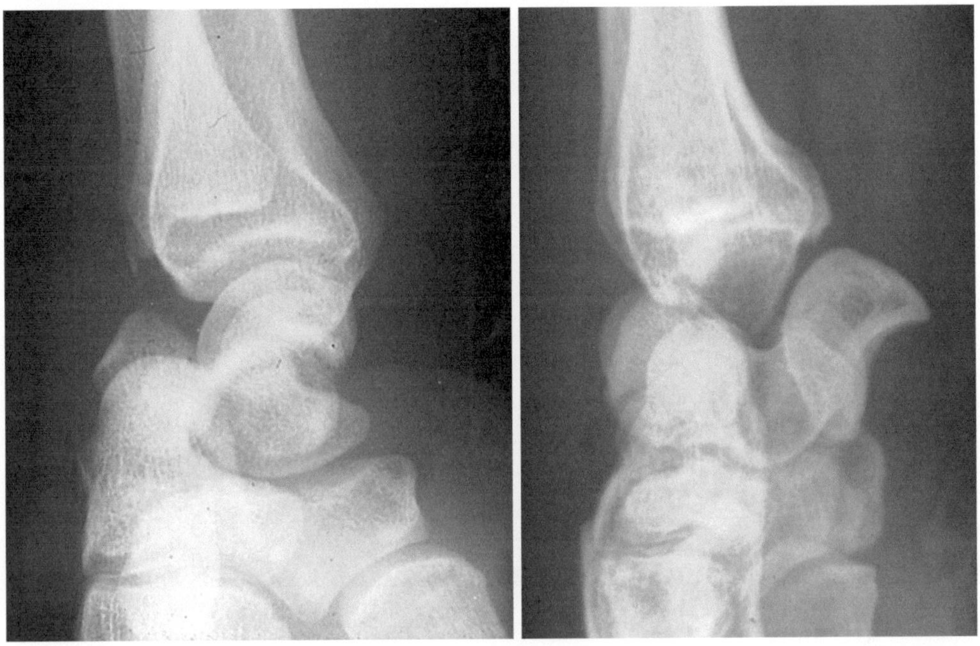

Fig. 26.3 Perilunate stage 1 (left) and stage 2 (right) dislocation

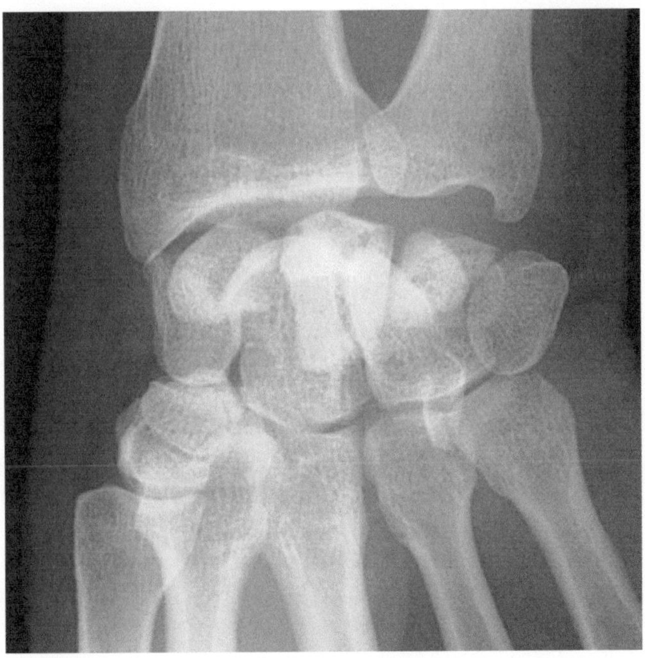

Fig. 26.4 Perilunate dislocation with scaphoid fracture

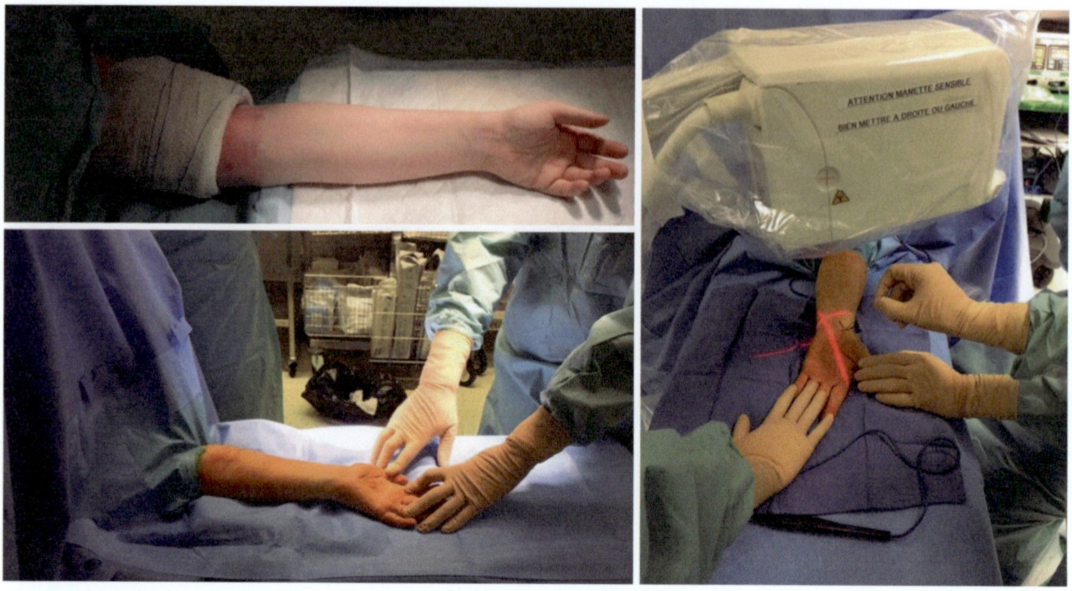

Fig. 26.5 Patient in supine position, tourniquet, and C arm are mandatory

exerts a posterior counterpressure. The lunate is reduced gently with the thumb and the wrist is moved in dorsiflexion. This manoeuvre should be easy, but traction is long (10–15 min). Surgical stabilization is ideally performed at the same time or in the following days, depending on the patient's condition, but can be delayed in the following days. Even if 40% of perilunate dislocations remain reduced, surgical stabilization is imperative in all cases.

Surgical Approach

Volar and dorsal approaches each have advantages and drawbacks. Herzberg reports that a combined volar and dorsal approach improves exposure, but increases the possibility of postoperative fibrosis and stiffness. Dorsal approach allows a perfect view on the first row which has to be reduced and fixed. Even if median nerve has to be released, it does not justify to perform a palmar approach.

Posterior approach is longitudinal on the skin. A retinaculum flap radially based allows an access to different extensor compartments. Arthrotomy can be performed in different ways (Fig. 26.6): we prefer the Herzberg "Z" approach (Fig. 26.7) in case of breaches in dorsal capsule and extrinsic ligaments or detachment of capsule and ligaments from the distal rim of radius in case of intact capsule (Fig. 26.8). The posterior interosseous nerve is resected due to the opening of the capsule.

Open Reduction Manoeuvres

After appropriate exposure of the dorsal carpus, the carpal bones are identified clinically as well as with fluoroscopy. Any free osteochondral debris are removed. After ligamentous injury scaphoid tends to go into palmar flexion, whereas triquetrum extends. The first phase consists of reducing the lunate, which can be very unstable, in pushing it between the radius and the capitate.

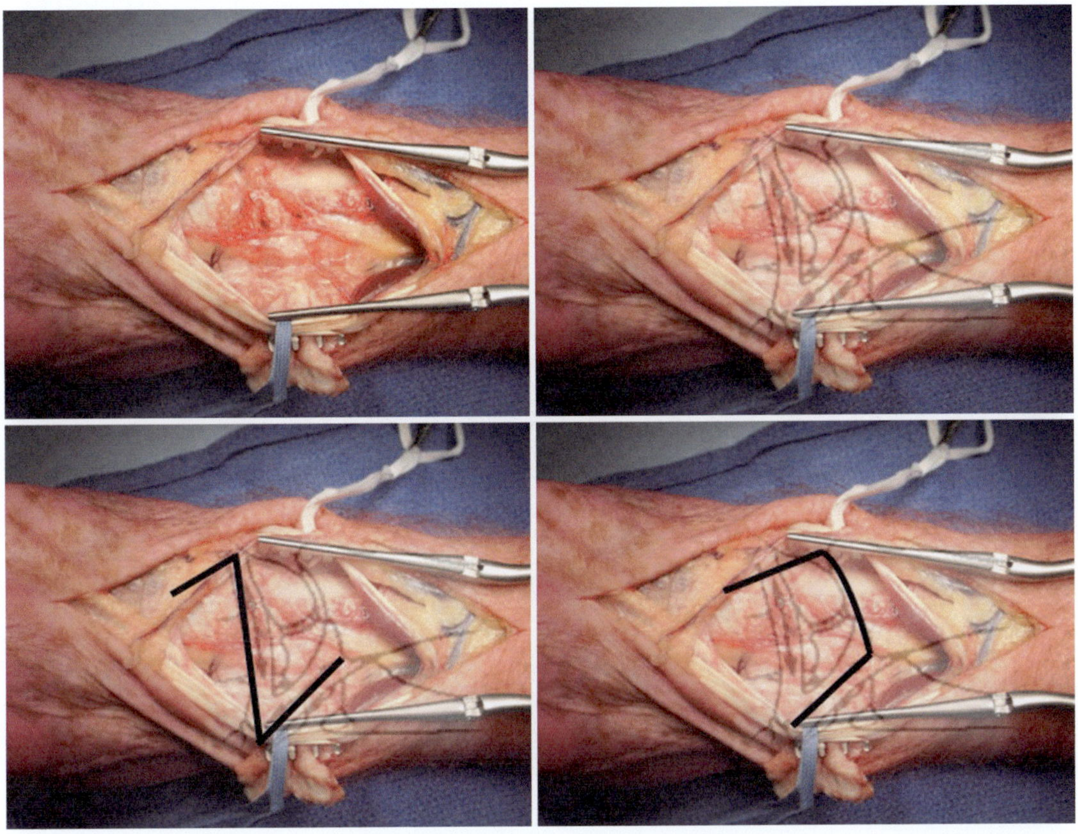

Fig. 26.6 Incision of capsule and extrinsic ligaments can be done following the direction of extrinsic dorsal ligaments (Z incision) or with a detachement of the capsule from the distal rim of the dorsal radius

If reduction is not easily possible, 1.4-mm Kirschner wires can be used as "joysticks" to manipulate each bone. After reduction, lunate has to cover the entire head of the capitate. Anchors are inserted into bones of first row (Fig. 26.9). The proper lateral position of the lunate under the radius and above the capitate bone must be verified under fluoroscopy, and this reduction is maintained in introducing 1.4-mm Kirschner wires to immobilize radio lunate joint (Fig. 26.10). Then, reduction of bone of the first row is done; the scapholunate and lunotriquetral joint are each immobilized by K wires. Those K wires will be put in place, checked, and left in place for 2–3 months and reconstruction of ligaments done (Fig. 26.11). Radiolunate arthrodesis K wire can be removed or left in place for 2 months. In cases where associated scaphoid fracture is present, first placing osteosynthesis of the scaphoid makes it possible to proceed to scapholunate pinning if the scapholunate ligament is intact. Postoperative immobilization is done for 2 months.

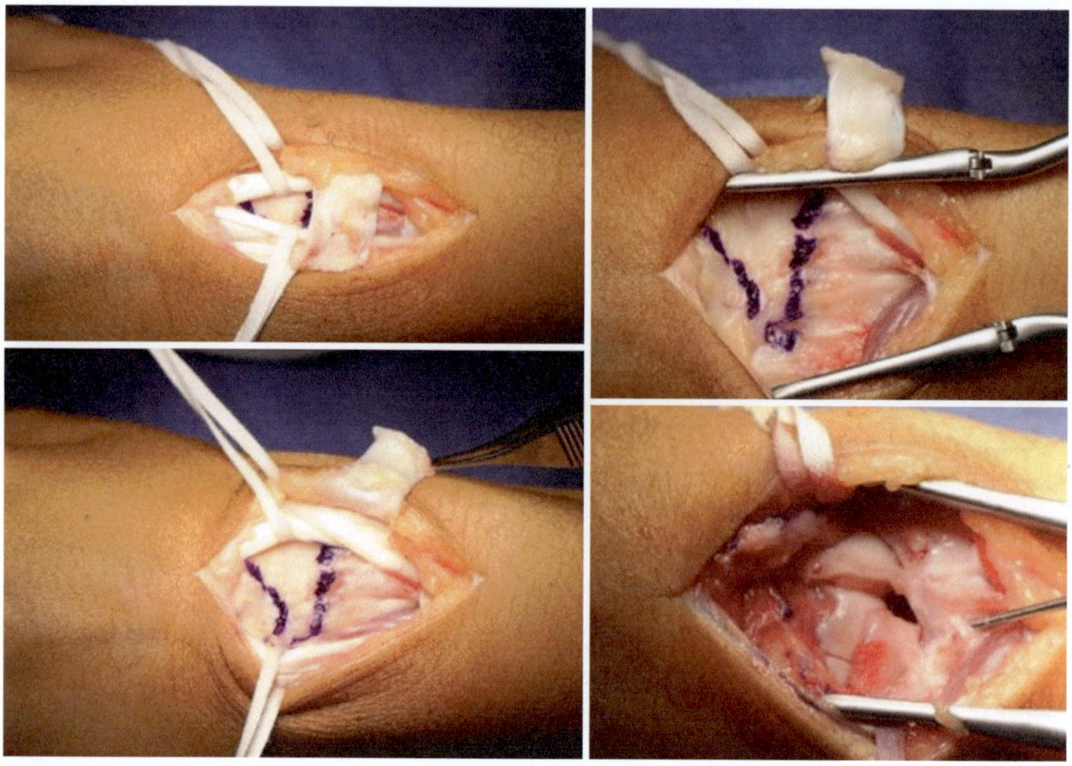

Fig. 26.7 Herzberg "Z" approach and view on the first row

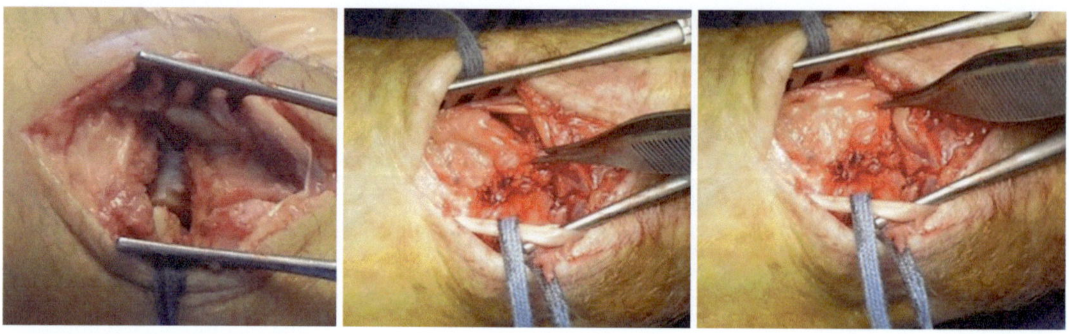

Fig. 26.8 Detachment of the capsule allow a "sur mesure" reinsertion by anchors more or less distally on the dorsal rim of distal radius

Summary of Tips, Tricks, and Pitfalls

- Advanced imaging is not necessary for diagnosis of perilunate dislocations among experts, but 2-D and 3-D CT might be helpful in evaluating of complexity.
- Manipulative reduction is mostly unsuccessful if not performed within the first few days.
- Closed reduction can only be maintained for a short period with cast immobilization.
- The optimal timing of definitive surgery for a manipulatively reducible dislocation is within a week after injury.
- The surgical approach should be based on the surgeon's preference and individualized for the patient.

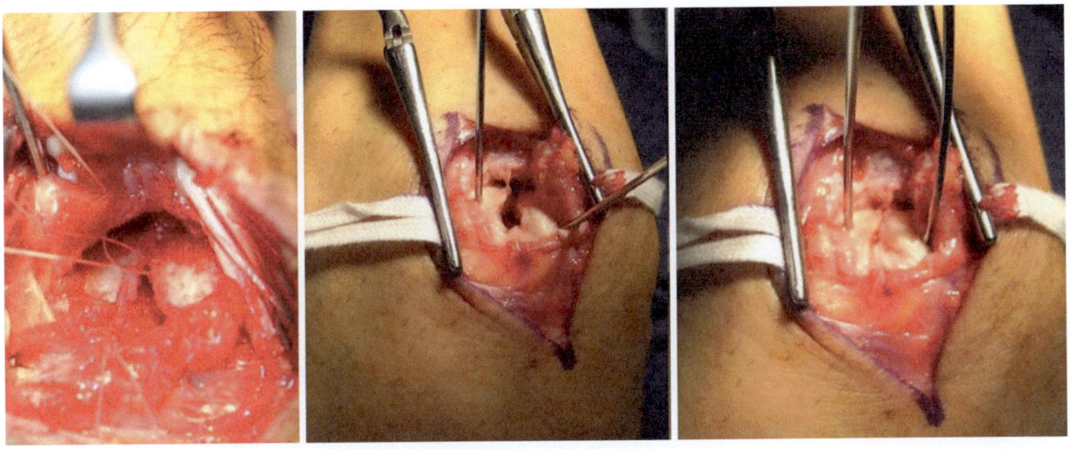

Fig. 26.9 Reduction of the bones of the first row is facilitated using Kirschner wire as "joysticks"

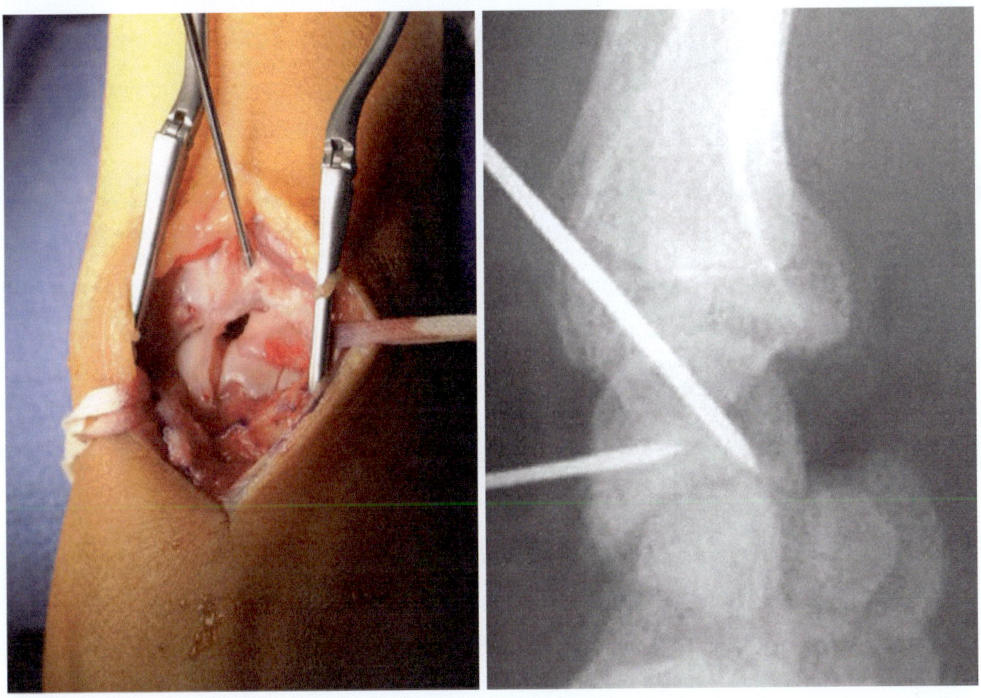

Fig. 26.10 A temporary fixation of the radio lunate joint allows to reduce anatomically the lunate

- The results of treatment with temporary screws and temporary K wires are comparable.
- The most important factors predicting impairment and disability are delay in treatment, open injury, and osteochondral fracture of the capitate head.
- Clinical outcomes are often substantially better than radiographic outcomes.
- There is no evidence to determine the best methods for reduction (open or closed), ligament repair or reattachment, or immobilization. Percutaneous reduction and fixation without direct ligament repair is appealing, but the little data published on this technique suggest that it is inferior to open techniques. Arthroscopy has to demonstrate now the benefit but probably will become.

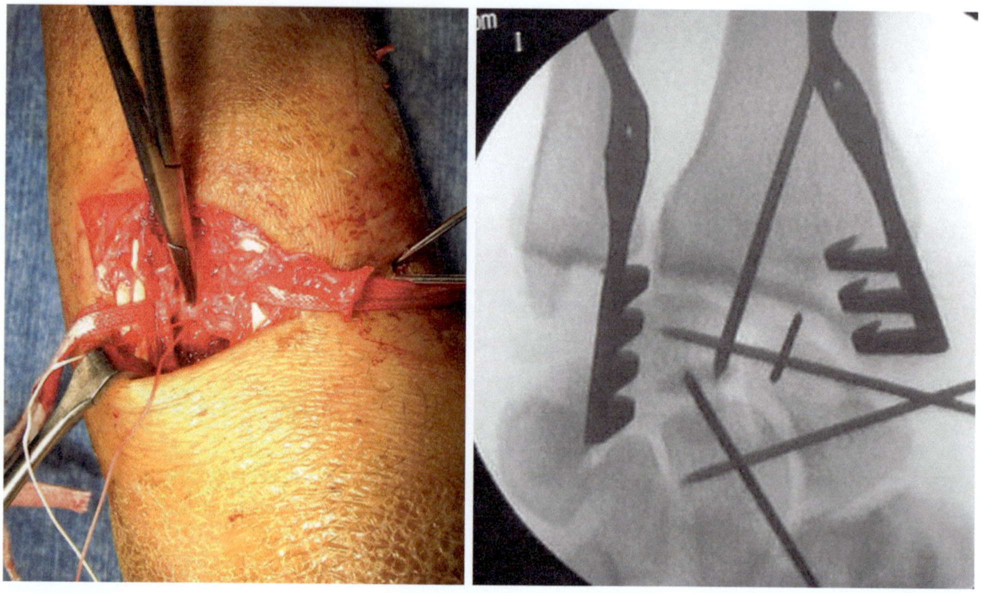

Fig. 26.11 Ligament reconstruction is not always possible, but suture anchor is a support for ligament healing

Further Reading

Herzberg G. Perilunate and axial carpal dislocations and fracture-dislocations. J Hand Surg [Am]. 2008;33:1659–68.

Buijze GA, Doornberg JN, Ring D. Perilunate dislocations. In: Bhandari M, editor. Evidence-based orthopedics. Hoboken, NJ: Wiley-Blackwell; 2012. p. 437–42.

Kremer T, Riedel K. Perilunate disclocations. In: Garcia Elias M, Mathoulin C, editors. Articular injury of the wrist FESSH instructional course Book. Stuttgart, Germany: Thieme; 2014. p. 52–60.

Obert L, Loisel F, Jardin E, Gasse N, Lepage D. High-energy injuries of the wrist. Orthop Traumatol Surg Res. 2016;102:S81–93.

Metacarpal Fractures

27

Sam Vollans

Anatomical Fracture Location

The annual incidence of metacarpal fractures has been reported to be 16.1 per 10,000 people [1].

Non-union is a rare complication of the nonoperative management of metacarpal fractures. It is however encountered more commonly following poor reduction and fixation of fractures. In addition, malunion, though often found in fractures treated nonoperatively, is most commonly asymptomatic. Some patients, however, have significant functional problems following malunion [2, 3]. The challenge, therefore, is to identify which metacarpal fractures require fixation to prevent symptomatic malunion and, in doing so, respect the biology and mechanisms of bone healing to prevent non-union.

Two factors will aid decision-making, displacement and stability. If a metacarpal fracture is displaced, then one needs to ask whether this displacement will cause unacceptable deformity, unacceptable function or post traumatic arthritis. If the answer is yes, the fracture must be reduced whether by closed or open techniques. If reducible closed, the fracture may be stable within traditional casts or splints and can be managed definitively in this way. If unstable however, then it must be stabilised through percutaneous or internal fixation to aid bone healing and allow early range of movement. If the fracture cannot be reduced closed, it requires open reduction and fixation. The specific indications for fixation of all types of metacarpal fracture are outside the remit of this chapter, but the above basic principles will serve as a general guide.

Below, we give examples of different metacarpal fractures requiring surgical reduction and fixation (shaft, head and base). We discuss the different techniques employed and the instrumentation required.

Metacarpal Shaft Fracture

Anatomical Fracture Pattern

The AP radiograph of the right hand shows a mid-shaft ring finger short oblique metacarpal fracture with a small degree of comminution (Fig. 27.1). The radiographs reveal shortening of the metacarpal with loss of the normal length progression of the metacarpal heads. This degree of shortening may lead to extensor lag and so is a relative indication for fixation. The length of the main fracture appears less than two times the diameter of the bone, so fixation with a plate is

S. Vollans, F.R.C.S. (Orth)
Consultant Upper Limb Surgery, Department of Trauma and Orthopaedics, Leeds General Infirmary, Leeds, UK
e-mail: s.vollans@me.com

P.V. Giannoudis (ed.), *Fracture Reduction and Fixation Techniques*,
https://doi.org/10.1007/978-3-319-68628-8_27

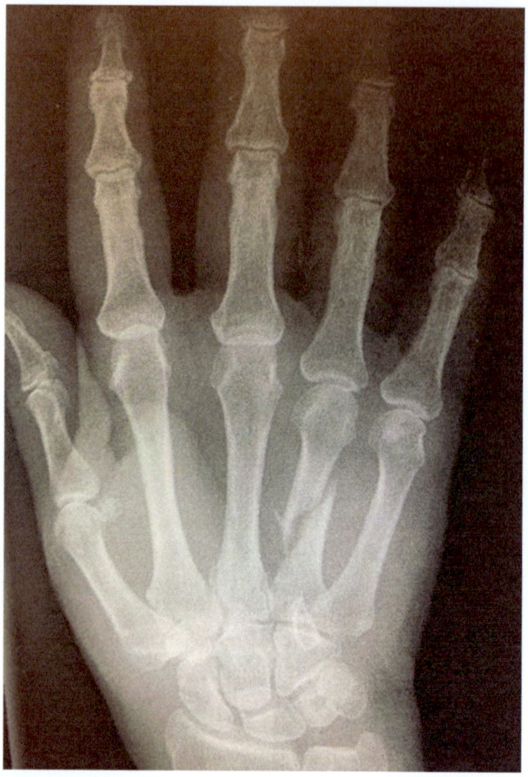

Fig. 27.1 AP radiograph* of the right hand showing a mid-shaft ring finger short oblique metacarpal fracture (*Radiograph and clinical photographs courtesy of Mr. B Thé, Consultant Hand Surgeon, Amphia Ziekenhuis, Breda, Netherlands)

indicated, with or without a lag screw. If the fracture length was longer (2–3 times the diameter of the bone or more), then fixation with two or three lag screws without a plate should be adequate to allow early mobilisation.

Pre-op Planning

The key to a successful clinical outcome is preventing post-op stiffness. For that reason, direct reduction and stability leading to primary bone healing without callous is what is required. Lag screw fixation is the gold standard for interfragmentary compression in the hand, with compression plating only reserved for transverse fractures and very short oblique fractures. In the case we present, we would attempt a lag screw between the two major fragments and neutralise the fracture with a plate, aiming for two screws on each side of the fracture (four cortices).

Theatre Setup

The vast majority of hand fractures requiring surgery can be treated as ambulatory day case patients, awake and with an appropriate regional block. The patient is positioned supine with an arm table. The surgeon is sat at the head end (since the dorsum of the hand naturally falls that way) with the mini c-arm or image intensifier brought in from the axilla when required. The assistant or scrub nurse can position themselves beside the surgeon with ease.

Surgical Approach

Metacarpal fractures are fixed via a dorsal approach. If a single metacarpal is to be fixed, an incision directly over the bone is utilised. If multiple metacarpals are to be fixed, a single incision between a pair of metacarpals can be used to access two bones.

The clinical photograph shows the incision directly over the ring finger metacarpal. The exposure continues to the side of the extensor tendon dividing and tagging the juncturae tendinum as in this case, which will be repaired at the end (Fig. 27.2).

If the fracture is a long spiral pattern, one must at least expose each end of the fracture site to ensure correct reduction of both length and rotation (Figure 27.3 shows the short oblique frac-

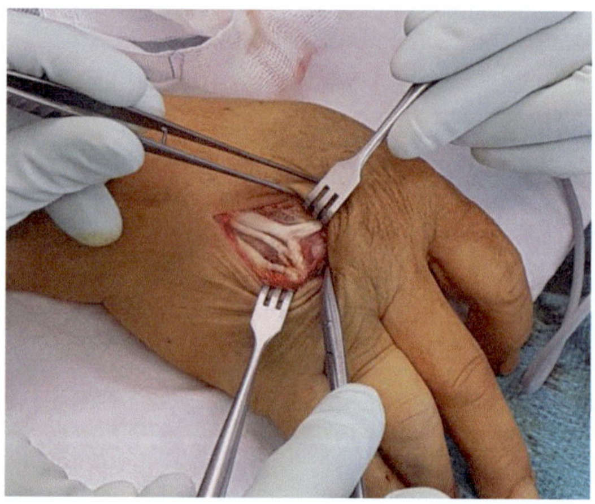

Fig. 27.2 Incision directly over the ring finger metacarpal (exposure continues to the side of the extensor tendon dividing and tagging the juncturae tendinum)

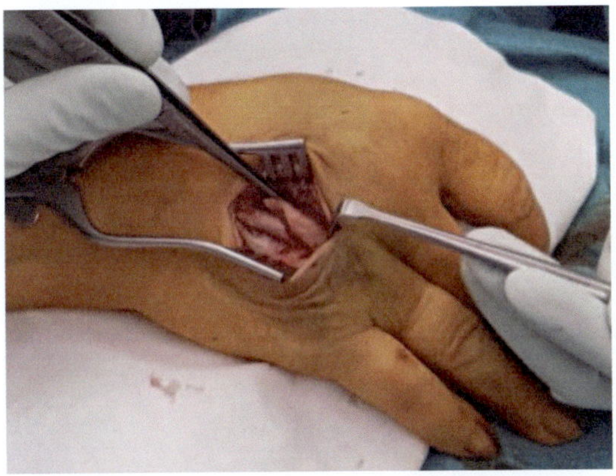

Fig. 27.3 Short oblique fracture has been exposed and cleared of haematoma to enable direct reduction techniques

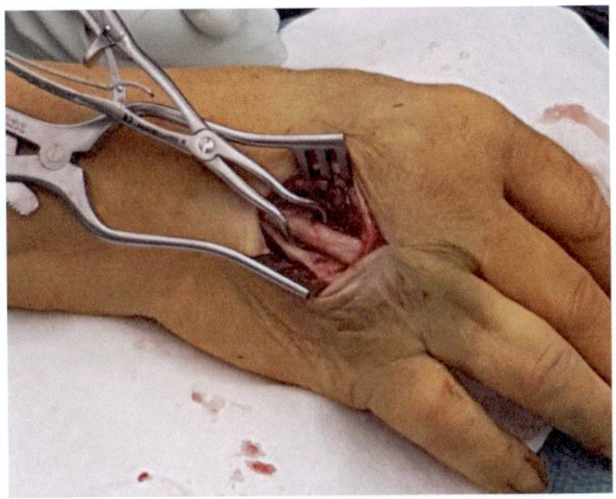

Fig. 27.4 Reduction of metacarpal fracture using one mini-fragment pointed reduction forceps

ture has been exposed and cleared of haematoma to enable direct reduction techniques).

Reduction Manoeuvres and Instruments

If planning to plate a metacarpal fracture as in this case, open reduction is usually required. This is because the hand is often quite swollen and the surround structures prevent insertion of a plate through smaller (minimally invasive) incisions.

The reduction is most commonly achieved by applying traction and then using one (for short oblique fractures) or two (for long spiral fractures) mini-fragment pointed reduction forceps, as seen in this case to hold the reduction out to length (Fig. 27.4).

Implant Insertion

With the fracture now reduced, a 2 mm drill is used to drill perpendicular to the fracture site through near and far cortices prior to over-drilling the near cortex with a 2.7 mm drill. This allows a 2.7 mm lag screw to compress the fracture which should now hold the fracture reduced and allow release of the bone reduction clamp. Finally, a mini-fragment plate is placed after having been pre-bent to match the convexity of the dorsum of the metacarpal, Fig. 27.5.

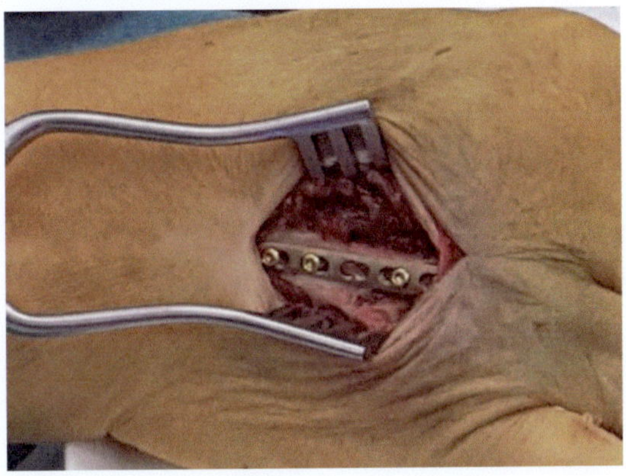

Fig. 27.5 Stabilisation of the fracture with a mini-fragment plate

Two bicortical screws are inserted to each side of the fracture in non-locking mode if the bone is of good quality as in this case. The final radiographs are seen in Fig. 27.6. The ulnar side of the hand will be protected for a week until the wound heals and then fully mobilised without restriction thereafter to prevent stiffness.

Metacarpal Head Fractures

In complex metacarpal head fractures, the principle is to trap smaller fragments between the bigger fragments rather than try and hold every fragment with instrumentation. Through an extensor tendon split, small elevators, dental

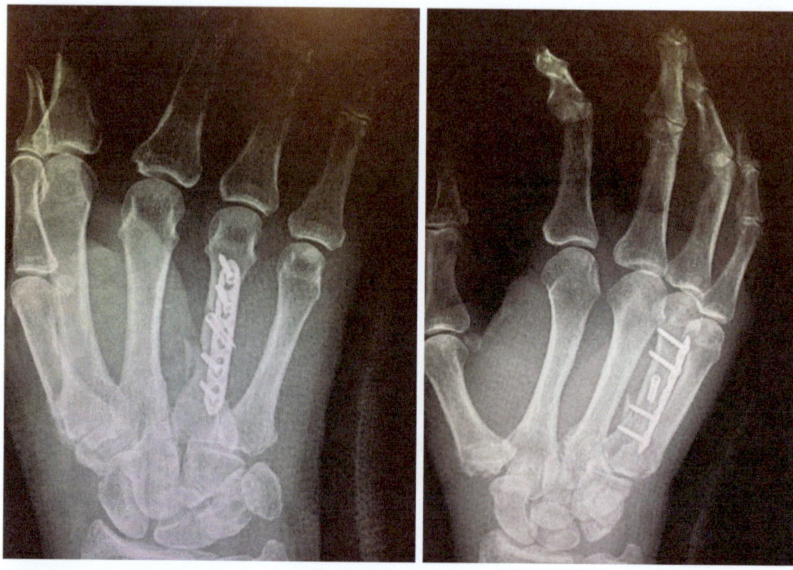

Fig. 27.6 AP and oblique radiographs of right-hand ring metacarpal demonstrating open reduction internal fixation (lag screw and mini-fragment plate)

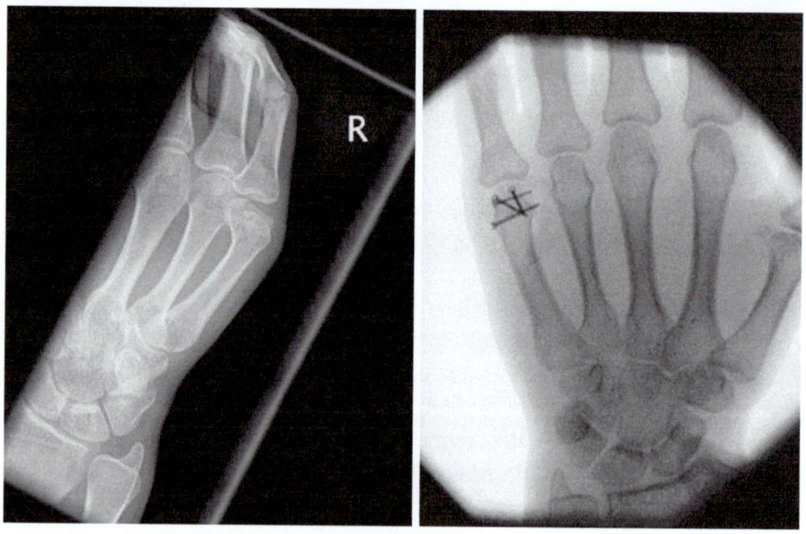

Fig. 27.7 Preoperative and postoperative radiograph* demonstrating little finger metacarpal head fracture and its subsequent fixation with 1.5 mm threaded screws (*Radiographs courtesy of Mr. D Dewar, Consultant Hand Surgeon, Leeds General Infirmary, Leeds, UK)

picks and 1–1.25 mm K-wire joysticks are used to position fragments prior to fixing them with 1.5 mm fully threaded screws (Fig. 27.7).

Metacarpal Base Fractures

Comminuted fractures at the base of the metacarpals, especially in the ring and little finger, are frequently associated with dislocations as can be seen in Fig. 27.8. In these cases restoration of the alignment of the carpometacarpal joint (CMCJ) and the length of the metacarpal is the priority. This is to allow healing of the intermetacarpal ligaments which provides stability. In these cases closed reduction is almost always successful with longitudinal traction and pressure directed palmarwards to the CMCJ base. The little finger CMCJ is held in joint via a percutaneous K-wire through the metacarpal base driven into the hamate. The ring finger fracture is additionally stabilised by transfixing the metacarpal shafts of the little and ring finger. This acts as an internal ex-fix construct to offload the comminuted fracture at the base of the ring finger, providing relative stability (Fig. 27.8).

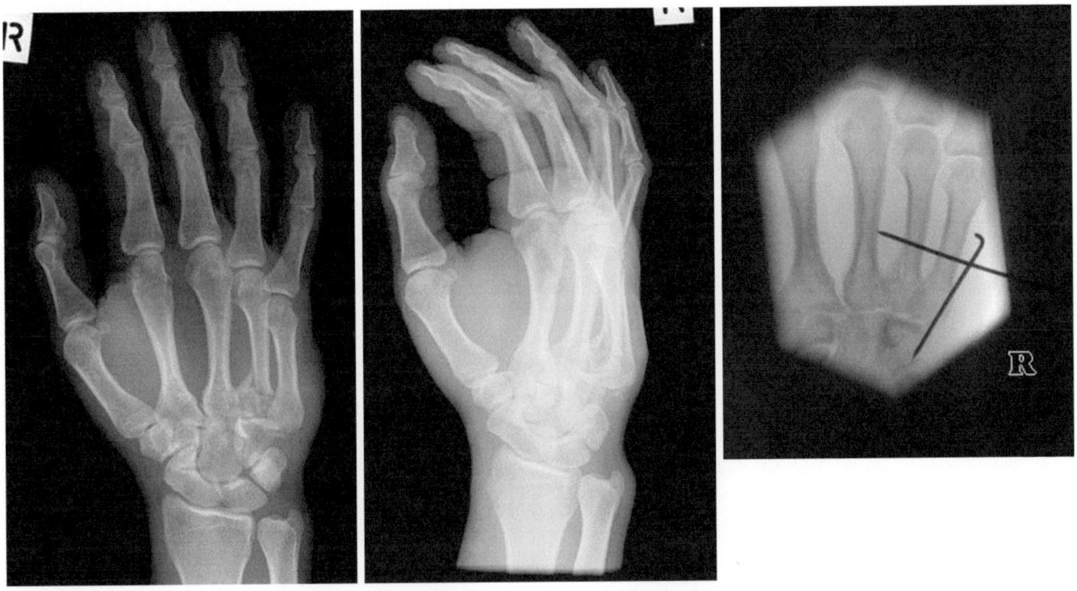

Fig. 27.8 Preoperative and postoperative radiograph* demonstrating a comminuted fracture at the base of the right ring and little finger metacarpals associated with dislocation. Following closed reduction, the little finger CMCJ is held in joint via a percutaneous K-wire through the metacarpal base driven into the hamate, while the ring finger fracture is additionally stabilised by transfixing the metacarpal shafts of the little and ring finger (*Radiographs courtesy of Mr. D Dewar, Consultant Hand Surgeon, Leeds General Infirmary, Leeds, UK)

Summary of Tips, Tricks and Pitfalls

- Since non-union is a feared complication of open reduction with internal fixation, the biology of bone healing must be respected. Fixing the fracture anatomically, with a sound construct as well as interfragmentary compression will more than likely lead to a good result. There are a number of tips and tricks to get this right.
- Firstly, only expose what you need to subperiosteally by starting at each end of the fracture zone, exposing the apices and reducing them as described previously. Only strip the central injury zone periosteum if required to reduce the fracture; otherwise preserve as much blood supply along the fracture edges as possible.
- Secondly, lag the fracture only once it has been reduced anatomically. A malreduced fracture fixed in distraction will almost certainly develop a non-union, and the metalwork will eventually fail.
- Thirdly, do not overbend plates to compress fractures (as one would with a forearm fracture to generate compression on the far cortex). In these cases the bone, whether lagged or not, will deform at the fracture site to conform to the plate rather than the plate conforming to the bone. This will result in either the volar or dorsal aspect of the fracture being held in distraction and risking non-union.
- Fourthly, plates must be pre-bent to match the contour of the bone exactly prior to applying them to the fixation construct.
- Finally, stress your fixation at the end of the case to confirm the patient can mobilise their hand from the outset to prevent stiffness.

References

1. Karl JW, Olson PR, Rosenwasser MP. The epidemiology of upper extremity fractures in the United States, 2009. J Orthop Trauma. 2015;29(8):e242–4.
2. Wong VW, Higgins JP. Evidence-based medicine: management of metacarpal fractures. Plast Reconstr Surg. 2017;140(1):140e–51e.
3. Melamed E, Joo L, Lin E, Perretta D, Capo JT. Plate fixation versus percutaneous pinning for unstable metacarpal fractures: a meta-analysis. J Hand Surg Asian Pac Vol. 2017;22(1):29–34.

28 Bennett Fracture and Fracture of Trapeziometacarpal Joint of the Thumb

Laurent Obert, Gauthier Menu, Daniel Lepage, and Francois Loisel

Anatomical Fracture Location and Treatment

A Bennett fracture is a fracture-dislocation of the thumb CMC joint. However, different types of fracture patterns can be described [1] (Fig. 28.1). In the Bennet fracture, the volar ulnar aspect of the metacarpal base remains attached to the volar oblique ligament which holds this fragment fixed while causing thumb instability. The adductor pollicis (AP) and AP longus are the primary deforming forces and combine to supinate,

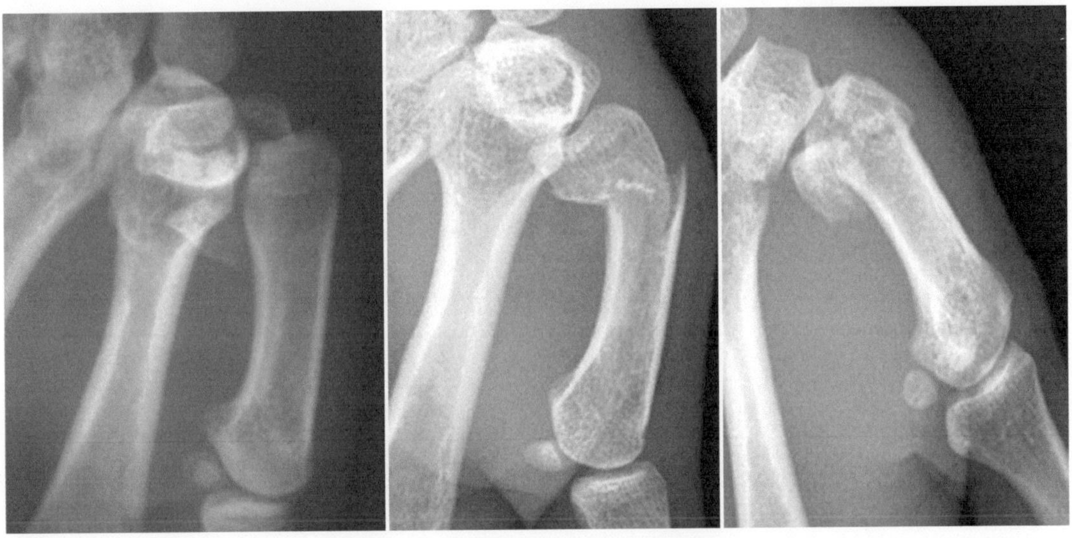

Fig. 28.1 Bennett fracture (left), extra-articular (middle) or articular and comminuted fracture (Rolando, right)

L. Obert, M.D. (✉) • G. Menu, M.D.
D. Lepage, M.D., Ph.D. • F. Loisel, M.D.
Orthopedic, Traumatology, and Hand Surgery Unit, University Hospital CHRU Besancon, Medical School, University of Bourgogne-Franche Comte, Research Unit: Nano Medicine, Besancon, France
e-mail: laurentobert@yahoo.fr; lobert@chu-besancon.fr

P.V. Giannoudis (ed.), *Fracture Reduction and Fixation Techniques*,
https://doi.org/10.1007/978-3-319-68628-8_28

adduct and flex the metacarpal shaft. The articular portion of the fracture must be fully reduced. Without stabilization, the metacarpal will tend to further displace.

Articular fracture can be treated by open reduction and fixation (direct or indirect fixation depending on the volume of bone) by lost key wire technique, screws or mini plate.

Preoperative Planning

Kapandji views allow to diagnose extra-articular or articular fractures. CT scan is mandatory to analyse the volume of bone fragments and to select the best option for fixation (Fig. 28.2).

Extra-articular fractures can be treated by closed reduction and fixation by Kirschner wire or temporary arthrodesis.

Patient Setup in Theatre

Standard table is used with the patient in the supine position. The surgeon stands on the side of the patient's head (depending on the dominant hand of the surgeon) while the image intensifier is coming from the opposite side (Fig. 28.3). An arm tourniquet is recommended for open approaches.

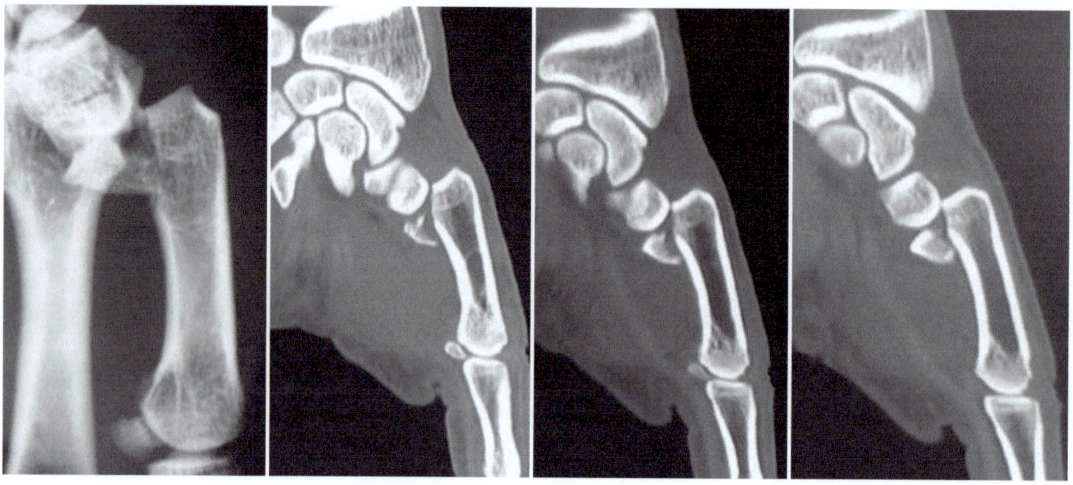

Fig. 28.2 Kapandji view and CT scan can be helpful to analyse the bone fragment and to decide the appropriate method of fixation

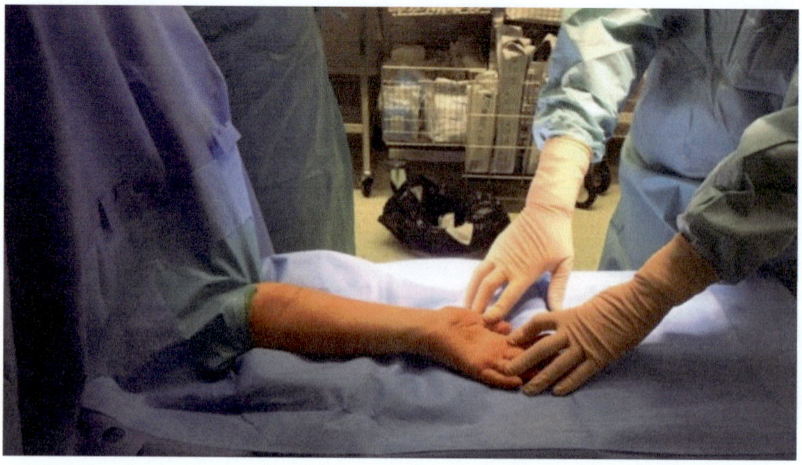

Fig. 28.3 Patient is placed in supine position with arm tourniquet. C arm is positioned from the surgeon's opposite side

Closed Reduction Manoeuvres

Axial traction, palmar abduction and slight pronation done by the assistant allow to reduce articular or extra-articular fractures. Comminuted articular fracture patterns usually require open reduction and fixation. Passive screw home torque technique method facilitates reduction in acute (fresh) cases (Fig. 28.4).

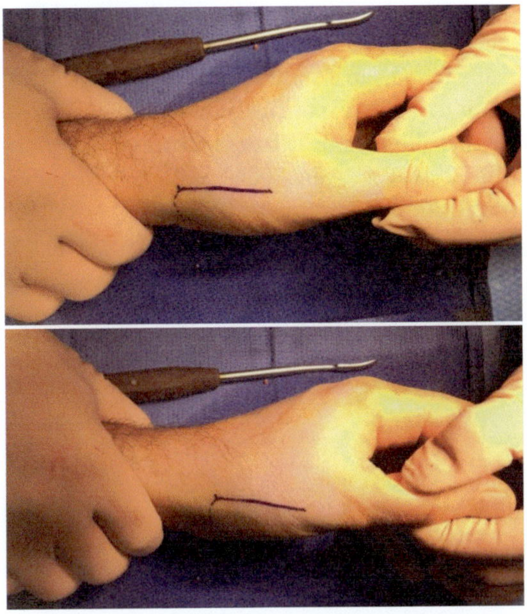

Fig. 28.4 Passive screw home torque technique consists of doing a thumb traction and a pronation manoeuvre

Closed Reduction and Fixation

Extra-articular fracture, damaged skin in the zone of incision and choice of the surgeon are the main reasons to choose this type of treatment. A 1.8 mm Kirschner wire is inserted percutaneously at metacarpal head level (Fig. 28.5) under X-ray control to reach the trapezium [2]. Temporary arthrodesis of TMC joint is done for 6 weeks protected by a thumb spica for 6 weeks.

Open Reduction and Fixation

Impossible closed reduction, articular fracture involvement and associated trapezium fracture are the main reasons to select this type of treatment [3]. A dorsal approach or an extended J approach to volar side is possible (Fig. 28.6).

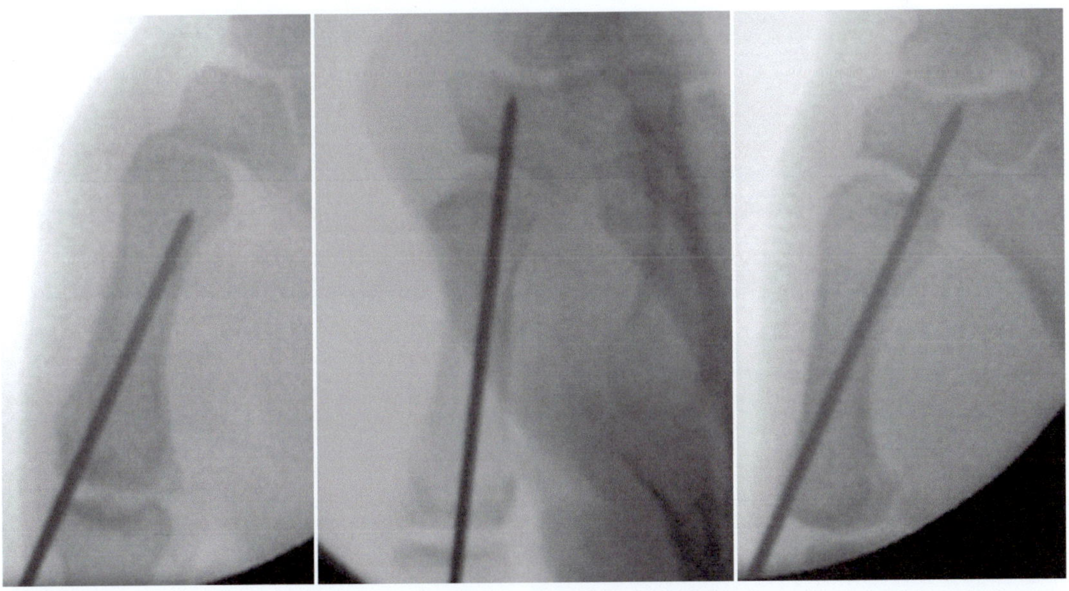

Fig. 28.5 Kirschner wire is inserted as distal as possible at metacarpal head level, crossing the joint for stability

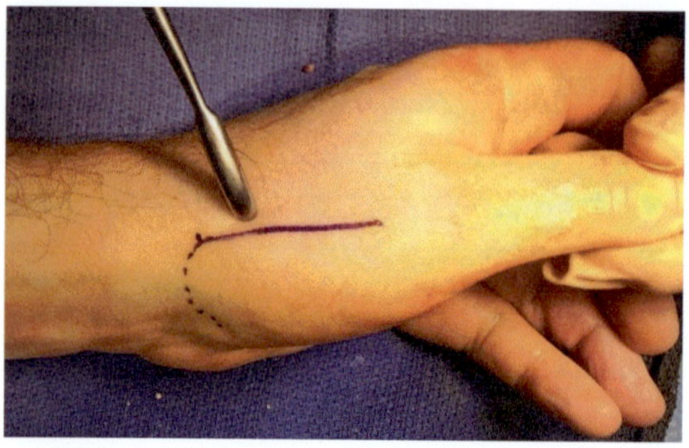

Fig. 28.6 A dorsal approach can be extended to volar approach

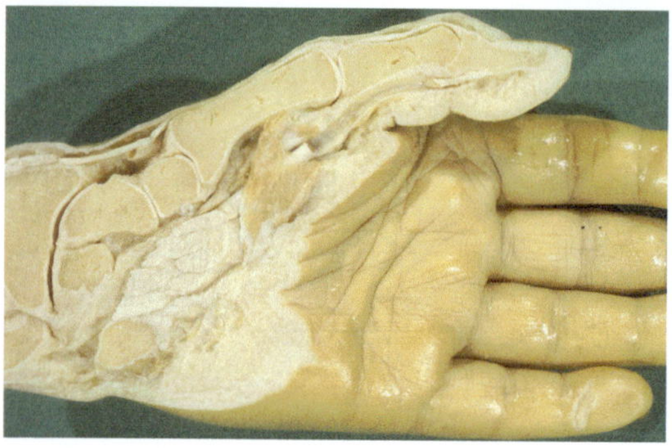

Fig. 28.7 Representation of the articular zone of the metacarpal base on a frontal anatomical view

Surgical Approach and Reduction Instruments

Dorsal approach is easier than volar which needs to strip the thenar intrinsic muscles (Fig. 28.7). Dorsal surgical approach is carried out without dissection of radial nerve but identification of EPB and APL (Fig. 28.8). A dorsal periosteal proximally based flap is raised (Figs. 28.9 and 28.10) to reach the joint, exposing the base of the metacarpal and allowing reduction of the articular surface (Fig. 28.11). Howard rugine (left) or AO rugine (right) allows to reduce the fragments (Fig. 28.12). Volar bone fragment is maintained by the rugine and fixed under X-ray control by K wires or

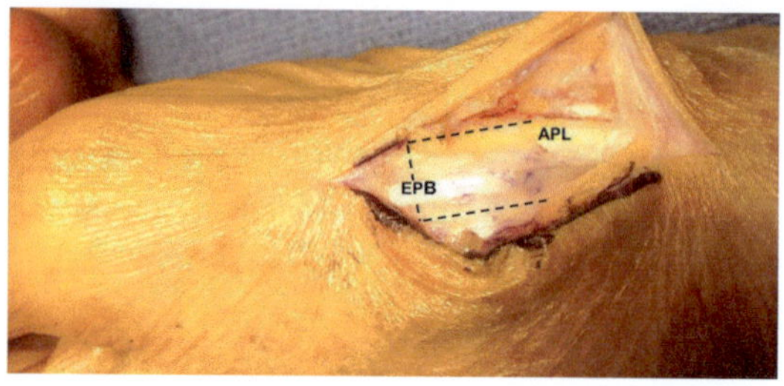

Fig. 28.8 Extensor pollicis brevis (EPB) is the landmark of the dorsal approach

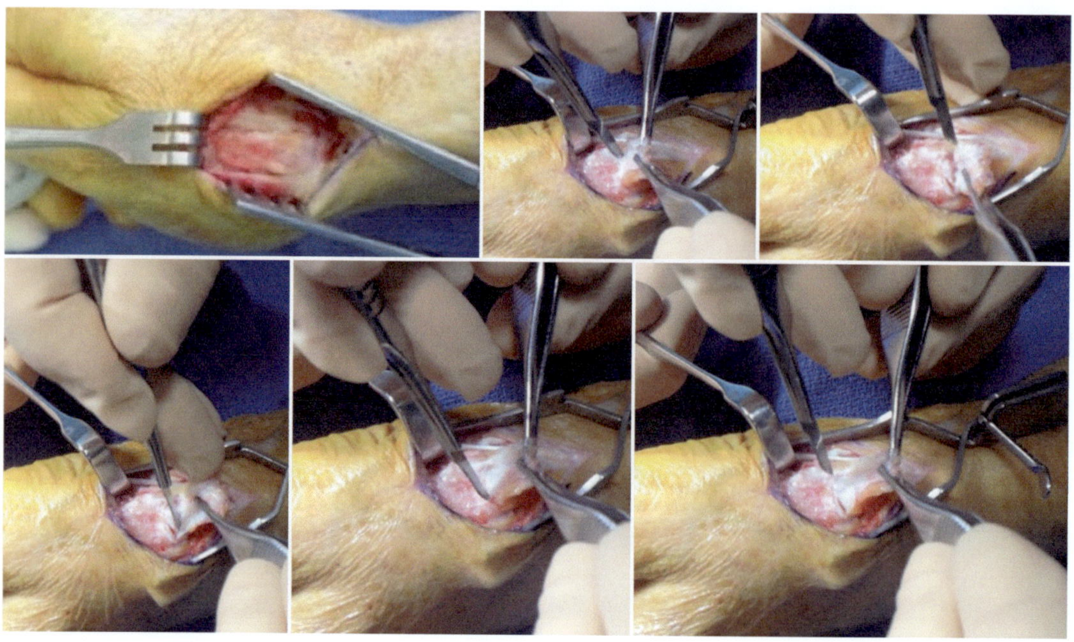

Fig. 28.9 The dorsal capsular-periosteal flap is raised as large as possible

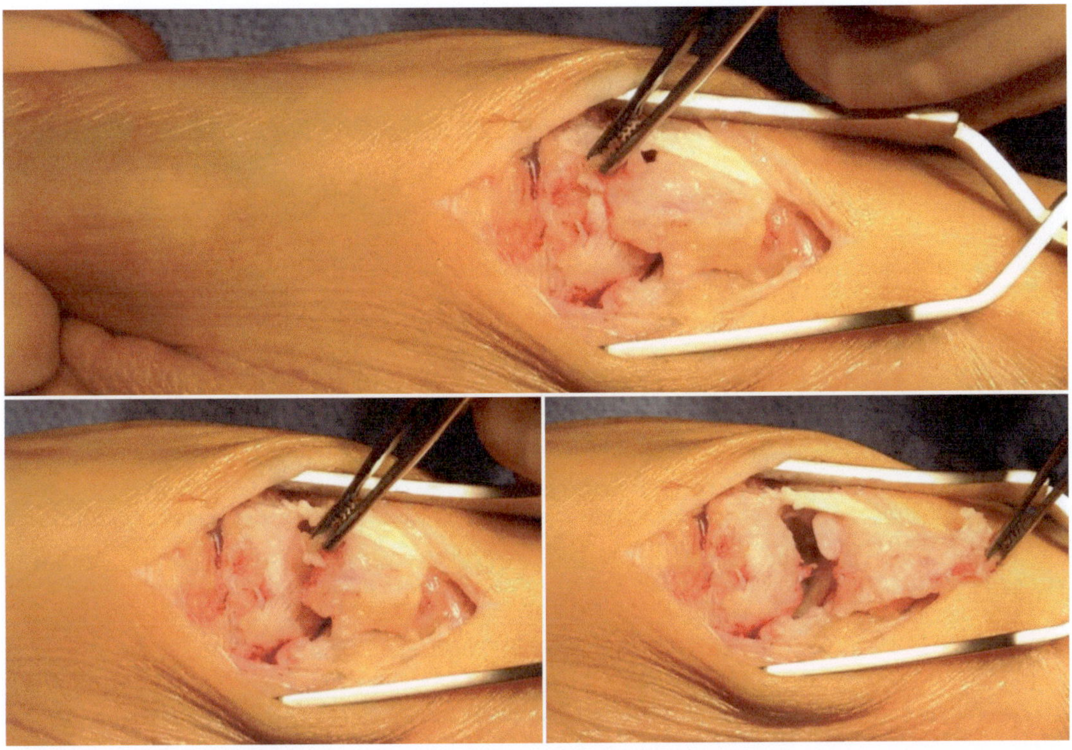

Fig. 28.10 The dorsal capsular-periosteal flap is raised with a proximal base

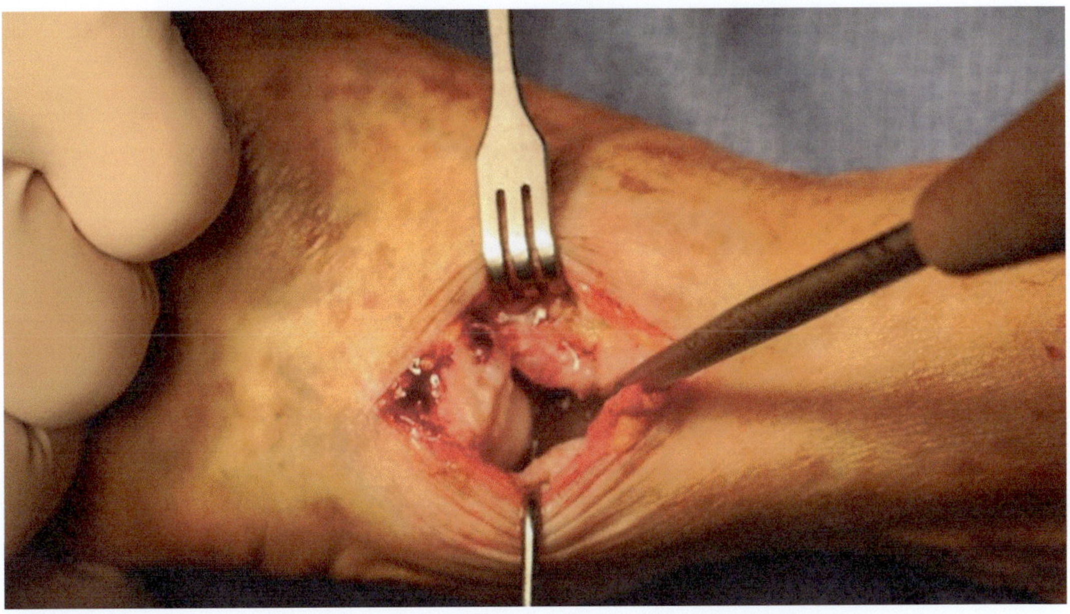

Fig. 28.11 The view on the articular surface is sufficient to reach and manipulate the articular fragment

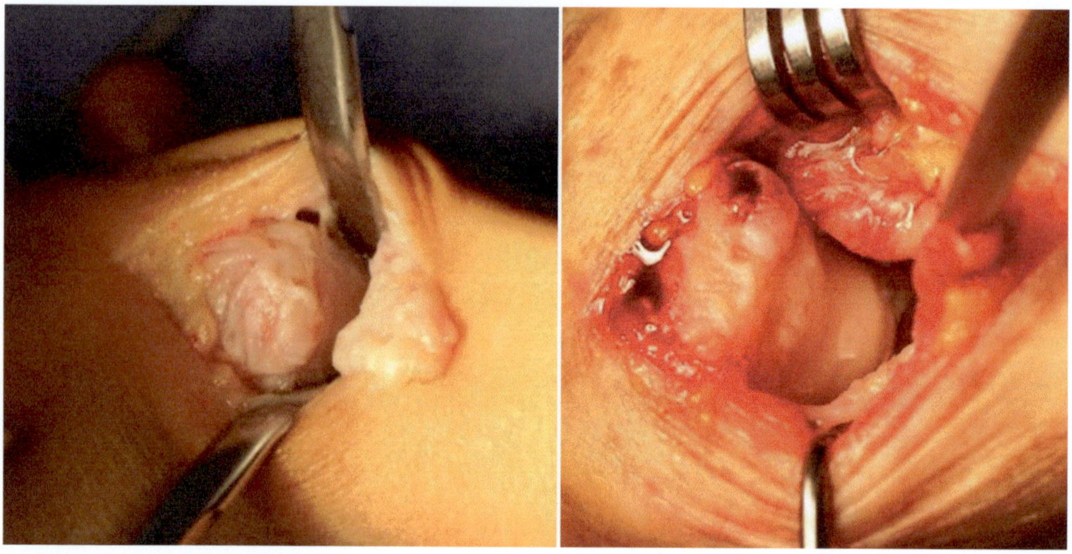

Fig. 28.11 (continued)

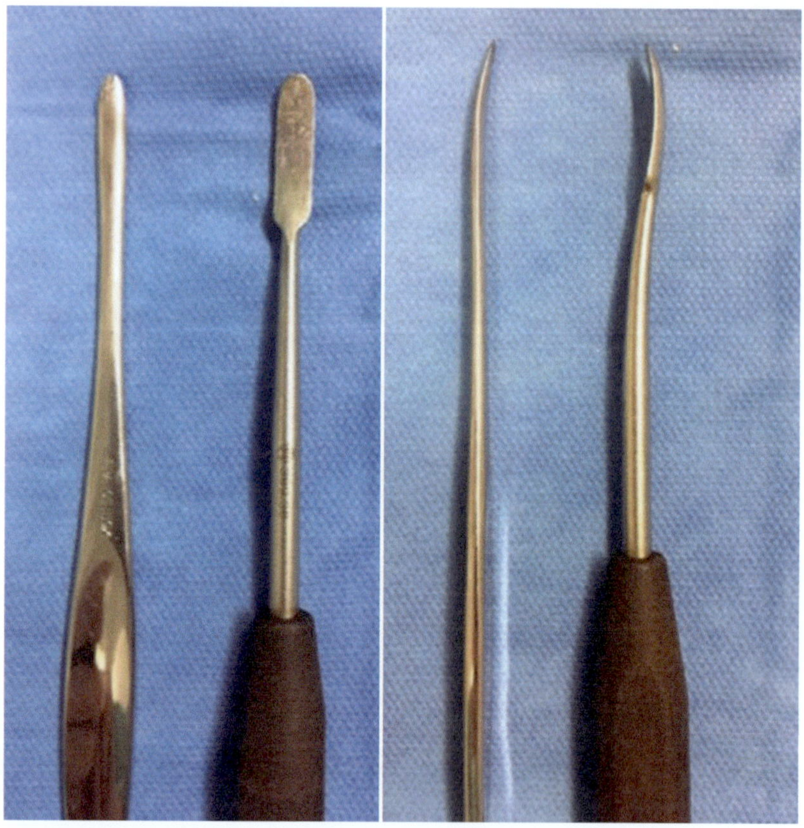

Fig. 28.12 The most appropriate rugine is used to manipulate and control the articular fragment

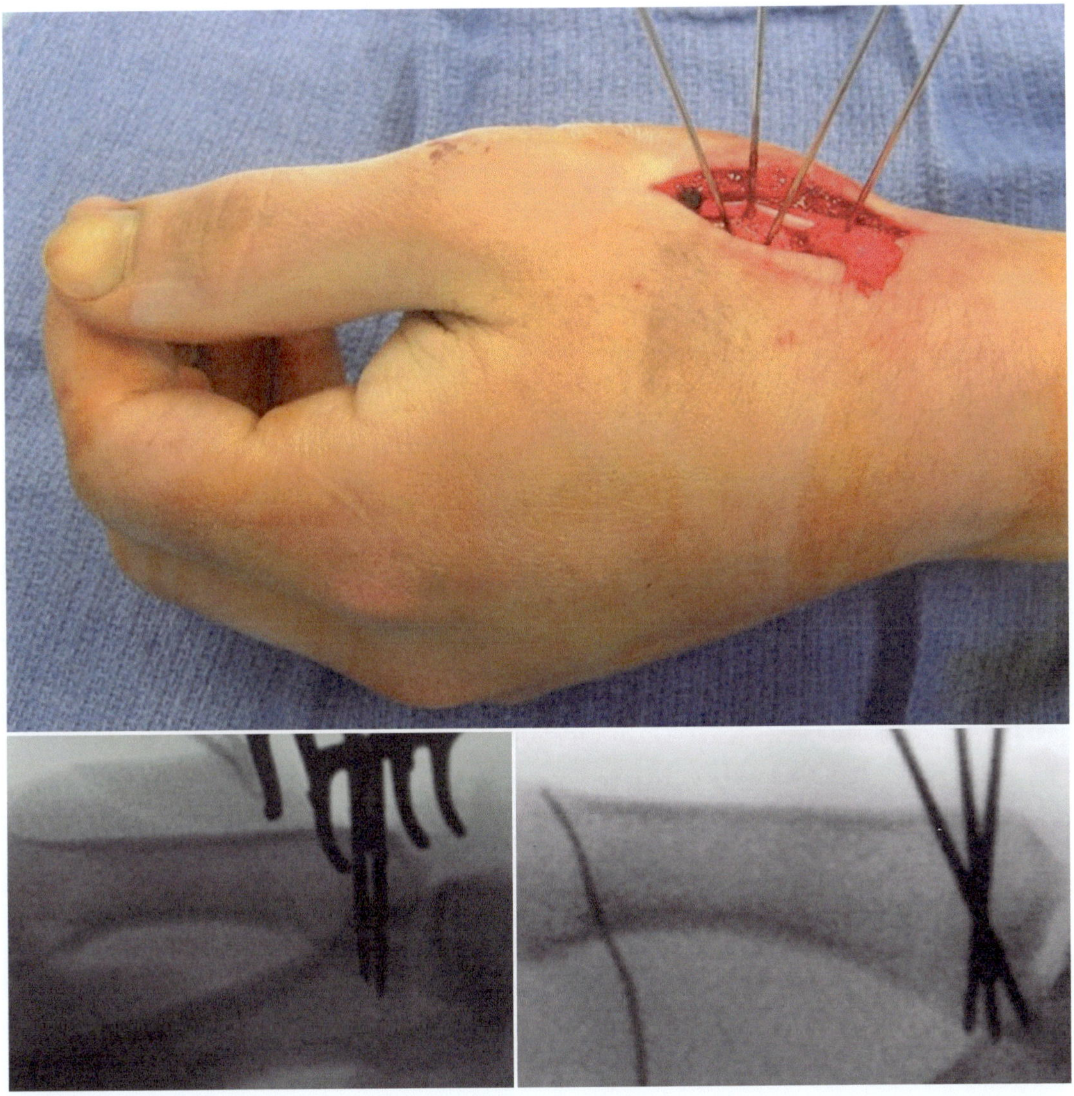

Fig. 28.13 Indirect fixation is controlled under X-ray with an appropriate length of threaded Kirschner wire

cannulated screws (Fig. 28.13). Periosteal flap is reinserted by anchors or transosseous suture on metacarpal bone. Kapandji view allows final assessment of fixation (Fig. 28.14). A thumb spica is mandatory for 4 weeks. Figure 28.15 demonstrates good functional results and a Kapandji X-ray view at 1 year of follow-up.

Summary of Tips, Tricks and Pitfalls

- Reduction and fixation are mandatory for fractures of first metacarpal base.
- Kapandji view allows to analyse the fracture preoperatively, intraoperatively and postoperatively.

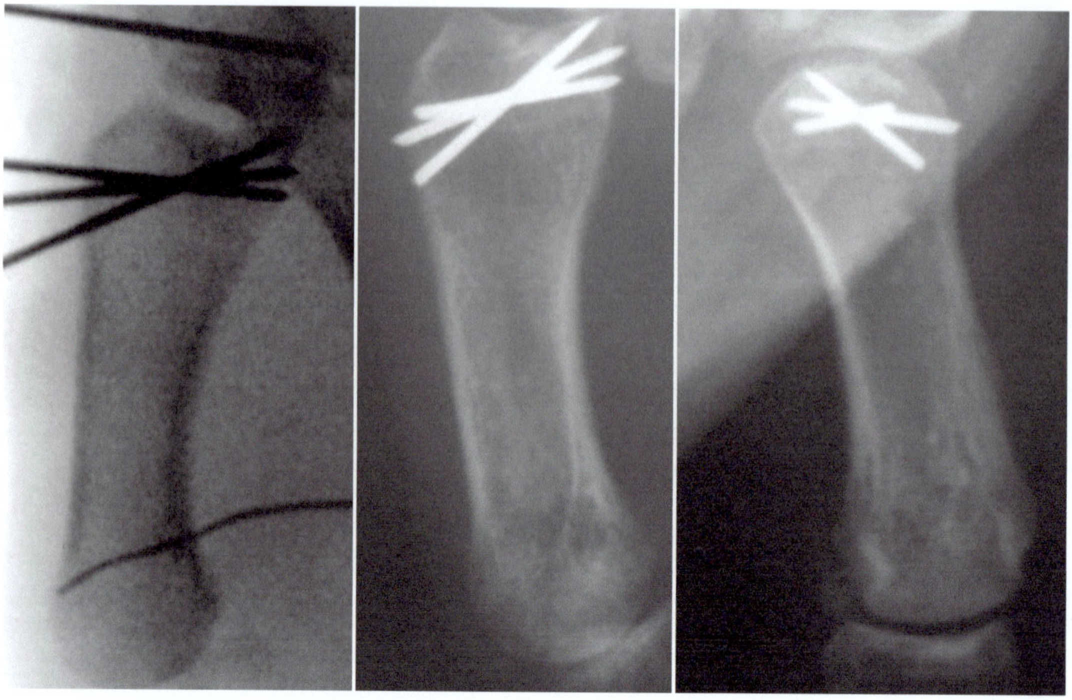

Fig. 28.14 The final check radiograph after fixation has to be done in the operating room

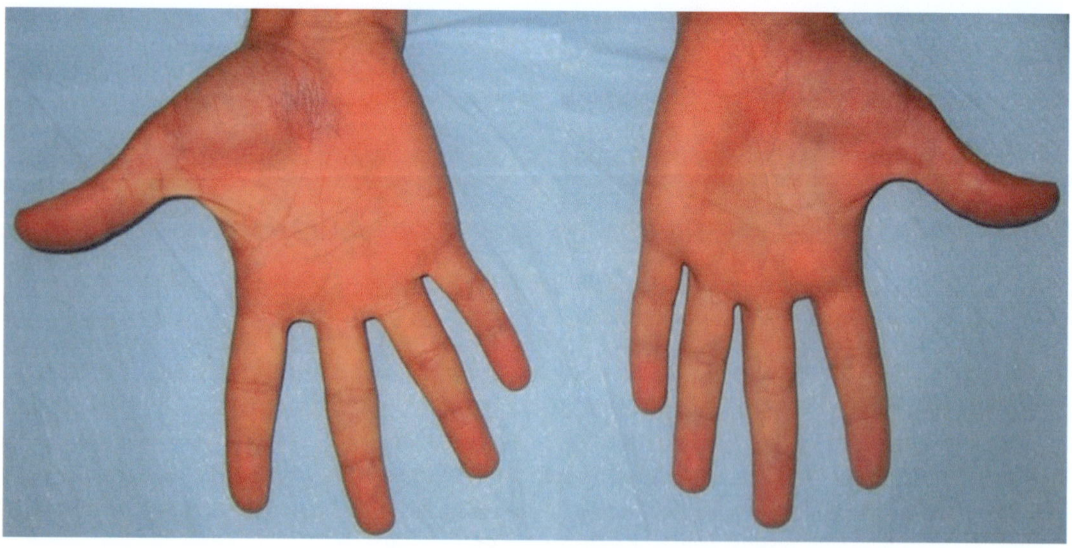

Fig. 28.15 At 1-year follow-up, clinical pictures demonstrating a full range of motion; radiograph shows maintenance of anatomical reduction

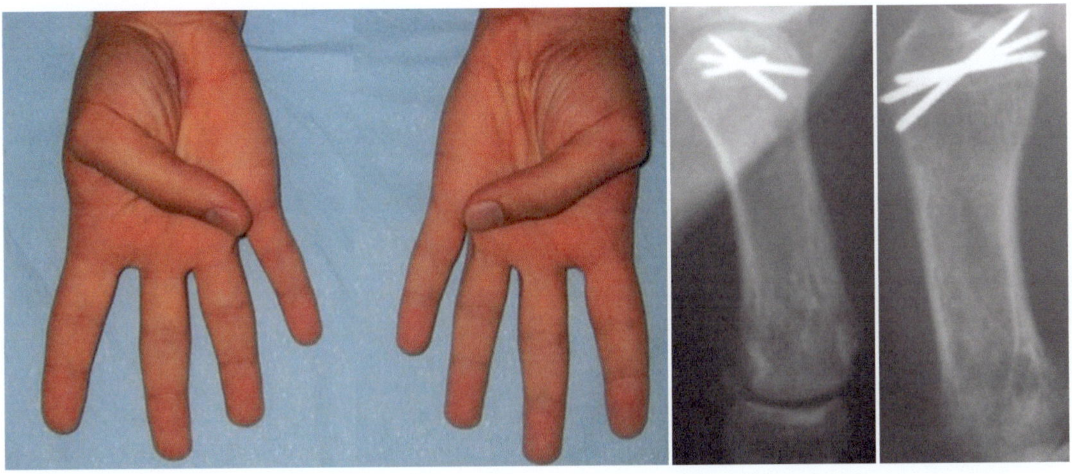

Fig. 28.15 (continued)

- The passive screw home torque technique method facilitates reduction in acute (fresh) cases.
- Dorsal approach using a periosteal flap remains a simple way to perform an anatomical reduction and fixation by pin or screw.

References

1. Kapandji A, Moatti E, Raab C. Specific radiography of the trapezo-metacarpal joint and its technique. Ann Chir. 1980;34:719–26.
2. Ollie Edmunds J. Traumatic dislocations and instability of the trapeziometacarpal joint of the thumb. Hand Clin. 2006;22:365–92.
3. Liverneaux PA, Ichihara S, Hendriks S, Facca S, Bodin F. Fractures and dislocation of the base of the thumb metacarpal. J Hand Surg Eur. 2015;40:42–50.

29 Hand-Phalanx Fracture-Dislocation (PIP Joint)

Laurent Obert, Margaux Delord, Gauthier Menu, Damien Feuvrier, Isabelle Pluvy, and Francois Loisel

Anatomical Fracture Location and Treatment

In case of fracture dislocation of proximal interphalangeal joint (PIP), the indication for surgery is a non-concentric PIP joint. If a concentric reduction can be achieved (flexing the joint), a dorsal block splint in flexion for several weeks can be advised. External fixation devices are available to maintain reduction whilst allowing early motion. If over 40–50% of the joint surface is involved, open surgery is mandatory to restore the joint congruity. Depending on the size of the fragment and preoperative delay, options include ORIF, volar plate arthroplasty and hemi-hamate arthroplasty or chondrocostal graft. We will present the ORIF technique for recent fracture and joint dislocation.

L. Obert, M.D. (✉) • M. Delord, M.D.
G. Menu, M.D. • D. Feuvrier, M.D.
I. Pluvy, M.D. • F. Loisel, M.D.
Orthopedic, Traumatology, and Hand Surgery Unit, University Hospital CHRU Besancon, Medical School, University of Bourgogne - Franche Comte, Research Unit: Nano Medicine, Besancon, France
e-mail: laurentobert@yahoo.fr; lobert@chu-besancon.fr

Preoperative Planning

AP and sagittal views are necessary to diagnose the dislocation which can be misdiagnosed. Dorsal or volar fragment will guide the surgeon to choose the right approach. CT scan is helpful to analyse the volume of bone fragments to choose the best fixation (Fig. 29.1). Articular fracture can be treated by open reduction and fixation (direct or indirect fixation depending on the volume of bone) by lost key wire, screw and temporary fixation of the joint for 3 weeks.

Patient Setup in Theatre

Standard table is used with the patient in supine position. The surgeon stands on the side of the patient's head (depending on the dominant hand of the surgeon). The image intensifier is positioned from the opposite side (Fig. 29.2). An arm tourniquet is applied.

Closed Reduction Manoeuvres

Axial traction done by the assistant allows to reduce the joint. A temporary fixation of the joint by Kirschner wire can be done under X-ray control.

P.V. Giannoudis (ed.), *Fracture Reduction and Fixation Techniques*,
https://doi.org/10.1007/978-3-319-68628-8_29

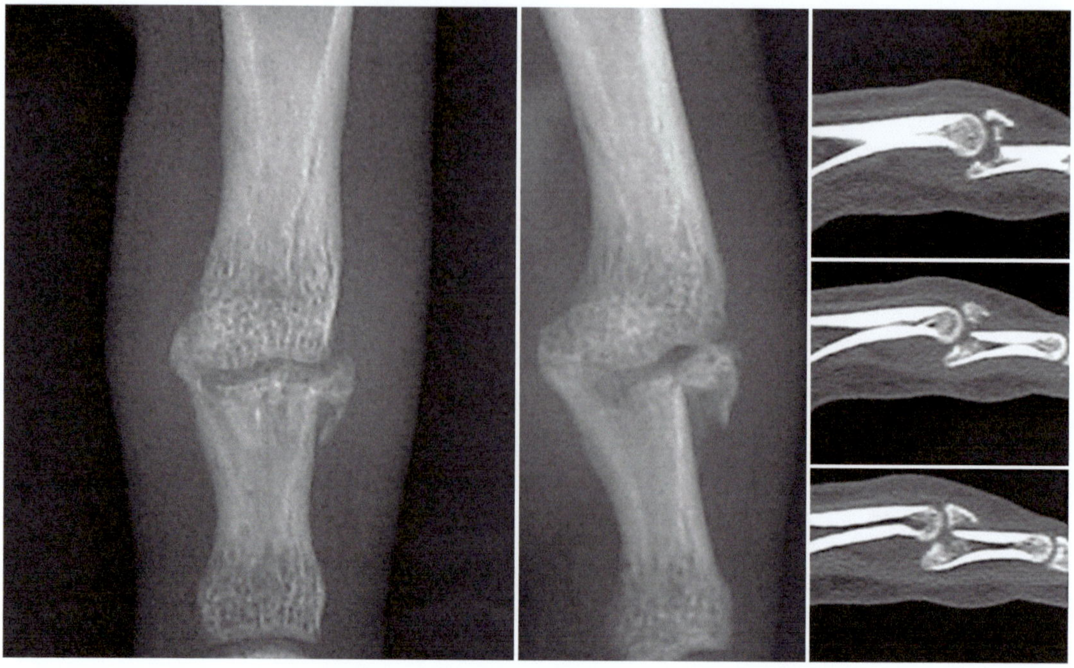

Fig. 29.1 CT scan demonstrates the number, degree of displacement and volume of fragments

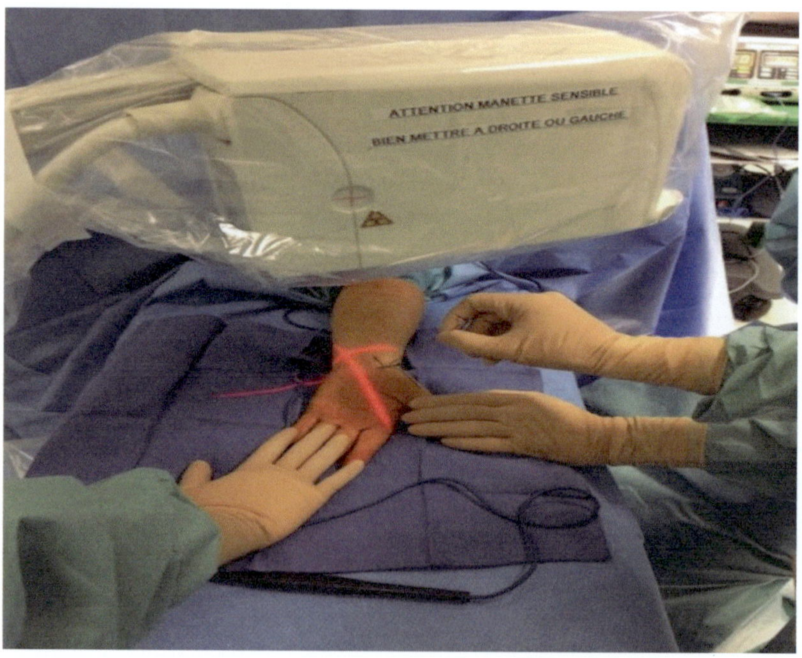

Fig. 29.2 Patient is placed in supine position with an arm tourniquet

Surgical Approach and Reduction Instruments

The use of a Ioban drape allows to remove the uninvolved fingers from the surgical field and to isolate the injured finger where a dorsolateral or a lateral skin incision centred on the PIP joint is made [1] (Fig. 29.3).

Dorsolateral approach is easier than volar and allows in all cases to control, reduce and fix the articular fragment (dorsal or volar). It is sometimes possible to reduce and to fix the fragment percutaneously (Fig. 29.4). If closed reduction is not followed by anatomical and concentric reduction of the joint, open reduction and fixation is mandatory.

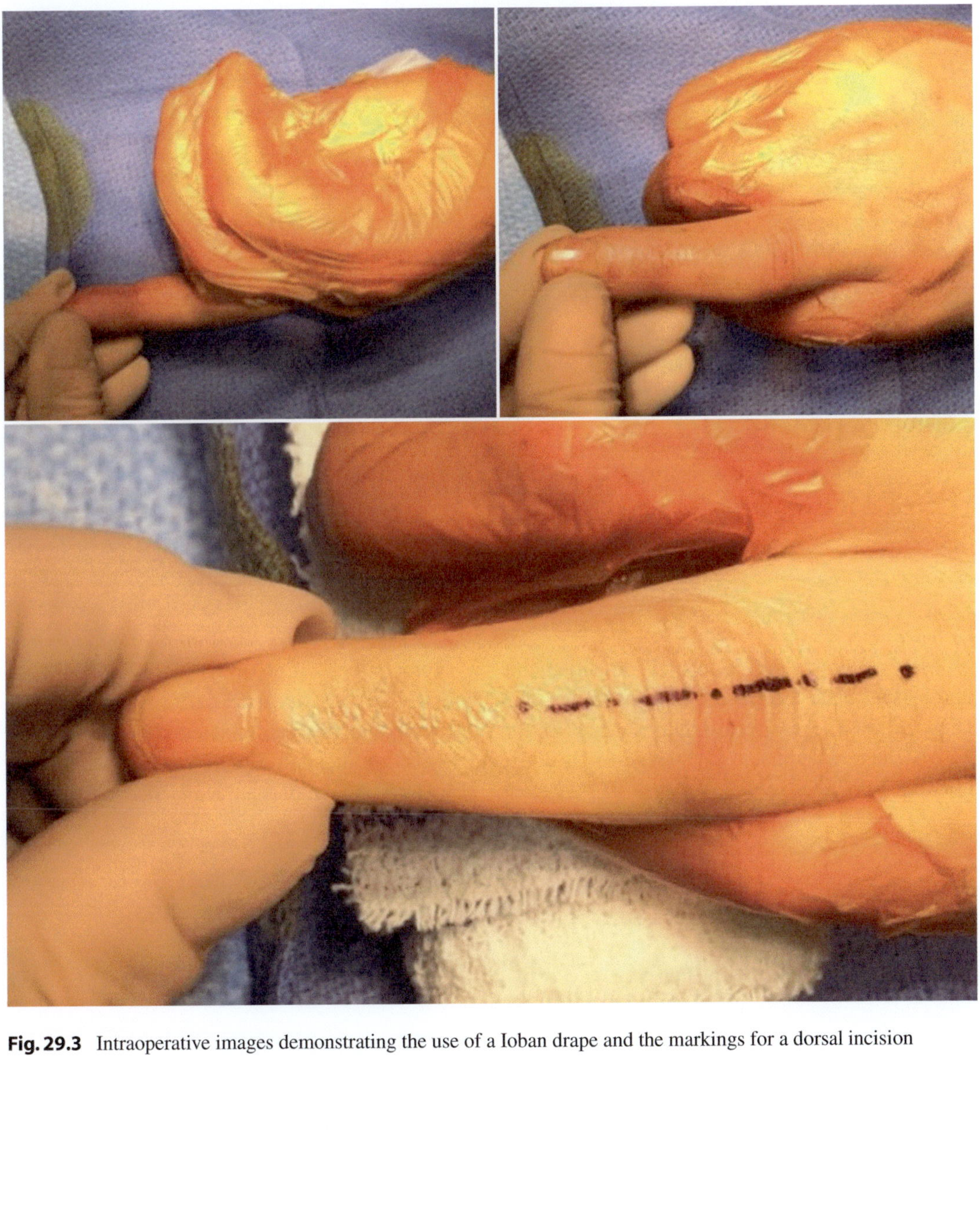

Fig. 29.3 Intraoperative images demonstrating the use of a Ioban drape and the markings for a dorsal incision

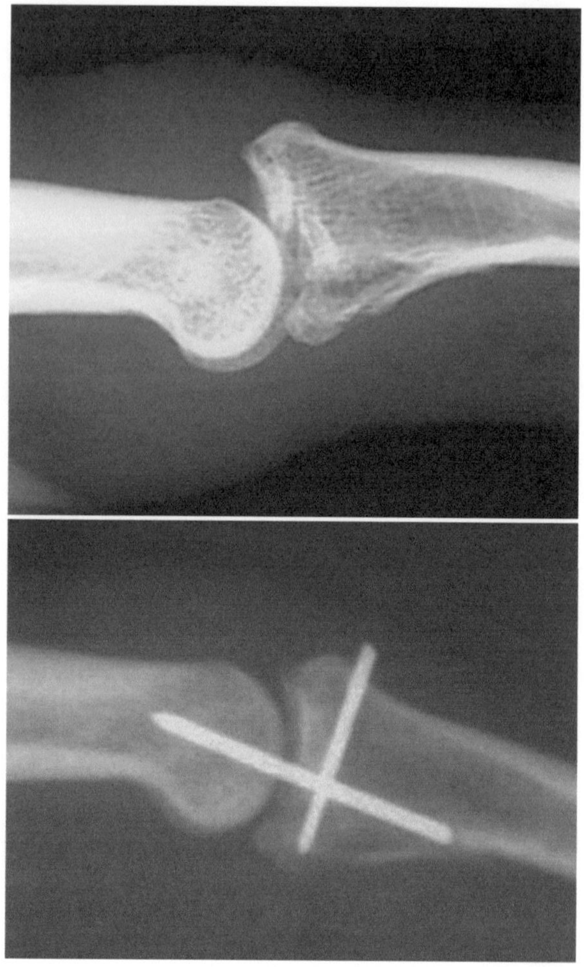

Fig. 29.4 Radiographs demonstrating anatomical reduction of the joint (fixation of the fracture by a Kirschner wire and of the articular fragment (palmar one) by a threaded K wire)

After a dorsolateral skin incision, ligaments and palmar plate are reflected to reach the joint (Fig. 29.5). The entire articular surface of the base of the middle phalanx is then perfectly under control.

Temporary fixation of the joint is done by 1.4-mm K wire for 3 weeks (Fig. 29.6). Articular fragment is maintained and fixed under X-ray control by a 1.0- or 1.2-mm K wire or cannulated screw (Fig. 29.7). Ligaments are reattached [2, 3].

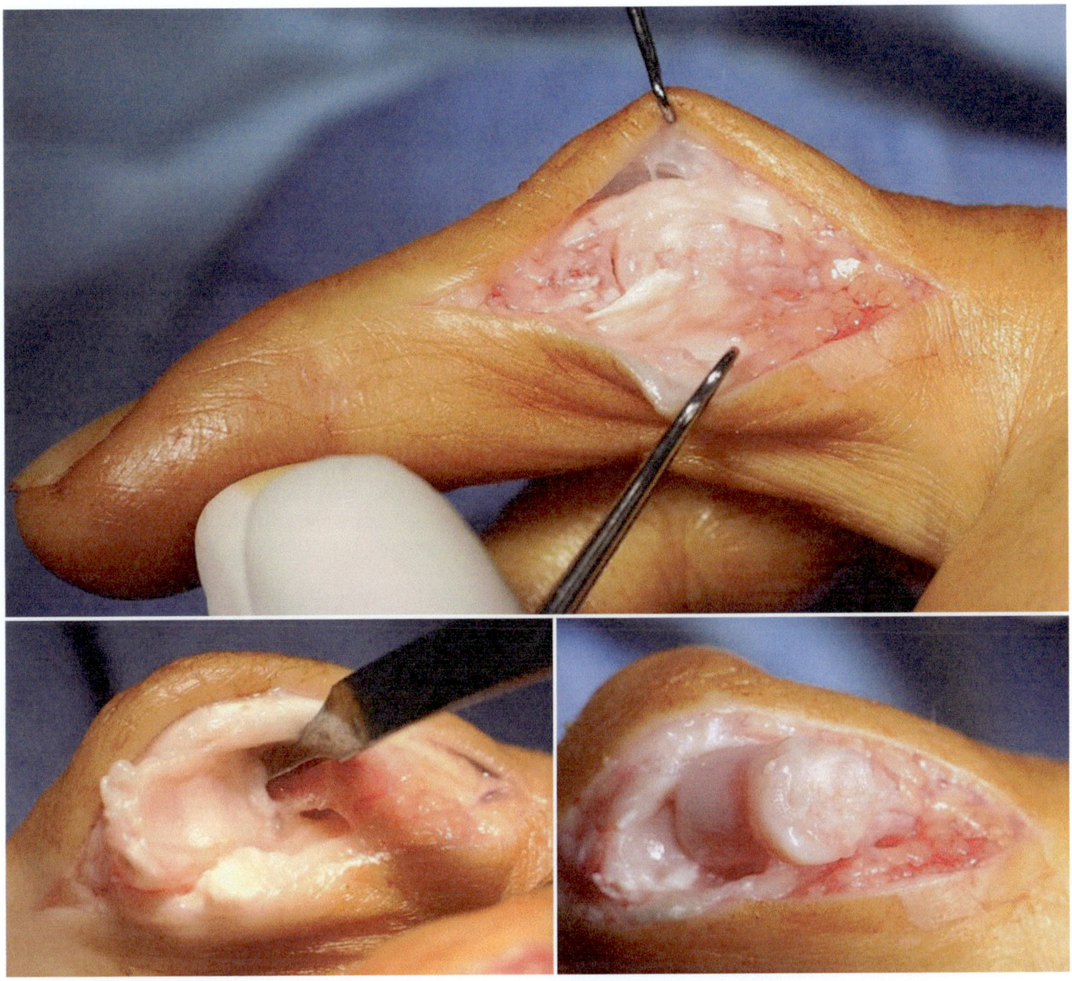

Fig. 29.5 Intraoperative images: using a dorsolateral approach allows to control the entire articular surface without tenotomy of extensor tendon

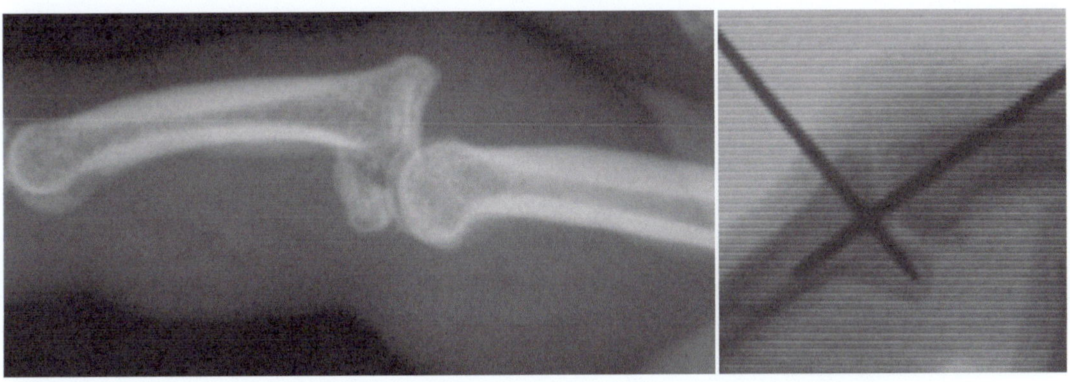

Fig. 29.6 Intraoperative images demonstrating that whilst reduction is not perfect, the joint remains concentric

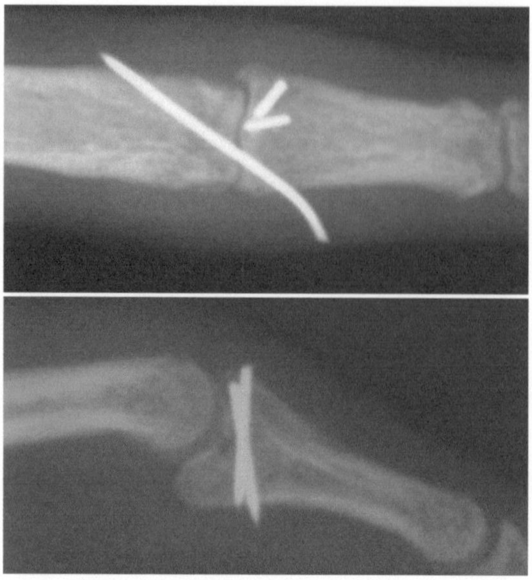

Fig. 29.7 Intraoperative images: although reduction of the fragment is anatomical in this case, the temporary K-wire fixation of the joint is mandatory

Summary of Tips, Tricks and Pitfalls

- Reduction and fixation are mandatory in case of articular fracture and non-concentric joint.
- Dorsal approach remains a simple way to perform an anatomical reduction and fixation by K wire or screw.

References

1. Verma MK, Bradley J, Jebson PJ. The Ioban drape: a simple method to improve finger surgery safety and efficiency. Tech Hand Up Extrem Surg. 2012;16(4):202–3.
2. De Haseth KB, Ring D. Management of finger fractures. In: Bhandari M, editor. Evidence-based orthopedics. Hoboken, NJ: Wiley-Blackwell; 2012. p. 987–92.
3. Oak N, Lawton JN. Intra articular fractures of the hand. Hand Clin. 2013;29:535–49.

Index

P.V. Giannoudis (ed.), *Fracture Reduction and Fixation Techniques*,
https://doi.org/10.1007/978-3-319-68628-8

MIX
Papier aus verantwortungsvollen Quellen
Paper from responsible sources
FSC® C105338

If you have any concerns about our products,
you can contact us on
ProductSafety@springernature.com

In case Publisher is established outside the EU,
the EU authorized representative is:
Springer Nature Customer Service Center GmbH
Europaplatz 3, 69115 Heidelberg, Germany

Printed by Libri Plureos GmbH
in Hamburg, Germany